A CULTURAL HISTORY OF THE SENSES

VOLUME 1

A CULTURAL HISTORY
OF THE SENSES
IN ANTIQUITY

Edited by Jerry Toner

BLOOMSBURY ACADEMIC
LONDON • NEW YORK • OXFORD • NEW DELHI • SYDNEY

BLOOMSBURY ACADEMIC
Bloomsbury Publishing Plc
50 Bedford Square, London, WC1B 3DP, UK

BLOOMSBURY, BLOOMSBURY ACADEMIC and the Diana logo are trademarks of
Bloomsbury Publishing Plc

First published in Great Britain 2014
This edition published 2019
Reprinted 2019 (twice)

Copyright © Bloomsbury Publishing, 2014, 2019

Jerry Toner has asserted his right under the Copyright, Designs and Patents Act, 1988,
to be identified as Editor of this work.

For legal purposes the Acknowledgments on p.xiii constitute an extension
of this copyright page.

Cover image: The Catechism with a Young Girl Reading and the Initiate Making an Offering,
North Wall, Oecus 5, c.60–50 BC (fresco), Roman, (1st century BC) / Villa dei Misteri,
Pompeii, Italy / Bridgeman Images.

All rights reserved. No part of this publication may be reproduced or transmitted in any form or
by any means, electronic or mechanical, including photocopying, recording, or any information
storage or retrieval system, without prior permission in writing from the publishers.

Bloomsbury Publishing Plc does not have any control over, or responsibility for, any third-party
websites referred to or in this book. All internet addresses given in this book were correct at the
time of going to press. The author and publisher regret any inconvenience caused if addresses
have changed or sites have ceased to exist, but can accept no responsibility for any such changes.

A catalogue record for this book is available from the British Library.

Library of Congress Cataloging-in-Publication Data.
A cultural history of the senses in Antiquity, 500 BCE–500 CE / edited by Jerry P. Toner.
pages cm
Includes bibliographical references and index
ISBN 978-0-85785-339-4 (hardback)
1. Senses and sensation—History. 2. History, Ancient. I. Toner, J. P.
BF233.C85 2014
152.109'014—dc23
2014005063

ISBN:	HB:	978-0-8578-5339-4
	PB:	978-1-3500-7784-3
	ePDF:	978-1-4742-3298-2
	eBook:	978-1-4742-3304-0
	HB Set:	978-0-8578-5338-7
	PB Set:	978-1-3500-7783-6

Series: The Cultural Histories Series

Typeset by RefineCatch Limited, Bungay, Suffolk

To find out more about our authors and books visit www.bloomsbury.com
and sign up for our newsletters.

CONTENTS

	LIST OF ILLUSTRATIONS	vii
	SERIES PREFACE	xi
	EDITOR'S ACKNOWLEDGMENTS	xiii
	Introduction: Sensing the Ancient Past *Jerry Toner*	1
1	The Social Life of the Senses: Feasts and Funerals *David Potter*	23
2	Urban Sensations: Opulence and Ordure *Gregory S. Aldrete*	45
3	The Senses in the Marketplace: The Luxury Market and Eastern Trade in Imperial Rome *Andrew Wallace-Hadrill*	69
4	The Senses in Religion: Piety, Critique, Competition *Susan Ashbrook Harvey*	91
5	The Senses in Philosophy and Science: Five Conceptions from Heraclitus to Plato *Ashley Clements*	115
6	Medicine and the Senses: Humors, Potions, and Spells *Helen King and Jerry Toner*	139

7 The Senses in Literature: Falling in Love in an
   Ancient Greek Novel   163
   Silvia Montiglio

8 Art and the Senses: The Artistry of Bodies, Stages, and
   Cities in the Greco-Roman World   183
   Mark Bradley

9 Sensory Media: Representation, Communication, and
   Performance in Ancient Literature   209
   Benjamin Eldon Stevens

   NOTES   227
   BIBLIOGRAPHY   235
   NOTES ON CONTRIBUTORS   253
   INDEX   257

LIST OF ILLUSTRATIONS

INTRODUCTION

I.1 Banquet scene from Pompeii showing fine clothes and draperies. 5

I.2 Fresco showing Hercules and a worshiper from a tomb from the Isola Sacra cemetery near Ostia. 9

I.3 Wall-painting showing a hunter facing a lion in the games. 15

CHAPTER ONE

1.1 The public banqueting area at Gabii. 32

1.2 Relief from Aminternum showing a public banquet. 35

1.3 Relief from Aminternum showing a funeral procession. 39

CHAPTER TWO

2.1 View of the Appian Way with remains of tombs. 46

2.2 Reconstruction of Rome showing juxtaposition of opulence and poverty. 49

2.3 Reconstruction of a public bath showing ornate decor and decorative marbles. 57

2.4 Marble statue of Messalina holding Britannicus. 60

2.5 Mosaic of the Triumph of Bacchus (Dionysus). 67

CHAPTER THREE

3.1 Egyptian style black obsidian bowl with white and pink coral inlays, lapis lazuli, malachite and gold, from Villa San Marco, Stabiae. 71

3.2 Indian ivory statue found at Pompeii, possibly of the goddess Lakshmi. 73

3.3 Mosaic from Pompeii showing a woman wearing a pearl necklace and earrings. 80

3.4 Pair of gold pins and pearls from Pompeii. 81

3.5 Fresco with banquet scene from the *Casa dei Casti Amanti* showing woman wearing see-through silk. 84

CHAPTER FOUR

4.1 Detail from the Column of Trajan showing the emperor wearing the veil of the Pontifex Maximus and performing libations at the altar. 93

4.2 Floor mosaic from the Beth Alpha synagogue showing instruments of sacred ritual, including the sacred lulav (palm branch), etrog (citron), shofar (ram's horn), and incense shovel. 99

4.3 Baptistry of Neon, Ravenna, showing sculpted columns and arches adorned with mosaics. 106

4.4 Christian liturgical instruments, Northern Syria, c. 500 CE: chalices, censers, wine strainer, a dove; silver, silver gilt. 110

4.5 Terracotta pilgrim flask, Egypt, sixth century CE, to be filled with perfumed holy oil at St. Menas' shrine. 112

LIST OF ILLUSTRATIONS   ix

CHAPTER SIX

6.1 Hippocrates and Galen, early thirteenth-century fresco, in the
Crypt of St. Mary Cathedral, Anagni, Lazio.   141

6.2 Roman vaginal speculum, 100 BCE–400 CE.   146

6.3 Bas-relief depicting surgical instruments, from the Catacomb of
Praetextatus, Rome.   149

6.4 A cast taken from an ancient Greek intaglio gem, depicting a
physician examining a patient while Asclepius, the god of healing,
stands nearby holding the symbol of medicine, a snake coiled
round a staff.   153

6.5 Imperial-age *ex-voto* depicting footprints uncovered in Italica,
Spain.   158

CHAPTER EIGHT

8.1 Bronze seated boxer, detail of face. Hellenistic period, late
fourth–second century BCE.   188

8.2 Detail from the color rendering of the "Alexander Sarcophagus,"
showing sophisticated and realistic uses of color to depict
the figure of a Persian fighter.   190

8.3 The Prima Porta statue of Augustus, c. 15 CE.   191

8.4 Jean-Léon Gérôme, *Pygmalion and Galatea* (1890).   193

8.5 Fresco showing a woman pouring perfume, Villa Farnesina,
Rome, late first century BCE.   195

8.6 Drawing of a scene from the "Pronomos Vase": Dionysus and
Ariadne surrounded by the actors and chorus of a satyr-play. Attic
red-figure krater, c. 410 BCE.   201

8.7a and 8.7b: Dioskourides mosaic (c. 125–100 BCE).   203

8.8 Digital reconstruction of the Theater of Pompey (dedicated
52 BCE).   206

Every effort has been made to trace copyright holders and to obtain their permission for the use of copyright material. The publisher apologizes for any errors or omissions there may be in the credits for the illustrations and would be grateful if notified of any corrections that should be incorporated in future editions of this book.

SERIES PREFACE

GENERAL EDITOR, CONSTANCE CLASSEN

A Cultural History of the Senses is an authoritative six-volume series investigating sensory values and experiences throughout Western history and presenting a vital new way of understanding the past. Each volume follows the same basic structure and begins with an overview of the cultural life of the senses in the period under consideration. Experts examine important aspects of sensory culture under nine major headings: social life, urban sensations, the marketplace, religion, philosophy and science, medicine, literature, art, and media. A single volume can be read to obtain a thorough knowledge of the life of the senses in a given period, or one of the nine themes can be followed through history by reading the relevant chapters of all six volumes, providing a thematic understanding of changes and developments over the long term. The six volumes divide the history of the senses as follows:

Volume 1. A Cultural History of the Senses in Antiquity (500 BCE–500 CE)
Volume 2. A Cultural History of the Senses in the Middle Ages (500–1450)
Volume 3. A Cultural History of the Senses in the Renaissance (1450–1650)
Volume 4. A Cultural History of the Senses in the Age of Enlightenment (1650–1800)
Volume 5. A Cultural History of the Senses in the Age of Empire (1800–1920)
Volume 6. A Cultural History of the Senses in the Modern Age (1920–2000)

EDITOR'S ACKNOWLEDGMENTS

I would like to thank Constance Classen for giving me the opportunity to exchange ideas with so many classical scholars interested in the growing sphere of sensory history. I would also like to thank her for her good-humored patience in dealing with me. Bloomsbury have done an excellent job in producing the series and I am grateful to their editors for guiding me through the production process.

Introduction: Sensing the Ancient Past

JERRY TONER

In his *True History*, the second-century Lucian tells us about his trip to the moon. "I am now going to describe," he says, "the strange and novel things which I noticed there." Not surprisingly lunar life had many differences to that of a Syrian within the Roman Empire. "When a man becomes old," he informs us, "he does not die, but dissolves in smoke into the air." Not only that but everyone shares the same diet: they roast figs on a fire but, instead of eating them, people sit around the hearth and sniff up the fumes. This olfactory offering serves them as food. Their drink is air that has been compressed in a cup until it gives off a moisture resembling dew. A handsome man on the moon wears his head bald and his body hairless; but at the same time he has a knee-length beard. These creatures have tails, which are like large evergreen cabbages. Their mucus is a pungent honey, and after hard work or exercise they sweat milk all over, which a drop or two of the honey curdles into cheese. The clothing of the wealthy is soft glass, and of the poor, woven brass, for the land is very rich in brass, which they work like wool after steeping it in water. Lucian hesitates to describe their eyes, fearing that they are so incredible that people will doubt that he is telling the truth. "But the fact is," he continues, "that they are removable." Their ears are the leaves of plane trees. Another amazing thing was a large mirror in the royal palace, hung over a well. Every word from Earth could be heard rising up through the well, and if you looked in the mirror, you could see every city in close detail. As Lucian says, "Anyone who doubts the truth of this statement has only to go there himself to be assured of my veracity."

Not having traveled to the Moon I cannot confirm or deny Lucian's observations. But what is clear is that Lucian's account of his ancient space travel relied heavily on the alternative use of the senses to generate an idea of how different lunar society was from his own. Lucian was not alone in placing emphasis on the importance of the senses. The ancient world, from classical Greece in the fifth century BCE to the end of the Western Roman Empire in the fifth century CE, used the senses to create and express a huge range of cultural meanings. Religious practices, for example, were fully embodied experiences, which used the senses to establish all kinds of religious meaning (see Chapter 4). Indeed, the senses were functionally significant to all aspects of ancient life, often in a way that was complexly interconnected. Antiquity was also a period of vivid sensations: cities stank, statues were brightly painted, brutal physical punishments were commonplace, and literature made full use of sensory imagery to create its effects. In a steeply hierarchical world, with vast differences between the landed wealthy, the poor, and the slaves, the senses also played a key role in establishing and maintaining boundaries between social groups. This steep social stratification meant that the juxtaposition of the awe-inspiring with the unpleasant was ubiquitous. Visually-dominating buildings such as the Colosseum were well-known places for reeking prostitutes to tout for business.

But the use of the senses in the ancient world was not static. The Roman emperors, for example, employed a powerful range of sensory effects in their architecture and the games to win over the people to their new form of autocratic government after the fall of the republic. New religions such as Christianity developed their own way of using the senses, and acquired their own particular set of sensory-related symbolism. These processes were slow and were often contested. There was rarely any simple agreement about what the senses signified. The aim of this introduction is to provide an overview of these structures and developments, concentrating primarily on the Roman world, and to show how their study can yield a more nuanced understanding of antiquity.

SYNAESTHESIA

Synaesthesia is a term that can often be applied to the ways in which the ancients used the senses. Synaesthesia represents a mixing of the senses, whereby different senses are used to stimulate each other. Antiquity was not a world which saw, as we in the modern West do, the senses as five clearly distinct registers, each with its own particularities. The ancient world was perceived in a way that mixed up the senses to create a rich and complex descriptive palette (see Butler and Purves 2013). Both Greek and Latin literature, for example, make frequent use of such sensory blends. Homer's "wine-dark sea" can be read as an image relating not just to the color, but to its sharp, pungent taste and smell. It may also give some hint of the unsettling feeling of being on a swell. Tasting, smelling, and feeling colors is not something that sits easily with the modern approach to the senses. In part, as Benjamin Eldon Stevens and Silvia Montiglio discuss in their chapters, this difference stemmed from the fact that reading ancient literature was itself a more varied sensory experience. Rather than being simply read, it was designed to be heard. It was natural, in such a context, to taste, hear, and smell what might to us seem purely visual descriptions. It is important to remember that the ancient world was largely oral and aural. Literacy levels were low, with perhaps less than 10 percent being functionally literate and much less than that able to read high literature fluently. Education was expensive and few could afford to allow their children the luxury of learning to enjoy such finery as poetry. But the necessity for literature to be read out aloud meant that writers had to learn to charm their listeners' ears. As Montiglio argues, a fundamental quality of good style was "vividness," the ability to make audiences see by means of words.

The senses were not seen as passive conduits through which perceptions flowed, but rather as directly influencing the physical body. The body, the mind, and the senses were all, therefore, interconnected. The science of Greek medicine was replete with sensory inputs. Humoral theory held that the body contained four distinct fluids, known as humors—black bile, yellow bile, blood, and phlegm—and physical illness basically reflected an imbalance between these fluids. The body was seen as permeable. So if an individual was placed in a certain environment then it would inevitably result in the appearance of certain conditions. This meant that it was vital to make sure that the body was only exposed to the right kind of sensations. The senses were not perceived as simple conduits for sensations to pass though. A smell, for example, was not understood as being a byproduct emanating from a thing or person. It was thought to have a direct affect on the recipient, which could influence the individual both physically and morally (Harvey 2006: 30). Bad air, therefore, could damage the individual if it entered the body through the nose.

Ancient Greek medicine, which was later taken up by the Romans, was deeply concerned with maintaining humoral balance by carefully controlling the physical sensations that were working on the body. An individual suffering from madness might be played music to bring harmony back to the humoral misalignment. Medicine was also not a unified profession. Rather, different "schools" of thought set out alternative uses of the senses to achieve their cures. So another text recommends sternutatories (sneezing powders) for the treatment of madness so that sufferers would sneeze out their imbalances. Other remedies included shaving the head to reduce the heat around the brain, as well as the application of a plaster compounded of such strong smelling elements as nitrium, spurge, pepper, and frankincense to overcome the brain's imbalances (Caelius Aurelianus 1.5.167). Oil of roses rubbed onto the head provided a calming medication for phrenitis, a supposed condition of the brain. One medical writer also advises that there should be no paintings or bright colors in the rooms of phrenitis sufferers in case such excessive visual stimulation encouraged hallucinations (Aretaeus *On the Causes and Symptoms of Chronic Diseases* 2.3) Female hysterics were so-called because it was believed that their womb was moving about inside them. They therefore underwent treatments that involved the use of strong odors to coax the wandering womb back into its proper place. A fetid fumigation was placed under the woman's nose to repel the ascending uterus, whereas an aromatic was applied to the vagina to attract it downwards. It is hard not to see the wandering womb as a metaphor for the dangers posed by any kind of female social mobility.

THE SENSES AND SOCIAL STATUS

Ancient societies were acutely alert to distinctions of personal status and rank. Indeed, for most people, their position as citizen or outsider, freeman or slave, their gender, and their wealth were of fundamental importance to their identity. The senses were one of the key ways in which people of different social strata established who they were. Controlling the spaces in which they lived allowed individuals to reflect their social identity. So the wealthy in the Roman world decorated their villas with a hierarchy of colors, with white being cheapest, then red and yellow, and blue and black being reserved for grand rooms to create an area of high value, luxury, and prestige (Wallace-Hadrill 1994: 31). In the same way, perfumed water was sprinkled on bathroom walls to establish this as a space that had a higher osmological value (Pliny *Natural Histories* 13.5). The rich in Rome collectively employed luxury goods to show publicly that they had a sufficiently developed sense of taste to appreciate such refined items. Naturally, a byproduct of this use of luxury was to mark them off from the masses below them.

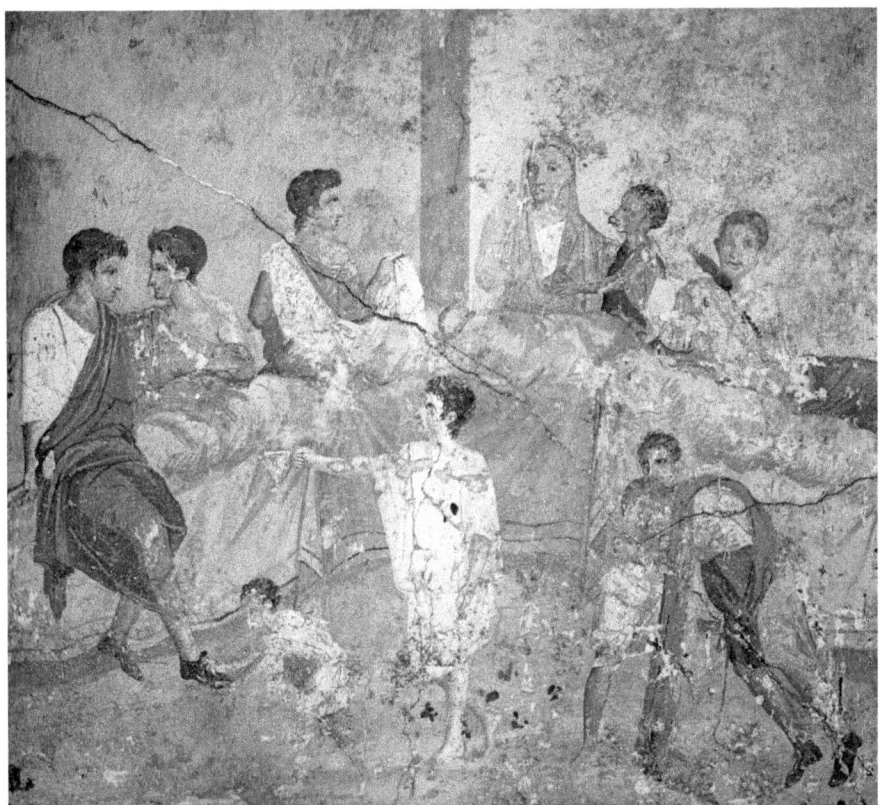

FIGURE I.1: Banquet scene from Pompeii showing fine clothes and draperies. The slaves are shown small scale to reflect their lower status. Wikimedia Commons.

The importance of controlling the senses for elite identity extended to codes of comportment for the body. Any release of foul odors might reveal a lack of health and status. Belching that had a foul or fishy odor was considered by some doctors to be a sign of melancholy. Similarly, flatulence was such poor behavior at dinner parties that it was taken as one of the warning signs of the imminent onset of mania (Caelius Aurelianus 1.5–6). The emperor Constantius II, when making his grand entry into Rome, made sure not to spit or wipe his nose, lest it should reduce his majesty (Ammianus Marcellinus 16.10.10). Defining what was acceptable behavior in this way established a *cordon sanitaire* around the culture of the elite. Taste became a means of social distinction, which was then itself used as evidence of the elite's cultural superiority.

Cultural exclusion of this kind cut off the masses. Most people in the ancient world were unable to afford expensive decorations or perfumes, nor did they care about the manners of the dining room. The popular culture was far more rough and ready. The average inhabitant of Rome undoubtedly lived in a world of powerful sensory experiences (see the chapter by Greg Aldrete). The streets of Rome were narrow, noisy, full of refuse, graffiti, animals, and people. People were crammed into small spaces and jerry-built houses. By necessity they spent more time outside in the bustle of the crowded streets and public spaces. Shoving and fighting seem to have been a common problem as people jostled to get on. The city air was polluted from the smoke of fires and dust. Certain neighborhoods were associated with particular smells, such as the area across the Tiber where the tanners worked. Other parts of town were characterized by the odors produced by the butchers or perfumers who congregated there.

The elite tended to associate unpleasant sensations of touch and smell with the people as a whole. In reality, many of the poor probably did smell strongly given that they lived crowded together and survived by carrying out manual work in a hot climate. Many will also have smelled in accordance with their trade. So tanners stank of hides, and fullers of the piss-pots that stood outside their establishments, urine being used in the processing of wool. Poor dental hygiene will also have meant that many had roaring halitosis. Physical work took a high physical toll on the body. It coarsened the hands and left bodies bent double with fatigue.

Touch was a particularly potent way of differentiating between social groups. Slaves were often branded and were subject to physical punishments in a way that citizens were not. In Roman law courts they were required to undergo torture in order to ensure that they spoke the truth. The marks on an individual's skin told their social contemporaries whether they were their equals or not. The scars of former beatings that remained on the backs of freedmen served as a permanent reminder of their previous lowly status. Some people took great pride in their scars, such as the men who hunted animals in the amphitheaters. But whereas they treated them as marks of valor, many others who had achieved modest upward social mobility were deeply embarrassed by the vestiges of their previous status. Former slaves who had been branded sometimes tried to cut out the scars or burned them to conceal their original meaning.

The elite, by contrast, were spared the whip. They used their wealth to ensure that they maintained space around themselves in their homes and by employing retinues to keep crowds at bay. The wealthy also used sound to establish social distance between themselves and the ordinary people. One writer claims that the worst kind of poor "make a disgusting sound by drawing back their breath into their nostrils" (Ammianus Marcellinus 14.6). The wealthy associated this kind of snorting with the grunting of animals and sex. It was the sort of thing you heard if you passed by a cheap brothel, where prostitutes serviced their clients behind the simple cover of a curtain. Ordinary people, by contrast, seemed to find such rude noises hilarious. In one joke, a sailor was asked where the wind was coming from and replied, "From the beans and onions" (*The Laughter Lover* 141). The humor stemmed from simple breaches in normal behavior, a kind of sensual subversion of high culture.

Ancient sensory discourse was also strongly bound up with morality. In the eyes of the elite, manual work coarsened the morals since it brought the laborer into contact with filth and dirt. In this way we can see that elite descriptions of the masses have less to do with reality than with the creation of sensory stereotypes. Hence bad breath was also attributed to sexual misdemeanors (see, for example, Martial 10.3; 11.30; 12.85). The physical and the moral became so intertwined that immorality stank. Brothels became notorious for their foul odor, as did prostitutes who worked in their filthy rooms. The fact that prostitutes disrupted the social order by using their bodies differently from how women were supposed to, meant that they were thought to smell like a corrupted body themselves. It was a way for society to link social outsiders with equally unacceptable sensations.

The close link between the senses and social status meant that the ancients made great efforts to manage the effect that they themselves had on others (see, for example, on dress, Edmondson and Keith 2008; Olson 2008). Rich Roman women could wear blond wigs, often imported from the fair peoples of what is now Germany and Holland. Such wigs were criticized as being unnecessary by the Christian bishop Synesius of Cyrene, in his *Eulogy of Baldness*, itself a rebuttal of Dio Chrysostom's *In Praise of Hair*. Most people understood that personal appearance did reveal a great deal about their social position and so there was a high level of demand for cheap goods that were thought to unduly enhance such an appearance, from fake gemstones and forgeries to cheap copies. Magic books told people how to make bronze look like gold (*Greek Magical Papyri* 7.167–86) and so imitate the wealthy. But the point of this was not to compete directly with the wealthy, but to appropriate some of the symbols of wealth in order to enhance status within a more humble social milieu.

The popular culture also made significant use of the senses to establish its desired outcomes. Magic spells and curses, for example, worked by confounding the everyday senses, playing with texture, color, and smell to subvert the normal sensory world. A "tested spell for invisibility" instructed: "Take an eye of an ape or of a corpse that has died a violent death and a peony plant," then "rub them with oil of lily" (*Greek Magical Papyri* 1.247–62 in Betz 1992). By specifying in exact, minute detail the ways in which particular items were to be used in the ritual, magic placed the individual in a new relationship both to the outlandish and to objects they encountered in their normal lives. The popular culture also openly celebrated physical fun, such as drinking and sex. The elite placed much more emphasis on control of the senses, but the ordinary people lived, for the most part, physical lives, focused largely on meeting material needs, so it is hardly surprising that their tastes were informed by the conditions of their subordination.

RELIGION AND THE SENSES

The ancient world placed great emphasis on the use of the senses to express all kinds of religious meaning. The senses were also an important way of communicating with and experiencing the gods. Rituals such as processions gave visual aspect to the divine order and were accompanied by music, dance, and spoken prayers. Touching cult statues with the hand or a kiss was an important way to transfer divine power to the individual. Various toilet-rituals centered on the washing, oiling, purifying, and dressing of the cult statue itself. Some religious rituals could be extreme. Lucian describes the rites concerned with the worship of the Syrian Goddess, where during festivals the most fanatical followers would gash their arms and turn their backs to be lashed, while the crowd played pipes, banged on drums, and sang sacred hymns (Lucian *The Syrian Goddess* 50–1). As the frenzy mounted some were so carried away by the intoxicating sensuousness of the drama that they committed "the great act"; that is to say that they stripped off, and with a loud shout picked up a sword and castrated themselves. They then ran wildly through the city, carrying their amputated genitals, which they would throw through the window of a house at random, and from this house they would be given women's clothing and jewelry.

Sacrifice was characterized by the smells it emitted: incense, flowers, burning flesh, smoke. Lucian describes the priest officiating at an animal sacrifice as "wallowing in gore." Wine was also sometimes poured onto the burning coals of incense to intensify the sensory experience. These wondrous scents were believed to attach themselves to those who had established a close relationship with the divine (Harvey 2006: 13). In the same way that the senses worked in ancient medicine to affect the body of the patient directly, so in religion it was

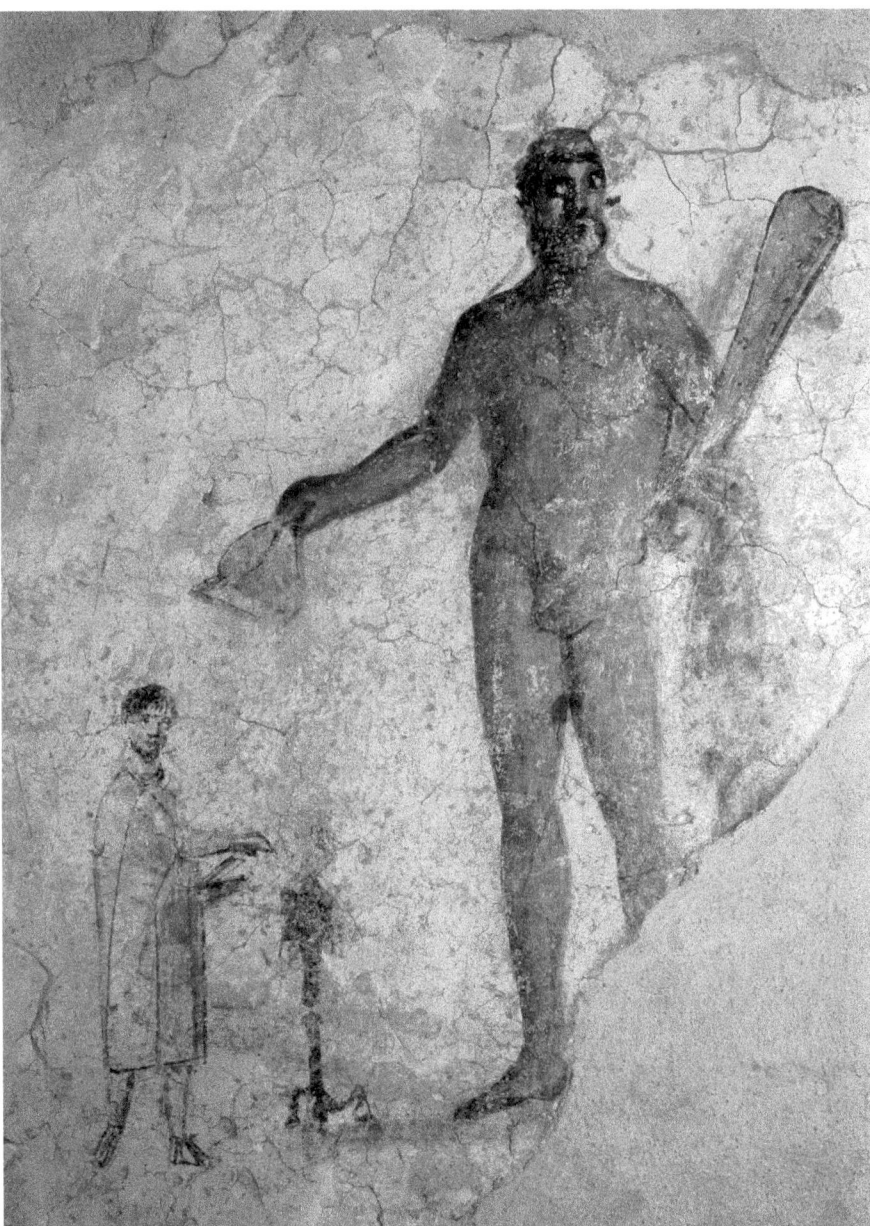

FIGURE I.2: Fresco showing Hercules and a worshiper from a tomb from the Isola Sacra cemetery near Ostia. Getty Images.

thought that the senses could have a palpable effect. At its most powerful, this revealed itself in the healing touch of the holy man. A woman who had suffered blood-loss for twelve years was cured by Jesus simply by touching the hem of his clothes. But in the wrong hands, the senses could become a potent weapon to entice people away from righteousness: the Christian heretic Arius seduced believers to his cause by composing catchy hymns (Philostorgius *Church History* 2.2).

The ancients sensed the divine in every aspect of their lives. This made contact with the sacred an intensely physical experience. Demons could enter the body simply through a yawning mouth. These demons were described by one saint as appearing like "bright phantoms" and "great howling arose" and they flew around his face like a swarm of bats (*Life of Hypatius* 18). When the possessed spoke in tongues it was because they spoke the language of these devils. One of main ways to influence the demonic powers was through the sounds of words. The incantations of magic spells represented the language of demons. Sharp, ringing noises, like those produced by wind-charms hung outside houses, were thought to ward off demons, perhaps because it was believed that the tinkling of brass was in fact the voice of a demon imprisoned within the metal.

THE SENSES AND THE GROWTH OF LUXURY

The spread of Roman power across the Mediterranean world meant that their empire incorporated an extraordinarily diverse set of cultures. The phenomenal growth of the city of Rome, to about one million inhabitants, also created a huge market for a greater variety of goods and imports from these new provinces. The Roman sensorium burgeoned as a result. There was, for example, a rapid increase in the numbers of pigments, dyes, gems, and different colored marbles, which significantly expanded the Roman chromatic spectrum. And traditional Roman behavior was transformed. The elite, made rich by the acquisitions of empire, were now in a position to spend vast sums on luxury. Modern free market capitalists might imagine that this was a wholly good thing. But for the Romans the increase in sensory pleasures created huge moral problems because it was seen as having a direct, harmful effect on the citizen body. Luxury represented a total onslaught against the senses since it reflected a coalescence of various sensuous experiences. It was feared that the tough military men on whom the empire had been founded would be weakened by exposure to softness and sensuousness. A moral discourse therefore arose which aimed to regulate such sensory excess.

Many Roman writers, therefore, condemned individual actions which broke the proper sensory order. Pliny, for example, complains that painting was by the first century thought worthless if it was not executed in a multitude of costly and exotic pigments (*Natural History* 35.39). The popularity of bathing was of particular concern. The fictional nouveau riche character, Trimalchio, is described by Petronius as luxuriating in the baths, his skin glistening all over with perfumed oil. He was being rubbed down, not with ordinary linen, but with towels of the purest and softest wool, and was then wrapped in a blazing scarlet robe (*Satyricon* 28). Everyone in Rome now seemed to have so much money that moralists fulminated that, "Everyone thinks himself impoverished and distressed unless the walls of his bathing area sparkle with marble, paintings and glass; or unless Thasian marble, once a rare sight even in a temple, lines the swimming pools and the water pours out of silver taps" (Seneca *Letters* 78.23, Loeb translation). Depilation had become more common among men, making their once hairy legs smooth and effeminate. Other "metrosexuals" were wearing balsam and cinnamon to perfume themselves (Martial 14.59; 3.63). Spices and perfumes were associated with the supposedly decadent Greek and Persian East, which added to their connotations of immorality. Even slaves allegedly had silver mirrors (Pliny *Natural History* 34.160). The emperors themselves were the most extreme examples of sensuous excess. Nero supposedly used to fish with a golden net, drawn by silken cords of purple and scarlet (Suetonius *Nero* 30).

All of this was, of course, wildly exaggerated for rhetorical effect. Vivid accounts of the sensory excesses of emperors, for example, can be seen as reflecting concerns about social change in wider Roman society. By concentrating on these supremely powerful individuals, Roman moralists were able to discuss concerns about societal change in a personalized and concrete form. Their hope was probably to try and influence, if not control, imperial misbehavior by establishing fixed norms about what was considered acceptable behavior for normal people in a civilized society. Whether it had any tangible effect is impossible to say.

Elite moral concerns about disruption in the sensory order also focused on the great city of Rome and its huge non-elite population. In the eyes of moralists, it was the city where the foulness of the people was most evident. The filth of the city was transposed onto the crowd: they became the *faex populi*, the shit of the people (Cicero *Letters to Atticus* 1.16). Juvenal complained that it was oriental influence that had degraded Rome with its foul-smelling and foreign-sounding pollutants: "For years now the Syrian Orontes has poured its sewage into our native Tiber—its lingo and manners, its flutes, its outlandish harps with their transverse strings, its native tambourines, and the whores who hang out round the race-course" (*Satires* 3.62–4, Loeb translation). Rome, with its sensory promiscuity, became the epitome of everything that was bad about empire.

EMPERORS AND THE SENSES

The transition from republic to empire at the turn of the first century saw a profound shift in the nature of Roman political and public life. The sole ruler, Augustus as he came to be known, was faced with unifying a society that had been fractured by decades of civil war. He turned to the senses to help him achieve this social reconciliation. Every sense was employed to entice and cajole the various strata of Roman society into a new spirit of concord and harmony. Luxury acquired positive moral connotations. This was not simply a matter of generosity. Making use of the perceived moral qualities of the senses, providing state-sponsored sensory excess in the baths and games was a way to improve both the life and the morality of the people. For it was believed that if the people of Rome had better sensory experiences then they would be directly affected by these influences.

Augustus later boasted that he had found Rome in brick and left it in marble. His extensive building program included gardens, his mausoleum, and the provision of spacious plazas. But these public spaces were not simply architectural. In the Colonnade of Livia stood a giant grapevine, whose shade cooled the crowds. Animals and curiosities were also put on display to satisfy popular interest in the wonders of the empire and beyond. Four elephants carved from highly polished obsidian stood in his Temple of Concord. The Campus Martius, where much of his building work was carried out, with its long, straight streets and clean lines of classical colonnades, contrasted with the jumbled mess of narrow alleyways of the city center. Stone pavements raised the walker from the filth of the street. In Agrippa's baths, glazed windows, polychrome marble and mosaics were used to create a dazzling internal space. Temples glistened with the varied hues of murals. Avenues lined with laurel and plane trees provided the shade that was synonymous with the life of leisure that had previously been the preserve of the rich. Flowers and bushes sweetened the air, and numerous ponds and fountains served to cool it. Public spaces were filled with classical bronze and marble statues, depicting heroes and mythological scenes.

Augustus' urban plan used stone and marble to demarcate prestige areas. Stone had always been associated with wealth and Augustus' extensive use of masonry for monumental effect gave out a clear impression of power, as well as representing the solid stability and endurance that made his regime different from the political chaos that preceded him. Its very smoothness symbolized the political concord that Augustus had established. At some point in the early empire, a marble map of Rome, the *Forma Urbis Romae*, was placed symbolically on a wall in the Temple of Peace. The empire itself brought access to new quarries: stones such as purple porphyry from Egypt, granite, honey-colored alabaster, and Phoenician snow-white marble all became available. The range of marble hues increased, from Phrygian marble that was spotted with violet, to stone with a reddish-yellow tint and green veins. It all acted as a sensory reminder of the empire and its benefits. But the use of stone had greater significance than this. For stone was often noted for its special ability to affect the senses directly and so also affect those exposed to it. By using masonry in specific settings, often carved with selected images, the imperial building program sought to morally uplift those who experienced it.

The same imperial use of the senses to create a context for social harmony can be seen in the games. These public festivals provided a feast of often-brutal entertainment, ranging from gladiatorial combat to chariot-racing and animal hunting. A religious ceremony preceded the games with the presiding magistrate leading in the garb of a general at a triumph, wearing a gold-braided purple toga, a tunic embroidered with palms, and with a bejeweled wreath of golden oak leaves resting on his head, holding an ivory scepter with an eagle's head. He was accompanied by musicians, statues of gods, and pictures of the emperor and his family. The crowd rose and cheered. The trumpets sounded to start the fights, with flutes signaling the first contests that involved sharp weapons. What is interesting here is the way that different sensory cues were used to guide the audience through the performance. Those watching knew what was about to happen and how they should react because of the sensory triggers implanted into the proceedings.

The games started with sacrifice. This sacrifice gave off the same divine odors that would occur at any sacrifice: of burning incense and smoke. But here it functioned to establish the close relationship between the gods and their emperor, who was seated in the place of honor. And once such a link had been emphasized, it made it clear that the spectators were experiencing an awe-inspiring encounter with the divine on earth. So when the emperor Caracalla entered Alexandria in 215 CE, "musical instruments of all sorts were set up everywhere... clouds of perfume and incense provided a sweet-smelling odor in the streets, and the emperor was honored with torch-light processions and with showers of flowers" (Herodian 4.4.8, Loeb translation). The emperors adopted the smells associated with sacrifice to enhance their aura of authority and divinity and thereby earn the respect, admiration, and awe of the spectator.

The spectacles were full of special effects. Fires and lights could light up the amphitheater to make dusk seem like day. Some of Nero's feasts lasted all night long and objections to the immorality that might result were met with the reply that the light would be too bright to allow any indiscretion (Tacitus *Annals* 14.20). Nero even employed the horrific gimmick of having the pitch-covered bodies of burning Christians illuminate nocturnal chariot races. Other visual effects were more subtle, with purple awnings casting a red shimmer on the pavement. Awnings were provided to help control the distribution of light within the amphitheater. Their popularity is attested to by the fact that adverts for shows often emphasize that awnings will be available. The benefits were partly practical, in that they kept spectators out of the scorching heat of the daytime sun, but also symbolic, in that they created the shade that was necessary for the leisurely life. Within the sensory scheme of the amphitheater, awnings also served to spotlight the stage so that all the action took place in the bright heat of the arena. The best fights were those where the combatants did not run away into the corners but where the "butchery was done in the middle where the amphitheater can see it" (Petronius *Satyricon* 45). The sand itself, the *harena*, helped establish visual focus by means of its glittering mobility.

The games were incredibly noisy. Musical accompaniment came from horns and trumpets, or on one occasion from hundreds of flutes. The screams of victims rang out. When 100 lions were slain at Probus' games, their roars sounded like thunder. One fictional account of a gladiatorial combat describes how, "there was noise everywhere produced by the equipment of death; here a sword was being sharpened, there someone was heating metal plates [used to check that a victim was really dead and not faking it], here rods were produced, there whips … The trumpets were blaring with their funereal sound … everywhere there were wounds, moans, gore" (Pseudo-Quintilian *Declamations* 9.6). When the emperor entered, a loud, formal acclamation greeted him, which acted as an audible register of popular support for the regime. Once the action had started, crescendos of cries arose according to the events in the arena itself.

The games were also full of color. At one of Julius Caesar's games, the gladiators appeared wearing silver armor, and at one of Nero's contests they were dressed in amber. The color, size, and sound of exotic animals imported into the arena from all over the empire overturned the normal sensory rules of sight, movement, and sound. Lions appeared with decorated, gilded manes, sheep entered the arena with purple and scarlet fleeces, and at Gordian the First's games 300 vermilion ostriches strutted across the sand. Inversion and variety were always popular. Thus, condemned criminals sometimes entered dressed in gold tunics, purple cloaks, and gold crowns, which then somehow spontaneously combusted. In some spectacles, the arena was transformed into a forest of trees, or a ship that broke up to release animals that started fighting each other, or the ground opened and up became a wood with fragrant fountains from which monsters emerged. These broad brush-strokes of bright colors and dramatic effects seem to have been popular with the crowd. In this regard, the games can be seen as appealing to the popular taste, rather than the more refined preferences of the educated elite. Instead the games worked on the senses to produce a powerful emotional effect, all of which the elite saw as merely sensational.

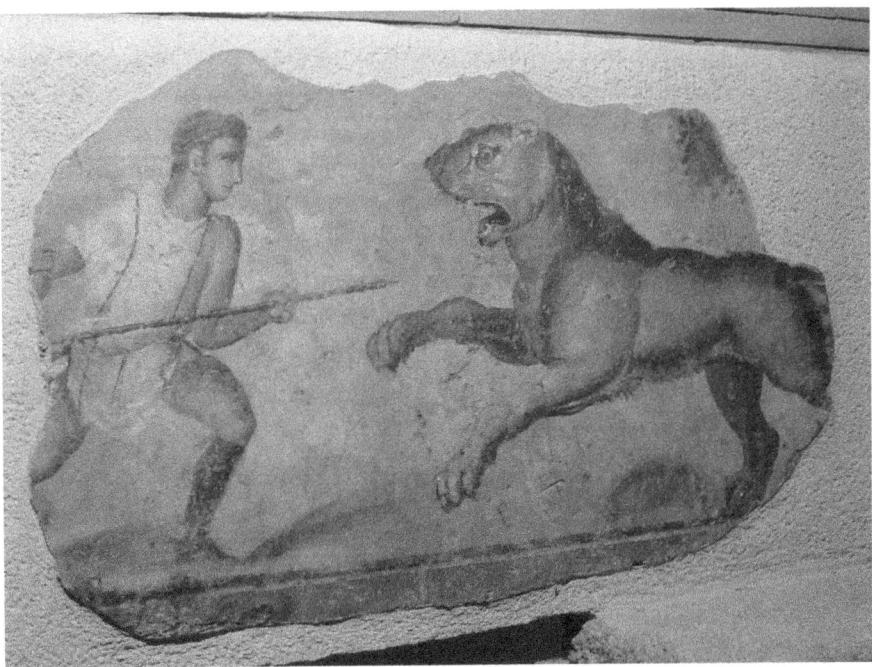

FIGURE I.3: Wall-painting showing a hunter facing a lion in the games. Wikimedia Commons.

Being a spectator was an intensely physical experience. The crowd waved, shouted, jumped, and clapped, as they stared intently at the contests before them. The thunderous applause for the winners echoed across Rome and could be heard well beyond the city walls. Citizens had to wear the heavy toga to the amphitheater, which must often have been extremely hot. In order to alleviate the oppressive conditions within the amphitheater, water was sprinkled to reduce the dust that was thrown up by contests and to cool the air. Perfume was sprayed onto the crowd to freshen the atmosphere. Fresh sand was spread in the arena to cover the blood-spattered traces of the previous combat and create a clean backdrop for the next fight. Cushions were sold to the public to make the stone seats more comfortable. The comfort of the crowd contrasted with the brutal public punishments that were being served up for their entertainment, which involved extremes of touch: wounding, whipping, and being ripped to pieces by wild beasts. Men who volunteered to become gladiators had to agree that they could be burned, beaten, and cut with iron, symbolizing their loss of freedom.

In the games, the emperors used the senses to express the nature of their rule in a physical form. The people, the elite, and the emperor coming together for shared pleasure in a luxurious environment emphasized the cross-social desire for political stability after the ravages of the late republic. But the central role that the emperor and his family played in the games also underlined how politics had changed. It showed exactly where power now lay: not with the senate, but in the hands of one man. The constant repetition of these images in the games, which were held increasingly frequently as the empire went on, made sure that everyone in Rome was aware of this political reality and, indeed, actively bought into it. Being a spectator taught Romans the etiquette for proper conduct in this new form of government: they should be enthusiastic and vigorously supportive, and at the same time obedient and firmly under imperial control. The games also showed spectators, by means of the carnage which often occurred, how utterly their lives were in the hands of the emperor.

THE SENSES AND RESISTANCE

In the games, then, the emperors deployed what they understood to be the affective properties of the senses to create an exciting distraction and vent for social unrest which could help restore the health of the body politic and re-establish social harmony. The enterprise was in many ways successful. When we look at amphitheaters across the Roman Empire we find significant uniformity in terms of design and the kinds of shows that were put on in them.

As such, these great buildings sat at the forefront of the Romanization of the provinces. The imperial use of the senses helped deliver a homogeneous template for how ordinary people could enjoy the benefits of empire and support the regime. Sensory symbols and practices, therefore, had an empire-wide unifying effect.

But by establishing a new sensory orthodoxy, the emperors also opened up the possibility of a new vocabulary of resistance and rejection. The acclamations by the crowd, for example, were an ideological device to deny the existence of any tensions between the emperor and his subjects. That is what the emperors wanted, and for the most part that is what they received. But sometimes the people did not simply clap and cheer as they were expected to. They would chant and clap in unison, and shout complaints and rude comments about the emperor. In more extreme outbursts of popular anger, the crowd rioted and threw excrement to underline the strength of their feeling. During riots in Antioch in 387, even statues of the emperor Theodosius were pulled down, smashed and covered in shit, then dragged through the streets. It was not a tactic that they could use too often, for risk of inciting a violent military response, but it was a way for the people to adopt the sensory language employed by the emperors but change the grammar of its expression.

In sixth-century CE Constantinople, groups of young male spectators in the circus used fashion to establish an alternative identity. They wore extravagant clothes with special sleeves on their tunics that billowed out when they waved their arms. They combined this theatrical display with synchronized clapping and chanting to maximize their group effect. They also wore their hair in a kind of ancient mullet, long at the back but cut short across the forehead, and grew Persian-style beards and mustaches. They called this the "Hunnic" look (Procopius *Secret History* 7.8). In this way, they established a close-knit group identity by using outrageous appearance and adopting a barbarian hairstyle. The relative freedom of expression granted to the crowd in the circus also meant that they had ample opportunities to express discontent as and when they felt like it.

What examples like this show is that, however much the emperors might have liked to control the senses, the ordinary people were always able to use them for their own ends. So while the emperors tried to keep purple as an exclusive color for themselves, its use remained widespread. People sometimes ignored the seating code in the amphitheater and wore colorful dress instead of the toga. Or they scratched graffiti into the stone. The seats in the amphitheater at Aphrodisias were littered with gameboards, phalluses, and signs of abuse. This indicates that imperial buildings should not be understood only from the emperor's point of view but also from that of the humble user. The Latin poet Ovid shows that elite authors could also delight in debunking the official culture. In his *Art of Love* (1.5 Loeb translation), he subverts the Augustan ideology of moral rebirth and uses the circus as a place to have an affair. The new sensory language of the emperors becomes the language of sensuousness:

> Sit right next to your girlfriend—no one will stop you—and squeeze up beside her as closely as possible. It's really easy to do. The seats are so narrow, you have to . . . Perhaps a speck of dust will settle on her breast (it often happens); make sure you brush it off with your hand. Even if there is no speck of dust, pretend—and keep brushing off nothing!

CHRISTIANITY AND THE SENSES

Many of those who used the senses to reject Rome were Christian. Ancient Christianity is often thought of as being an entirely non-sensual, non-physical religion. The early Christians certainly seem to have shown little interest in the sensuousness of the Roman Empire in which they lived. As a small, marginal, and largely ignored religious group they had sought to differentiate themselves from the surrounding religious milieu by adopting an alternative sensory vocabulary. These early Christians were more focused on the Second Coming than on employing the senses to help them develop a closer relationship with God. It is, therefore, in their apocalyptic literature, which looked forward to Judgment Day, that we find a far greater focus on the senses. Images of heaven and hell contained vivid details of the awe-inspiring or terrible sights and sounds which would be found there. But as the small Christian community steadily grew during the first centuries of its life, this new religion developed its own way of using the senses, and acquired its own particular set of sensory-related symbolism. Whether it was in the increasing use of scents as part of their rituals and processions, the dramatic use of light in churches, or the imagined fragrance of the afterlife, the senses came to sit at the heart of how Christians defined themselves and the structure of their communities.

Sacrifice, which included a range of offerings, lay at the heart of Roman pagan religion because it acted as the channel of communication between the human and the divine spheres. The smell of incense was habitually used to initiate contact with the gods, who were thought to delight in its sweet odor. The early Christians had refused to partake in such sacrifice, even if it only entailed the burning of incense. In the occasional persecutions of Christians by the Roman authorities, those Christians who gave in to Roman threats and torture and did make such sacrifice were dismissively known by other Christians as "incense-burners." But the Christians found it far easier to accept the idea that the presence of God resulted in a beautiful aroma, perhaps because of the more ethereal qualities of smell. Smell therefore provided a means to gain access to God. Nor was it surprising that some of this divine odor rubbed off on those individuals who had been fortunate enough to experience God directly. To smell God was to smell of God (see Toner, forthcoming).

Smell in particular of the senses, therefore, played a critical role in helping Christians to evaluate the moral qualities of individuals, acts, and spaces. This was particularly true on account of the close association that existed in the ancient world between human sexual behavior and smell. Perfume and desire, immoral sex acts and stench, were thought of as natural bedfellows. This moral aspect to smell was of vital importance because it was believed that the senses could act as entrances to the individual's inner being, the senses being likened to the five gates of a city. In this way, the senses could admit spiritual qualities into the body, which could have a powerful moral effect. It also allowed the Christians to define what they were *not*. By moralizing the senses, they were able to establish a new sensory order to replace what they saw as the debased sensorium of pagan society. Rome became a place which stank of luxury and vice. Accounts of Christian martyrs focused on the sweet smell they gave off while being burned to entertain their Roman oppressors. The purpose of such accounts was, through their repeated retelling, no less than to create a group united in opposition to the Roman state.

We should not assume that these extreme texts reflect the realities of daily religious life for most Christians. In reality, common practices such as interfaith marriage made it impossible for Christians to maintain rigid boundaries between themselves and pagans. The restrained stimulation of the senses, rather than outright rejection, came to be portrayed as the key to living a Christian life within a non-Christian environment. Writers such as Tertullian, Clement of Alexandria, and Origen all insisted that Christians must accept the physical world and seek to understand and know God better by means of sensory experience. God, they argued, had created the senses as part of the material world. It was only if the Christian were to become bound by the senses that he or she would end up their slave.

Constantine's conversion to Christianity in 312 CE brought a sea-change in the social environment in which Christians lived. Suddenly finding itself with the most powerful patron in the Roman world, both wealth and converts poured into the Christian Church. The fact that the Roman Empire now had a Christian head also meant that the physical world lost much of its stigma. The emperor's conversion implied divine approval for the secular state on earth. Among the many changes this transformation brought was a significant increase in the degree of authorized sensory engagement by the Christian community. This new-found acceptability of the physical world meant that the body could be embraced as a site for experiencing the divine. The use of the senses, therefore, acquired a fundamental role in creating a new form of Romano-Christian identity. Such a transformation did not happen overnight. But by the fifth century, when Christianity was firmly embedded in its official status, both public and private Christian ceremony had become comfortably soaked in stunning attire and incense.

Yet Christians continued to voice concerns over what they saw as sensory indulgence even after the empire had become Christian. A fifth-century peasant monk in Egypt, for example, wrote a letter complaining about the bath tax locals had to pay: "We don't want to wash—we have no bread to eat; we have no care for anything of that sort when our children are starving and naked." As he says, those who are forced to build them, unlike the Romans, "do not wash in baths." Here baths are seen as an unnecessary luxury when children are starving for want of food. A disregard for personal hygiene might also serve as a sign of ascetic devotion: When St. Theodore of Sykeon emerged after two years in a cave, "his head was covered in sores and pus, his hair was matted and an indescribable number of worms were lodged in it; his bones were all but through the flesh and the stench was such that no one could stand near him" (*Life of St. Theodore of Sykeon*, Chapter 20, in Baynes and Dawes 1948). Christians rejected the sensory world of the empire and its concomitant sensuality in favor of the "odor of sanctity." These Christian sources from the late Roman Empire show the limits of the Christian accommodation with secular power. However, looking at the incense-filled censers and holy oils which accompanied the ceremonies and processions of late antique orthodox Christianity, and served to give olfactory reminders of the new relationship between God, His Church, and His emperor, it is hard not to see a paganization of Christian practice. Such sensory convergence caused grave concerns in many Christians, who feared a corruption of the true faith. However much, then, Christian moralists might rail against the disgusting sights and smells of pagan practices, in contrast to the holy fragrance of their own, this anger probably reflected their unease at the similarity which certain Christian and pagan sensory practices had come to acquire.

For more than a millennium, therefore, the senses sat at the heart of ancient cultures, from classical Greece to the fall of Rome. That is why any attempt to understand the beliefs of these societies, how they operated in practice, and how they developed, must necessarily involve a detailed analysis of the ways in which the senses permeated their world. It is this detail which the following chapters provide, each showing the ubiquity, centrality, and uniqueness of the senses in different aspects of life in antiquity. For whether it was philosophy or literature, religion or urban life, art or medicine, the ancients inhabited a world that needs to be closely sensed to be the better understood.

CHAPTER ONE

The Social Life of the Senses: Feasts and Funerals

DAVID POTTER

INTRODUCTION

In the winter of 290/91 CE Diocletian Augustus met his colleague Maximian Augustus at Milan. There was a ceremonial entry into the city, on a day when one important sensory experience for all involved must have been chill. Few in the vast crowd that assembled to see what no one had seen in years—the two rulers of the world in one place at one time—heard either of the emperors speak. At times, and at a distance, they could see them speaking to each other in a friendly way, but they were not privy to the conversations. Some people, if they had been close enough to the parade, might have smelt the torches that would have been carried, even in broad daylight, before their rulers. They would have seen the soldiers—maybe there were cavalry units bearing the dragon banner adapted from the Persians which hissed in the wind—heard the tramp of their feet, the martial music with which they marched through the city. They would have seen images of imperial victories on the far-flung frontiers of the empire, images of northern barbarians bowing before Maximian and the submission of Persia's king to Diocletian. They had seen the splendid clothes the emperors wore. The emperors held still, like their images with which people were familiar, as they entered the city, looking neither left nor right, though possibly ducking as they entered the city gates to symbolize their physical superiority (perhaps though this was only a trope developed for a notably short emperor on his visit to Rome some sixty years later). But the great mass of people were not invited to pass into the imperial audience hall, they were not invited to dinner, so they would not taste the food prepared for the emperors themselves. If there was a banquet offered for the crowd—we are not told there was one—they might have scented its preparation and tasted of the emperor's largess that way, but it would not have been the emperor's food, consumed with those privileged few who were permitted into his direct presence. To share the emperor's food, to hear him speak, to touch his very clothes, those were things that only the members of the imperial entourage or the leaders of the community could hope to do. Distinctions of sensory experience shaped the sense of class, privilege of rank, and worth that day. The average person was simply not good enough to hear the emperor's voice, touch his clothes, eat his food, smell his perfume, or see him in an intimate setting.[1]

Sensory control mattered for imperial ceremonial, but do we also see in these moments a more general commentary on the senses? Power may have been expressed by sensory deprivation, but was that deprivation determined by some ranking of senses from greater to lesser—some would now argue that the modern world has elevated sight and sound above touching, tasting and smelling (see Smith 2007: 1–18). If the importance of a sense was related to the emperor's ability to restrict someone's access to him through that sense, such a scheme would have left sight at the bottom, for that was the one of the five senses most open to the masses. If you were really important you could hear the emperor's voice, share his food, possibly even smell his perfume, and touch his clothing—and be seen to do so. You had to be very important to touch the emperor.

Even if touch achieved a somewhat more important role in Diocletianic spectacle, the strongest impression that emerges from the description of imperial arrival (*adventus*) ceremonies is that it was the mixture of senses that mattered most of all. Such a view would be very much in tune with views expressed by various writers on the senses, though not by all. In reviewing discussions of the senses to gain an impression of what might have been expected to be a good or bad sensual experience, it is plain that we are exploring the parameters within which a discussion was held, possible terms that might be used rather than uncovering hard and fast rules, even amongst those who could agree on (or care about) general theories of perception. Those theories of perception begin to emerge into our view during the late fifth and early fourth centuries BCE in the work of Plato and Aristotle. People who moved in Aristotle's circle, for instance, might agree with his association of a "proper sensible" with each sense—"resisting the hand" (hardness) for touch, savors for taste, sound for hearing, odors for smell, and light for sight (Harvey 2006: 104; see also [Simplicius] *On Aristotle's On the Soul 2.5–12* 159 and see Huby and Steele 1997: 196). Both Plato and Aristotle did also try to rank the senses, Plato making sight the most important, while Aristotle claimed that touch and taste were of lesser significance in that all animals made use of them (Harvey 2006: 101–3). Not everyone would agree. Cicero, for instance, seemingly reflects a tradition, also evident many centuries later in the work of Augustine, in which the senses were on a par (Cic. *Or.* 3.99; Aug. *Mus.* 38). In general terms theories of sense perception were essentially tactile—one perceived something because one encountered its sensible manifestation. Even diametrically opposed systems of thought—e.g. Stoic and Epicurean—could agree on this point, though for the Stoic the mind processed impressions of things the sense organs encountered, while for Epicureans sense organs did the processing on their own.

When it came to evaluating touch, the discussion tended to be framed by concepts derived from both religion and philosophy (Ar. *De anima* 2.6.418a 11–14; Ptolemy *Optics* 2.13, tr. Smith). In the one case there was the basic dichotomy between pure and impure, both of which tended to be defined by physical contact or lack of same. The other was connected with Empedocles' theory of earth, wind, water, and fire as the four elements of being. Aristotle and Theophrastus, for instance, argued that the organs for sense other than touch consisted of air and water (Huby and Steele (trs.) *Priscian on Theophrastus* 29). That being the case Aristotle located the sense of touch in the flesh, which he felt to be composed of earth. That was why he was tempted to assert that touch wasn't a "primary" sense organ, "even if we sense immediately on contact with it." ([Simplicius] *On Aristotle's On the Soul 2.5–12* 162; 161; see Huby and Steele 1997: 202, 199).

The situation with touch was a bit more nuanced outside the school of Aristotle, especially in discussions associated with concepts of impurity and cleanliness. In Latin the primary meaning of *sacro* was to "set something aside" for the service of a god, while the verb *polluo* implies a physical act of making something impure. To be *sacer* was either (in its most basic meaning) to be consecrated to a god, or to have forfeited everything to a god through a criminal act; to be *sacrosanctus* was to be untouchable (a good thing in this case).[2] To make something *consacratus* was to set something aside for the use of a divinity; a *fanum* was property that was consecrated; something *profanes* was, in its mildest sense, to be unused in a religious setting, or, more harshly, to be unclean; to be *purus* was to be free from dirt, contamination or admixture; to be *impurus* was to be physically dirty or engaged in sex (OLD s.v. *consacratus; fanum; purus; impurus*). One could turn a perfectly innocent statement into something quite offensive, as Cicero points out, depending on how fast one spoke, so that an audience might hear *illam dicam* (no doubt with a gesture at the person in question) as *landicam* (Cic. *Fam.* 9.22.2 with Douglas 1996: 3). In the Greek world one was not supposed to offer sacrifice unless one was *hagnos*, or pure, a view related to the notion that while divine bodies were pure, human bodies were not. Just how one could become *hagnos* varied from place to place, but in general terms, one who had been in contact with a corpse or been having sex ought to stay away from the gods—at Metropolis in Ionia, a man could be *hagnos* twelve days after the death of a family member, two days after sex with his wife, and three days after sex with a prostitute. At Maionia, the intervals were five days after the death of a relative, three days after the death of another, the same day, if properly cleansed (in public) after sex with one's spouse, three days (again with public washing) after sex with a prostitute. At Olympia, sex in the sanctuary was strictly prohibited (*LSAM* 29 (Metropolis); *LSAM* 19 (Maionia); Minon (2007) n. 4 (Olympia) with Vernant 1991: 49; Parker 1983: 144–50; Potter 2003: 408–9). The regulations of the Yahwist cult that emerge from Deuteronomy and Leviticus make it plain that priests are not meant to come into contact with death, that bodily secretion disqualified one from approaching the divine and even from remaining in the army camp at night—as the army was God's army one could not defile the ground upon which it resided.[3] In this case though the distinction was not so much clean and unclean as things lacking blemish because they are "whole," and actions that detract from "wholeness." Still the crucial point is that these are distinctions arising from physical actions.

Hearing and seeing appear often to have been considered as a pair, both conducive of pleasure and central to understanding of mimesis. In the *Hippias Major*, Plato's Socrates compares the pleasure obtained through the observation of fine decorations and artworks with that of hearing fine sounds, music, pleasing speech, and stories (Plat. *Hipp. Maior.* 298a; *Rep.* 601a–b; 603 b–c), while in the *Republic* he deals with the problem that while a good artist can produce images that look like things that are real, they are not, they deceive people who judge things by their colors and shapes. Whereas Plato is suspicious of the power of imitation, others applaud it. In the third century CE (probably), Aristides Quintilianus asserted that the virtue of musical performance excited the emotions through both melody and actors' gestures—though he also notes that people's emotions might be aroused differently according to age and gender—children sing through pleasure, women in grief, and old men through divine possession. Such was the power of music that people needed to make sure they used it in the right way, with properly authorized melodies, rhythms, and dances (Aristid. Quint. 4–6). If one looked at things the wrong way or at the wrong things, one could become perverted, as was Hostius Quadra, the infamous libertine of the Augustan age who had himself surrounded by mirrors so he could watch himself having sex. Seneca noted that Augustus felt that his slaves should not be punished for murdering him (Sen. *Quest. Nat.* 1.16). This warning tracked Lucretius' observation that desire could pervert vision by influencing a person to see beauty where there was none, even though this might have reflected his personal understanding of pleasure—he also equated orgasm with death and compared it with a battle wound. Such talk resonated with concern that what one could perceive was perceived correctly (Lucr. 4.1155).

One test for correct perception was symmetry. Plotinus noted that we perceive beauty through what we see and what we hear; what we understand to be beautiful is that which is symmetrical and appropriate, hence the linkage between sight and sound that are judged by the same measure (Plot. *En.* 1.6). Much earlier, Cicero had suggested that correct perception arose from nature— the painter did not have an actual image of Minerva in front of him when he painted the divinity, rather an image of what was beautiful. So too with speech—a person had an innate ability to perceive the rhythmic principles that gave pleasure (*Orator* 2.7–9; 53.178; 55.183–4). Eyes, he would write, would judge the beauty and order of colors and shapes as well as moral qualities, agreeing with Plato that the sight of beauty could inspire an aspiration for virtue, while the ears judge the variety of tones and intervals, the qualities of instruments and voices, evidently according to a common scale (*De Nat. Deor.* 2.57.145–6; *De off.* 1.4.14 quoting Plat. *Phaed.* 250d). In this, his view was similar to Philodemus who noted that with hearing all people had the same capacity to grasp the same tunes and experience similar pleasures, even though with other senses people might differ in their perceptions according to their predispositions (*Mus.* 115.44).

Perception was connected with the way sight was understood. Although some, Epicureans for instance, might adopt an intromissionist understanding of vision (one perceived emanations of atoms), most mature thinking on the subject asserted an extramissionist model of vision (Lehoux 2012: 106–32; Smith 1996: 21–35, 49–55). One's perception of an object depended on the ability of reasoning faculties to interpret the stimuli, since perception depended upon the interaction of color, light, and "visual rays" (Ptolemy *Optics* 2.16–17). Sight thus contained a subjective element, with misperceptions arising both from the processes of seeing and of perceiving—visual power accounted for why some people could see better than others, while perception depended upon the ability to perceive what one was seeing. For instance, in viewing a horse-drawn chariot one does not perceive that the wheels are moving at a different speed to the horses because one does not perceive the constituent parts of motion as being separate (Ptolemy *Optics* 2.142; see also Lehoux 2012: 126).

In more practical terms, vision appears to have been the sense most closely associated with understanding power on the human plane. This is perhaps nowhere more obvious than in the theater, where the stratified society of a city met to enjoy the illusions of the stage. Front seats were best in the Greek world and women were excluded from male entertainments, both athletic and dramatic (street theater and mime were another matter and in the Roman period female performers became significant). Still the basic sense was that one saw society the way it should be. The point was made even more strongly in Roman contexts, where first the *leges theatrales* and then laws governing seating at the circus as well as in the amphitheater defined the social order, though in this case one in which women and slaves could be admitted (albeit most often in the cheap seats).[4] It was sight that also allowed people to experience different places—hence the importance of painting, both at triumphs and on other occasions where imperial virtues were illustrated, often coded with complex meanings (for instance, depictions of barbarian villages without the massacre of their inhabitants symbolized integration within the Roman system, while depictions of atrocities represented no interest in finding new Romans; Dillon 2006). No visual spectacle was ever so powerful as that enacted, wordlessly, by Diocletian, when, on May 1, 305 CE, he removed the purple cloak from his shoulders on the very platform outside Nicomedia where once he had been proclaimed emperor to announce what he hoped to be the dawn of a new era of order in his empire (Lact. *DMP* 19).

Roman imperial art and Diocletianic visual spectacle were relatively straightforward when compared to some spectacles of earlier ages, especially those that had evolved in the context of the Ptolemaic court that aimed to create a nearly divine atmosphere on earth. The grand procession of Ptolemy II, with its intermixing of divine statues and humans clad as if they were mythological characters was intended to blur the line between the kings and the gods. So it was that a four-wheeled cart, drawn by 180 men carried a 15-foot statue of Dionysus pouring a libation followed by a procession that included two massive Delphic tripods, the priest of Dionysus, the guild of artisans, and "satyrs, having golden crowns and dressed in scarlet," some carrying a golden oinochoe, others a karchesion. They followed "two Silenoi in purple cloaks and white sandals" between whom walked physical representations of the concept of time in the form of

> a taller man, six feet tall, in a tragic costume and mask, who carried the golden horn of Amaltheia. He was called Eniautos. A beautiful woman of the same height followed him, adorned with much gold jewelry and a magnificent [costume]; in one hand she carried a crown of persea, in the other a palm branch. She was called Penteris. Four Horai followed her elaborately dressed and carrying her fruits.[5]

Cleopatra's later displays when she greeted Antony in Cilicia, with their own evocation of her divinity, and Antony's own imitation of Dionysus at Ephesian and Alexandrian processions are in the same visual tradition (Plut. *Ant.* 24–8). In Antony's case the coded message that he could stand in for the pharaoh played into the hands of his Roman enemies who saw such spectacle as being fundamentally un-Roman, as living men, even those who might claim the special favor of the gods, would avoid such overt identification.

Just as sight and hearing tend to be joined in classical discourse, so too tend to be smell and taste. Both are linked with the social gradation of food, and the moral evaluation that accompanied the advertised consumption of certain types. In Ptolemaic Egypt, accounts connected with visits to villages by royal officials show that villages were expected to provide foodstuffs appropriate to the rank of their inspectors (Verhoogt 2005: 62–5). In Classical Athenian thought, the *opsophagos*, or person who indulged in the most expensive of foods, was routinely denounced as an anti-democratic hedonist—such menu items included delicacies such as boiled feet, heads, ears, cheeks, intestines, stomach, snout, and tongues prepared in an overtly non-Homeric way, by boiling; a nasty send-up of Thyestes' feast as fine dining has him commenting on the innards of his children as if they were those of a pig. These foods, in imperial Alexandria, were prepared in what appears to have been a series of gourmet shops, the *ephthôpolooi* (Ath. *Diep.* 94c–6e with Wilkins 2000: 12–24). The association of stewed innards with luxury may have reinforced a mainland Greek identity that appears to have been reinforced by literal tastes for more simple food preparations, by way of contrast with the stews prepared by "Italian" and "Sicilian" cooks, a prejudice that appears to be visible in Delian houses which provide evidence for ethnic differences in food terms (Romans liked their stews).

In this case, careful study of cooking utensils on Delos shows that characteristic Greek cooking vessels were placed directly over a fire, while characteristically Roman cooking vessels are constructed either for use in an oven or to act as ovens when placed over a fire (Olson and Sens 2000: liv–lv; Peignard-Giros 2000). Scent, however, had purposes beyond taste in defining appropriate space, the difference between human and divine (Potter 1999: 171–2).

FEASTS

Within the range of beliefs about the senses, the exploitation of sensory experience in private and public life varied enormously according to context, and in what follows we shall explore the theme in conjunction with two collective rituals—banquets and funerals. My point will not be to catalog all the sensory aspects of these events, but rather to illustrate a range of ways in which ritual could activate sensory awareness. By activate, I mean to draw particularly upon one or another sense to achieve meaning; since all witnesses will obviously be employing all their sense in basic daily functions, I am interested in how one or the other appears to be a particular focus of attention.

Before discussing the activation of the senses it is necessary to consider public actions taken to prevent that activation. Both funerals and banquets were, in different ways, the object of laws aimed at limiting elaborate personal expenditure, largely as a way of preventing such events from becoming excessive public displays (which would happen in the long run as democratic institutions failed to constrain the ambitions of the dominant classes of the ancient world). In the case of dining, ridicule of the sort that appears in Aristophanes might have served to quell some excess, as might the notion that gustatory excess was somehow barbaric—the sort of thing that Persians engaged in. On the Roman side, more formal legislation was the order of the day: a *lex sumptuaria*, a law limiting private spending on dinners, appears to have been a specifically Roman legislative act (Rosivach 2006: 1–2). Such laws look much like moral lectures in their efforts to restrict the amount of silver on display, the placing of limits on expenditure for market-bought food according to the day of the week, insistence on specific indigenous menu items, some dispensation for things grown on the host's property, and bans on the artificial fattening of poultry. Athenaeus claimed that only three people ever actually observed these limits. It is not clear how he knows this. Still, the underlying issue is one that is in common with other discussions of the senses, that what is good is "natural," and that "mixing" is at variance with the natural order (hence also a sign of sophistication).[6]

Just as private dining habits were taken as an indication of character, so were public dinners taken as symbolizing community values. Group feasting as a form of community formation is attested as far back as Homer, whose image of heroes sitting down to their simple meals at which each person was served an equal portion of food perhaps reflects the ideology of Homer's eighth-century society.[7] It may also be a style of dining fossilized in the Spartan *syssitia* whereby members of the mess contributed food and dined together as a way of building community, and in the custom by which the meat of sacrifice was divided by lot.[8] The massive dinner that Alexander held at Opis to represent the reconstruction of the community briefly shattered by the Macedonian mutiny over the appearance of Persians equipped as Macedonian soldiers was another such event (Arr. *Anab*. 7.11.8–9; see also Diod 17.115.6 on the massive funeral feast for Hephaestion with Schmitt Pantel 1997: 458–9). In that case it is especially unfortunate that we cannot know what was on the menu—were there Eastern delicacies to supplement standard Macedonian fare? Certainly there would have been a lot of wine. At Athens, the first day of the Apatouria, the annual festival that concluded with the admission of new members to a phratry, involved a public banquet for the phratry's men. The meal seems to have been plentiful, as, it seems, does the drink (Lambert 1993: 152–62). One other thing that was important about these events is that they excluded women. Places where free women were allowed into public feasts that ought to have been for men only were doomed and, by the Hellenistic period, there were a number of moral tales available stressing the negative effects of mixed dining in public—one of these cases was that of the Etruscans, noted by Theopompus (Diod. 5.40.3–4; *FGrH* 115 n. 204 with Schmitt Pantal 1997: 453–4).

In Homeric banquets, the inclusion only of men of equal status deliberately excluded others, an exclusion made all the more obvious by the scent of meals cooking that people could not eat. In the classical period, the primary venue for public dining was the religious festival, which both offered a socially exclusive vision of society and, through the large-scale activation of scent, was thoroughly noticeable in the urban environment. The scent, at least in Athens, may also have conveyed further meaning as the food preparation appears to have been relatively straightforward, with the meat provided by the hundreds of bovine and caprid sacrificial animals—the cuisine of sacrifice in fact seems to have had a deliberately archaic air, possibly emphasizing the antiquity of the rites themselves. The sorts of delicacies mentioned as features of private feasts in, for instance, Aristophanes' comedies—items such as hare and chaffinch as well as roasted nuts—do not seem to have been on the menu (though, in the absence of direct evidence either for the way food was cooked or distributed it

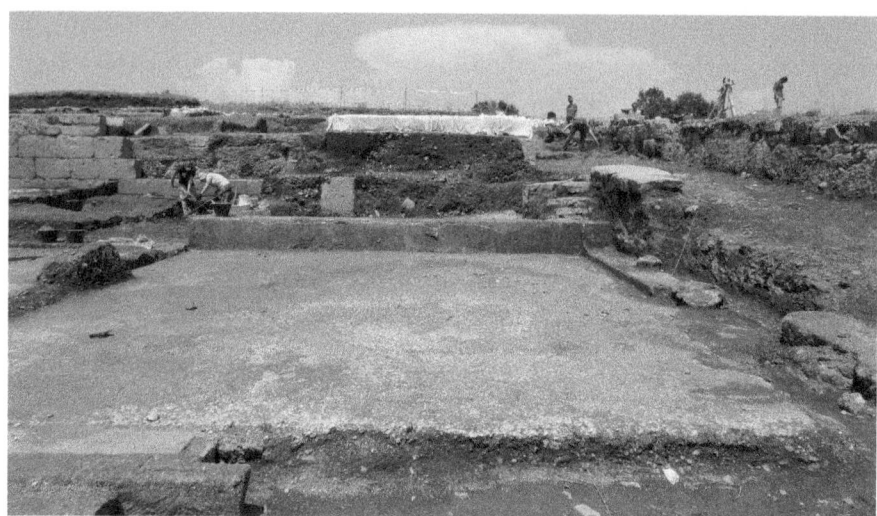

FIGURE 1.1: The public banqueting area at Gabii, from a private collection.

is impossible to be absolutely certain on this point) (Ar. *Pax* 1136–7; 1149–50 with Olson 1998 ad loc.). Changes in food preparation could also have special meaning as, for instance, at an Attic festival for the *Horai* (seasons) where all the sacrificial meat was boiled as roasting was thought to symbolize heat and draught, which people wished these divinities to prevent (*FGrH* 328 F. 173 with Parker 2005: 204).

If the religious festivals of a city such as Athens served to offer an idealized version of society (albeit highly gendered—there were two festivals for women in addition to the many for men), the situation changes somewhat in the years after Alexander when public feasts, funded as liturgies by members of the upper class, were supplemented by further acts of private benefaction. The menu for such events also seems to have been a good deal more varied, as might the guest list have been. The purpose was also rather different, for if traditional sacrificial banquets were intended to stress the notion of community under the gods, euergetical banquets served to stress the magnificence of the donor, his taste and sophistication. We cannot be sure how the tradition began, but public feasting had an important place in Near Eastern ritual well before Alexander arrived in the East at the head of the supremely sympotic Macedonian court—and it may be relevant that euergetic feasts were not, as far as we can tell, intended to be displays of public drunkenness.

Banquets presented in conjunction with cult celebrations or sponsored by kings usually restricted participation to citizens (in the case of cult celebrations) or people in whom the king was interested. Banquets presented by private individuals could have somewhat broader reach as a benefactor wished to send a message about his importance to a more generously defined (if still largely male) audience. A case in point are the dining activities sponsored at Cyme around the end of the first century BCE by a man named Cleanax who invited, "by public announcement citizens, Romans, *paroikoi* and foreigners into the *temenos* [of Dionysus] and entertained them lavishly." This same man "offered a banquet to the people," when celebrating the marriage of his daughter, who may well have been one of very few women present.[9] When he was *prytanis* "he entertained, magnificently and for many days, both the citizens and the Romans; also, for those who dwell in the city, on the regular day, fixed by custom, he offered the necessary sacrifices, including an offering of wine infused with milk, for all inhabitants, free and slave" (*SEG* 32 n. 1246 lines 32–6; see also Hadot 1982: 176–8). This last event, by way of contrast to feeding of the privileged, being concerned as it was with the spirits of the dead, involved everyone in every household. In general terms, public feasts came increasingly to be under the control of private benefactors who used them to reify their views of a properly ordered society (van Nijf 1997: 187).

In the Roman world, there were public dinners accompanying some rites very early in Roman history—the festival of the Latin League seems to have included the status-driven disposition of a sacrificial bull. We are told that the different cities—forty-seven in all—brought various foods ranging from lambs and cheeses to (evidently) cakes, which may have been shared equally but that each representative took "an appointed" part of the bull, an act that appears similar to the differential distributions of meat amongst members of a sacrificial party that appears, for instance, on a fourth-century BCE sacrificial calendar from Cos (Dion. *AR* 4.49.3 with e.g. Rhodes and Osborne 2003 n. 62 lines 46–54; see also Donahue 2004: 54–5). Another archaic ritual, that of the Arval Brethren, involved the brethren dining away from public view, symbolizing the important point that the state cult was in the hands of special people. If the menu that is later attested derived from early iterations, then it would seem that the Arvales had a relatively simple meal involving bread, vegetables, honeyed wine, and possibly some lamb at one of them. A relief showing a meal at which the Vestals were present likewise appears to have had rather simple fare (for Arval meals see Scheid 1998 n. 100: 114 with Schied 1990: 441–676; for the Vestal banquet see Dunbabin 2004: 73–4). It is a pity we don't know what was on the menu in 311 BCE when the *collegium* of flautists who played at public sacrifices was banned from holding a public dinner in the temple of Capitoline Jupiter and went on strike to Tibur (their banquet was restored). What we do know is that a public banquet was being held so that a group within the city could publically celebrate themselves (Livy 9.30.5–10 with discussion of other traditions in Oakley 2000: 397–8). A very different context for public dining appears in the account of Tiberius Sempronius Gracchus' victory over Hanno outside Beneventum in 214 BCE, after which, upon the invitation of the townspeople, he allowed his men to celebrate a public banquet (he later dedicated a picture of the event in the temple of Libertas) (Livy 24. 16.14–19).

Gracchus' victory celebration suggests that there were already occasions for massive public feasts, and there is even more evidence in the course of the second century for the spread of various forms of dining, both luxury and mass. On the luxurious side we have sumptuary legislation passed to limit expenditure at the banquets patrician families held during the Megalensian games. On the side of mass feeding, in the same period, it appears that large-scale feasts were sponsored in conjunction with the Cerealia. What we cannot know for certain is what inspired Antiochus IV to lay on 1,000, then 1,500 *triclinia* (dining couches) for events he held at roughly the same time that patrician expenditure was being restricted at Rome (Pol. 30.26.3; for the context see Potter 2011: 176–7). The choice of Italian dinner equipment, along with the decision to offer a gladiatorial exhibition, suggests he was looking to Roman examples, and the particular context—an imitation *munus*—might suggest that public feasting was coming into vogue at this point in conjunction with *munera*, privately organized spectacles whose content was not dictated by tradition. It is against this background that we may have to reinterpret the significance of Caesar's massive celebration, which included huge feasts for the Roman people. Rather than being something new, it would seem rather to have been simply an "upscaling" of things that were being done already. Just as Crassus, in his consulship and possibly with a view to discomfiting Pompey, who was his colleague in that year, had laid out 10,000 *triclinia*, Caesar in 46 would lay out 22,000 *triclinia*. We do not know who was entitled to a place on the couches; the number of possible diners exceeds the number of people left on the grain rolls after his reform in the previous year, and it is possible that he may not have been thinking of feasting a mere 198,000 people as some images of public feasts reveal. Certainly, more than the regulation three persons would take a place, but those who did not have space on a couch might have had seats around tables nearby, which was by that time a well-established way of denoting status.[10] In 22 BCE Augustus tried to limit the expansion of banqueting, ending some and cutting expenditure on others (Dio 54.2.3).

Although interested in limiting expenditure on regular occasions, Augustus was willing to splash out on special events; his *ludi saeculares* would include public banquets after each of the major sacrifices all around the city, while in

9 BCE, Tiberius, celebrating an *ovatio* over the Dalmatians and Pannonians, offered a banquet for citizens (presumably senators) on the Capitolium and "at many places throughout the city." Livia and Julia hosted a banquet for what Dio describes as "women" (possibly indicating the matrons who were invited to events at the *ludi saeculares*).[11] One occasion upon which it appears that people of very different social backgrounds were seated together was at a feast Domitian held at the Colosseum to celebrate the Saturnalia—but that may be an exception that proves what seems to be a rule. The Saturnalia was an event that supported the social order by eliminating typical boundaries (Statius *Silvae* 1.6.43–50 with Donahue 2004: 21–2). It was also rare in that large-scale public banqueting seems to have become a rarity at Rome after the early years

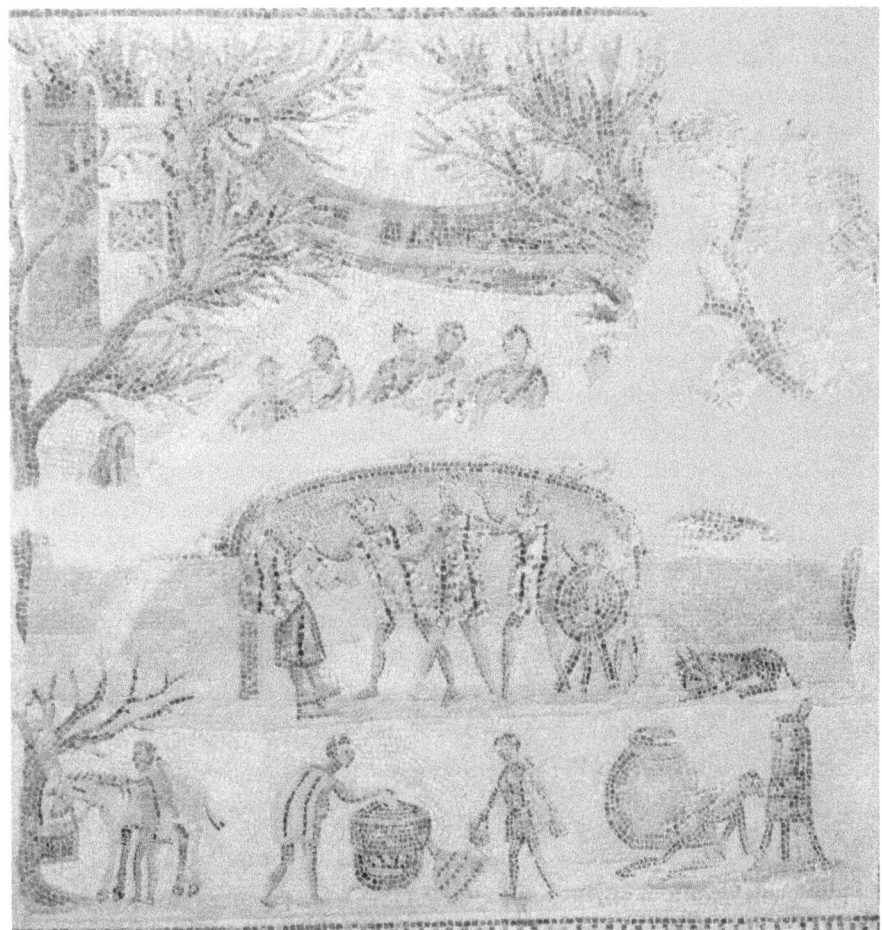

FIGURE 1.2: Relief from Aminternum showing a public banquet, from a private collection.

of Augustus. Possibly, with a million or more people living in the city and a quarter of a million on the grain rolls, it had just become impractical—and, with the development of massive entertainments in the Circus Maximus (much improved under Augustus) and Colosseum, unnecessary (Donahue 2004: 80).

Even though Augustus was trying to limit expenditure at Rome, it is clear that people in Italy and the provinces were watching for precedents they could follow to illustrate their own good breeding. The influence of some Augustan practices, well outside of Rome, may be evident in a second-century CE decree from Boeotia, honoring a wealthy man named Epaminondas of Acraephia who, amongst other things, served honeyed wine (*mulsum*), hurled *missilia* (tokens that could be exchanged for gifts) into the crowd, and held separate meals for men and women. In the context of a Caesarea celebrated along with a local festival,

> he invited to all the breakfasts the children of the citizens and the slaves of an appropriate age while his wife, Kotila, offered breakfast to the women of the city, their daughters and the slave girls of appropriate age; he did not even leave out the travelling merchants and the people helping with the festival, inviting them to breakfast after the official opening of the festival, which no one had ever done.
>
> *IG* 7.2712 with Oliver 1971

A sign of the very rapid reaction to events in Rome might be provided by the feasts put on by a man named Gamala at Ostia, which, as was the case with Epaminondas' benefactions, appealed to different audiences (D'Arms 2000: 198–200). Hundreds of inscriptions give greater or lesser degrees of detail about municipal feasts, some including all male residents, others only members of a colony implanted within another urban environment, others citizens only, and in some cases even including people in the area (*vicani*). Food would at a minimum include honeyed wine and bread (*crustulum*). Generally speaking, the higher one's status on such occasions, the better one ate—just as was the case in the contemporary Greek world (Donahue 2004: 92–145). The crucial point is that sensory deprivation—the obvious refusal to allow a person to participate in the full experience available to others—was a fundamental aspect of social structuring.

FUNERALS

Funerals tended to activate sight and sound to reify the concept of sadness, while using scent to eclipse the reek of a dead body—the last thing that anyone of any means at all wanted to have at a funeral. The earliest description of a funeral that we have in the twenty-third book of the *Iliad* stresses, on the day of the actual burial, the sound of the Myrmidons as they led the lament, the gushing blood of the sacrifices, the smoke of the pyre made from wet wood, and finally the roar of the flames, burning into the night as they consumed the body of Patroclus. The body itself had been washed to occlude the evidence of the violence with which Patroclus' life had ended, and scented to hide what may be implied in Homer's description of the care the gods were taking of Hector's corpse—the increasing evidence of decay as the days passed. Excavations on Cyprus, and, especially at Lefkandi on Euboea, have shown that some aspects of Patroclus' funeral existed in the real world, and here again we must imagine not just the scent of the pyre, but the howls of death, animal and in some cases human, and the scent of freshly spilled blood, that accompanied a leader of society into the grave (Coldstream 2003: 349–52; Popham *et al.* 1993: 1–4, 19–22). Then, of course there would have been the scent of roasting flesh, as a prelude to the funerary banquet—the clash of sounds and scents between those connected with departure and social continuity are significant aspects of the way death's meaning was encoded.

In the ancient world the sensual social division in death is especially notable, particularly in Roman contexts, though it is by no means absent in Greek contexts either. The worst thing that could happen to a person was to be buried as an unattended corpse in a public grave, surrounded by the reek of death (Hopkins 1983: 208–10).

At conventional funerals in, for instance, classical Athens, the first sense to be activated by death was touch. The house where the person had died was polluted—if the death could be imminently predicted the house might be declared off limits even before the death. A special water beaker would be placed at the door so that people leaving the house could wash themselves— the water would come from the unpolluted house of a neighbor. Within the house it was the women's duty to wash and anoint the corpse, placing it in clean clothing with a crown. The funeral bier would be spread with branches and leaves; ideally the house would be swept so that the polluted dirt could be placed at the tomb. On the third day, the body would be carried out to the tomb, preferably early in the morning to avoid accidentally polluting people who might encounter the procession to the place of the funeral (the preceding discussion is dependent upon Parker 1983: 33–4). Ordinarily, in the classical period, the body would be burned so that the its scent would be taken up in the scent of the funeral pyre, as in the archaic period, though it would seem that, where there might be a public commemoration of the deceased in a given year—as at Athens—private funerals would have taken care of the corpses independently of the rites of commemoration, where citizens would attend, dressed for mourning and the space would be divided by gender as women and men would grieve individually. At other times and in other places, throughout the Greek world, inhumation was vastly preferred to cremation, and there was considerable concern about the reuse of tombs by unauthorized persons. States were supposed to take care that respectable corpses were not mistreated. From a sensory point of view the dominant sense throughout is touch, for touch is intimately connected with the contagion of pollution.

Rome's immense size brought with it special problems in dealing with the dead, and it is reasonable to assume that these problems may also have beset very large cities such as Carthage, Antioch, and Alexandria. In Rome's case it has reasonably been estimated that some 9 million people died between 100 BCE and 200 CE: the poor, unattached and indigent, those who had come to Rome in the false hope of better things, those living in the huts of the impoverished —*ergasteria* and *turgaria*—or slaves of cruel masters who abandoned them in their last days. Body parts could become a problem: it was a matter of extreme ill omen that wolves were found tearing apart a body in the Forum, or when a dog dropped a human hand beneath Vespasian's dinner table.[12] In the republic bodies were supposed to be buried outside the city gates. In 38 BCE the senate ordered that bodies be burned and that the crematoria be no closer than two miles from the city (Dio 48.43.3 with Bodel 2000: 132; Patterson 2000: 92). Those whose remains could not be cared for became *cadavera* as opposed to *corpora*. Those who handled the bodies of the dead, *libitinarii*, were based by the Esquiline gate near the temple of Juno Libitina and burial grounds for the poor were located south along the Via Labicana and the Via Praenestina, well away from the tombs of the wealthy on the Via Appia. The *libitinarii*, despite their crucial calling, were expected to wear special clothing and were excluded from polite company. Efforts to differentiate status in this group between those who laid out bodies (a more respectable occupation) and those who dragged them away seem to have collapsed by the early imperial period. Outside of Rome, at Isola Sacra, there are remains of some 600 burials either just in the ground or in terracotta sarcophagi (Carroll 2006: 69). These bodies were most likely buried by the authorities who were charged with removing the bodies of the indigent at night. Only the socially untouchable would be witnesses to the disposals of the bodies of the poor, whose end would be otherwise unwatched and unmarked. They were consigned to oblivion.

Funerals for Romans of higher status were governed by specific rules limiting expenditure, allegedly borrowed from the laws of Solon. While these rules, which we know largely through Cicero's discussion in his *Concerning Laws*, were primarily designed to control costs at aristocratic funerals, they enable us to understand what the "proper" handling of the dead would be. As in the Greek world, pollution fell immediately upon the household and property of a person who had died—the household would go into mourning for a period of nine days during which time the body would be disposed of, unless the deceased was a young child, whose body, like that of an indigent person, would be removed at night. In the period of mourning no family member could sacrifice to the gods. After the moment of death, a close relative would close the eyes of the corpse and family members would call the name of the deceased on a regular basis until the funeral. The body itself would then be prepared for viewing (and, when possible, perfumes would be burnt to control the reek of putrification). On the day of the funeral friends would take the body out of the house to the place of burial beyond the city walls. There, a family member or friend would deliver an elegy and the body would be burned, with the ashes to be collected and placed in the tomb, or the body itself laid to rest (see in general Lindsay 2000: 60–8). Those who accompanied the body would then enjoy a feast (sometimes involving a great deal to drink) (Carroll 2006: 45–6, 71–3).

Cicero once opined that it was in accordance with nature that differences in wealth should cease with death (Cic. *Leg.* 2.59: *quod quidem maxime e natura est, tolli fortunae discrimen in morte*; see also Dyck 2004: 326–7; 4, 5, 6). This may not have been his most accurate observation. The style of a funeral depended very much on who someone was. In the case of grand funerals, a good deal more attention was paid to sensory stimulation than was the case in those for members of the lower classes, where the suppression of senses other than sight and sound was a notable factor until the activation of taste, after the

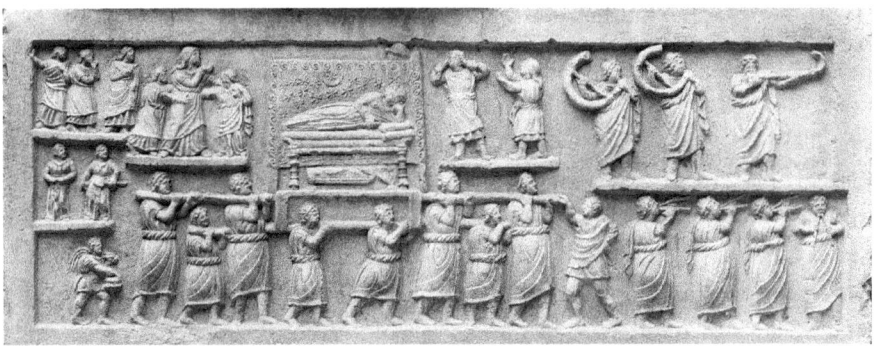

FIGURE 1.3: Relief from Aminternum showing a funeral procession, from a private collection.

deceased's body had been disposed of. Even before the imperial period, Cicero noted that some aristocratic bodies were buried within the *pomerium*, and events were expected to start in the Forum itself (Cic. *Leg.* 2.58 with Dyck 2004: 400–2; see also Flower 1996: 97–109). For grand events of this sort, scent would seem to play an especially important role despite a theoretical ban on especially scented behavior in the ancestral law of the Twelve Tables (*Leg.* 2.60). The funerals of Nero's second wife, Poppaea, and of the dictator Lucius Cornelius Sulla, were notorious for the extraordinary quantity of scent consumed on the pyre (Potter 1999: 181–2). It may also be that while the practice of public incineration developed as a penalty in capital cases in the Roman Empire, heavy perfuming was especially important—it indicated a body properly dealt with, while the smell of roasting human flesh was associated with hideous punishment. The power of this association is perhaps no better stressed than in the account of the death of the Christian teacher, Polycarp, executed in the reign of Antoninus Pius. Witnesses claimed that his body smelled like bread baked in an oven and then frankincense. The smell of bread evoked, for Christians, thoughts of the Eucharist, that of frankincense a sacrificial offering, which Polycarp had become (*P.Poly.* 15.1–16.1 with Harvey 2006: 12).

Vision was also important. The body of the deceased was marked out from that of the living by its attire—usually white for the corpse and black for the mourners. As Artemidorus says: "For a sick man to wear white clothing signifies death due to the fact that dead men are carried out in white. But a black garment signifies recovery. For not the dead but those who mourn the dead wear garments of this sort."[13] So too in the commemorative rites for Lucius Caesar at Pisa, at the altar erected in his memory, public sacrifices were to be made by priests dressed in dark togas, and the beasts offered were to be a black ox and a black sheep wearing black fillets, and when news of Gaius Caesar's death arrived, everyone was to change their clothes until news came that the funeral rites were complete (*ILS* 139, 18–21; 140, 20–3 with Rowe 2002: 111–19). The peaceful accomplishment of these rites, as with the later rites celebrated for the deceased Augustus (albeit with the inclusion of the release of a bird from the funeral pyre to symbolize the deceased's union with the gods) were intended to stress orderly continuity. Tacitus comments that on the day, people thought of another funeral some fifty-eight years earlier which had ended very differently, but then Antony and others had inverted all the cues, visual and auditory, at the funeral of Julius Caesar for effect (*Ann.* 1.8.6). Things that were not supposed to happen were that the deceased would speak (even through an actor), demanding vengeance at the end of the laudation, and wax images of the deceased, revealing the bloody wounds inflicted by assassins were not supposed to pop up from the funeral bier and twirl around in front of the audience (for the events of Caesar's funeral see Sumi 2006: 104–11).

The importance of such a message, again delivered primarily through visual media, is made especially plain in Herodian's description of Severus' deification (which, despite what Herodian has to say, was likely devised for the special circumstance of an emperor who had died away from Rome, just as, much earlier, the Roman funeral of Germanicus had to be arranged to take account of the fact that the body was cremated at Antioch) (Tac. *Ann.* 3.4). In this case we are told that a wax image of the emperor was placed on golden drapes resting on a high couch in front of the palace, with the male leaders of Roman society sitting in black woolen cloaks on the left. Notable women were dressed in white, with no necklaces or gold jewelry, which "signified they were in mourning." After seven days, during which time doctors made pronouncements on the image's health, the image was pronounced dead, at which point the leaders of the equestrian order, along with young men from the senate, took the image along the sacred way into the Forum. In the Forum, probably in front of the rostra, a chorus of young men and another of women from important families sang hymns, after which the image was moved to the Campus Martius where it was incinerated in a fast-burning, heavily scented fire (Herodian 4.2, see also Price 1993: 56–105). The fire was accompanied by a funeral procession. This procession, like the one to the pyre, involved some significant changes from earlier periods—in the case of the final procession it involved the equestrian order, on horse, a Pyrrhic dance, which was by this time, through a bogus etymology, associated with funeral pyres, and chariots bearing people who wore masks of Romans—both emperors and famous people—from the past (Herod. 4.2.9 with Ath. *Diep.* 12.630d and C. R. Whittaker's note on this passage in his Loeb edition).

Assuming Herodian is correct about the order of events (which is not always a safe assumption), there would have been some notable variations on the most recent imperial funeral in 193 BCE, that of Pertinax, also celebrated with a wax corpse, though in this case the reason was that the actual body had been disposed of in the immediate aftermath of his assassination some months before. On this occasion our witness, Cassius Dio, places all the action in the Forum in a special shrine Severus had constructed. He tells us that while the body lay upon its bier, a young man was employed to keep flies away with peacock feathers. Interestingly he says that this was just what would happen if a person slept (did he too have a peacock feather-waving attendant?). Severus and senators approached the body along with their wives and then separated so that the men were sitting in the open air, the women in the porticos. It was then that images of famous Romans of the past were carried by while choruses of men and boys sang dirge-like hymns, and images of subject nations and then the city guilds were also paraded. Finally there were images of other men, soldiers, horse and foot, both under arms, racehorses and offerings to the deceased from the emperor, the senators and their wives, distinguished equestrians, communities, and civic corporations. When this procession had passed, Severus delivered a eulogy to the acclamation of the senate. When he had finished and the loudest acclamations had come to an end, all the senators lamented together as priests and magistrates brought the bier down from its perch. These men carried it to the pyre, walking behind the senators who beat their breasts or played dirges on flutes. Once the procession had arrived at the pyre, Severus' and Pertinax's relatives bade the corpse farewell before taking their place on a tribunal surrounded by benches for the senators, who joined the emperor in watching the elaborate maneuvers of the magistrates, equestrians and soldiers. When this was done, the consul lit the pyre, and the old emperor joined the gods in a mass of Eastern scent (Dio 74.4.1–5.5).

Again, assuming Herodian described something that actually happened, the differences between these seemingly similar ceremonies are striking—most notably in the depression of the role of the senate and the elevation of that of the equestrian order. This would have been entirely appropriate in the new regime, most of whose most significant members were equestrians, while the actions of the doctors appear to have been designed to mime the emperor's final illness, stressing the point that he died of natural causes. At Pertinax's funeral, by way of contrast, the senate's dominant position was stressed, as was the discipline of the army under the new regime (something of a sore point, one might surmise, given the role of the now-discharged praetorian guard in Pertinax's death). Similarly, at another funeral in 337 BCE, a very different visual spectacle revealed essential truths about the system.

The funeral in question was that of Constantine. Constantine was not cremated. His body, transported to Constantinople from the imperial estate outside Nicomedia, where he died, must have been preserved in some way, for it would be kept on display until Constantius II could make the journey from Antioch to oversee the funeral (this was the first sign that Constantine's plans for the succession would be put aside because there was no self-evident reason why Dalmatius, Constantine's nephew and one of his designated heirs, could not have run the event himself if he had the support to do so). In Eusebius' politically charged version, it was the military that took charge of the body, laying it in a golden coffin shrouded in purple, which was duly taken to the capital and placed in the palace's most splendid audience hall. There it was placed on a high pedestal surrounded by candles on golden stands, offering "a wonderful spectacle for the onlookers of a kind never seen on earth by anyone under the light of the sun from the first creation of the world" (Eus. VC 4.66.1 tr. Hall). Then it appears that every day until the funeral:

> The commanders of the whole armies, the *comites* and all the ruling class, who were bound by law to pay homage to the emperor first, making no change in their usual routine, filed past at the required times and saluted the emperor on the bier with genuflections after his death in the same way as when he was alive.
>
> VC 4.67.1, trans. Hall

They were followed by members of the senate and other important folk, then by the common people. So far the behavior is largely recognizable as a continuation of earlier ceremonials, with pride of place now going to military and court officials in a city where the "senate" was no more than a glorified town council. Things changed on the day of the funeral when Constantius II, newly installed in power, led the funeral cortège, consisting of soldiers only from the palace, to the mausoleum Constantine had built across town near the Church of the Twelve Apostles and whose remains would be collected to join his own. His sarcophagus was facing the entrance. As a Christian he had to await the Second Coming and thus the notable scent of ascension had to be omitted.[14] Instead of becoming a god, he became a relic.

Funerals, imperial or otherwise, activated a particular set of the senses, those most closely associated with the description/recognition of status. The degree to which this was the result of deliberate selection or simply "the way things worked," depends upon the degree to which other public acts might activate other senses, especially touch, given that the activation of taste could to some degree depend (in ancient theory as in human reality) upon the activation of scent. The sensitivity of the planners of major events to the sensual messages that they were sending was perhaps more visible when codes were broken than at other times—you cannot break a code that does not exist. The sophistication with which these codes were handled, the cultural weight they bore, is evident at every period of antiquity, and the changes in the way that the senses were activated over time tend to reflect quite closely broader sociopolitical developments. The ways that Constantine and Diocletian departed the political scene are perhaps the most striking examples of how sensitive the sensory aspect of spectacle could be. Diocletian wished to depart as a symbol of a reordered world in which one ruler could pass on power to another. Constantine wished to depart in a way symbolic of the fundamental change his life had made to the intellectual orientation of the Western world.

CHAPTER TWO

Urban Sensations: Opulence and Ordure

GREGORY S. ALDRETE

APPROACHING ANCIENT ROME: A STUDY IN CONTRASTS

Imagine a traveler approaching the outskirts of Rome along one of the empire's great roads, such as the famed Appian Way. Even before setting foot in the city proper, he or she would have encountered several strong visual and olfactory stimuli that would have served as appropriate introductions to both the positive and negative aspects of the Roman urban experience. First, representing the wealth and grandeur of Rome, our visitor would have encountered a veritable forest of often extravagant marble tombs lining the last few miles of the approach to the capital city.[1] These mausoleums ranged from simple, upright, inscribed stone slabs to elaborate house-like marble structures containing the ashes of Rome's great aristocratic families. Reflecting the intense competition for status among the members of this class, their tombs were frequently built using the finest imported marbles and decorative stones, and would have been adorned with high-quality statues or reliefs of those interred. Some of these larger tombs were surrounded by beautiful park-like manicured gardens, replete with marble benches for visitors or mourners to take their ease upon, and marble tables where they could eat an annual feast in honor of the dead. Expertly carved inscriptions boasted of the deceased's life and accomplishments. A visitor from the countryside would no doubt have felt awe at the sumptuousness of these tombs for the dead, many of which would have surpassed, in both richness and size, anything in his or her home village.

Our traveler would soon have been confronted with some less pleasant reminders of the big city, however. While many tombs were immaculately maintained, others were neglected and crumbling, or covered in unsightly graffiti. Some of these had been broken into by Rome's large homeless population and converted into impromptu shelters, while others had materials crudely stripped off them for reuse in other monuments. Since the cremation of bodies took place outside the city boundaries, and because a city of Rome's size would have produced around 90–150 corpses per day, there would have been funeral pyres burning more or less constantly in this region, and the whole area would have lain under an unpleasant pall of smoke. The air would have been permeated with the acrid smell of burnt wood and flesh, and every surface would have been coated with a nasty layer of greyish ash.

Even more disturbing, Rome's colossal population seems to have used the zones just beyond the city gates as convenient dumping grounds for garbage of all kinds. In addition to the refuse and excrement that appears to have been deposited here, there were bodies of the poor or homeless who could not afford any form of interment. It has been estimated that Rome produced 1,500 such corpses annually, and to these would have been added innumerable animal

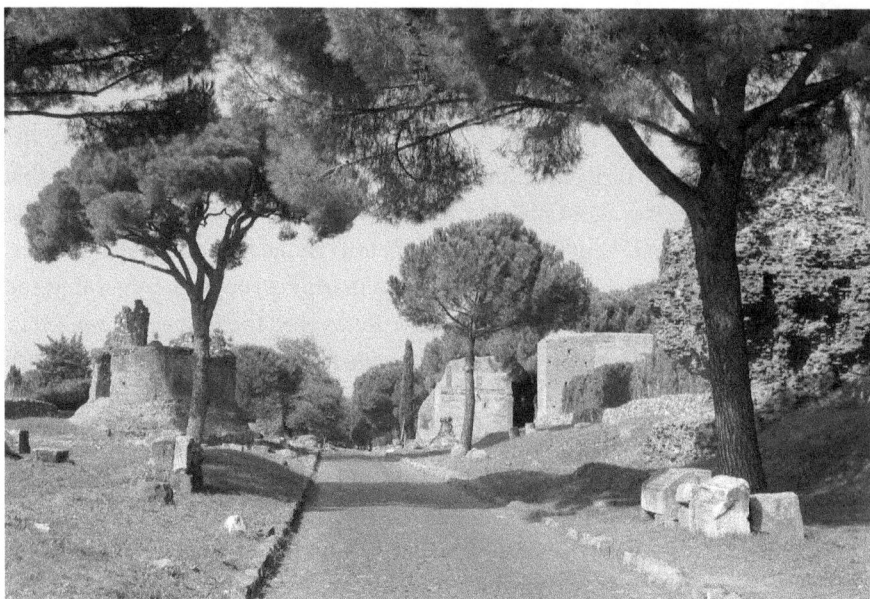

FIGURE 2.1: View of the Appian Way with remains of tombs, from a private collection.

carcasses. Much of this unwanted material apparently ended up in great open-air pits, known as *puticuli*, whose name suggestively was believed to derive from a word, *putescare*, meaning "to rot" (Varro *Ling.* 5.25). These pits (or similar ones) have been excavated just beyond the city walls on the Esquiline hill, and disclosed a revolting mixture of refuse, excrement, and both human and animal corpses and offal. The excavator described the contents of these pits as having been "reduced to a mass of black, viscid, pestilent, unctuous matter," and the stench was allegedly still so vile after 2,000 years that the workers had to be allowed frequent breaks (Lanciani 1888: 65).

Outside Rome's boundaries, a number of official inscriptions have been discovered declaring that bodies or ordure had to be carried and dumped beyond the location of the marker, but the very presence of these stones seems to suggest frequent violations of this injunction (*CIL* 6.31615; *CIL* 6.31614). On one of these markers, a perhaps exasperated official had hand-scrawled an additional warning: "Haul your shit farther on if you don't want trouble!" (*CIL* 6.31615). Similar tomb inscriptions that command "Don't piss here" further testify to attempts to discourage or prohibit such practices, but nevertheless, along with the visual splendor of the tombs, the very first strong sensory impression that ancient Rome would have made on visitors would have been the stench of burning bodies, rotting garbage, and human excrement. Like the god Janus, ancient Rome presented its inhabitants with a two-sided visage, and the sights and smells that greeted a traveler approaching the city nicely encapsulate both sides of the Roman urban experience.[2]

This side-by-side juxtaposition of the awe-inspiring and the unusual with the commonplace and unpleasant would continue once one had passed through the gates and begun to wander around the city. On the one hand, Rome was an impressive place, exhibiting unheard of architectural and technological achievements and wealth, a city which functioned as a trophy case displaying the raw materials, art works, and loot garnered from its conquests—this is the gleaming marble city full of massive edifices familiar from its recreations in the historical movie epics of the 1950s and 1960s. On the other, it was intensely crowded, loud, dirty, smelly, chaotic, and dangerous.

Rome was the largest and most imitated city of the ancient world, so this chapter will attempt to recreate how ancient cities in general were experienced through the five senses by using it both as a representative exemplar and as a site in which many of the most distinctive characteristics of ancient cities were present in their most extreme forms. The chapter will survey how ancient Rome would have been interpreted by the five senses, focusing primarily on two aspects of this experience: perception and negotiation. First, it will consider what it was actually like to live in ancient Rome, and will concentrate on exploring what sensory perceptions would have been specific to, or typical of, urban life. It will also consider how the positive and negative aspects of urban sensual experience made the city a place that both fed the senses (often to excess) and necessitated their relief. In the ancient world, all aspects of life were profoundly shaped and stratified by class, status, and gender, so this chapter will next explore some examples of how sensory experiences differed according to these categories. Finally, it will examine how certain specific sensory stimuli or data, especially sound, would have been used by urban inhabitants to negotiate the landscape of the ancient city and understand what was happening in it.

VIEWING THE CITY: THINGS THAT TOWER, THINGS THAT GLITTER

Once inside the gates of Rome, a visitor would have found his neck becoming sore from repeatedly gazing upward at man-made structures that towered above him. The multi-story apartment buildings (*insulae*) in which the majority of Rome's inhabitants lived, although shoddily built, would have impressed with their sheer height. These wobbly structures, often soaring to 70 or 80 feet of stories haphazardly piled one atop another, and with rickety wooden extensions and porches dangerously overhanging the narrow streets, were proverbially prone to collapse (on Roman *insulae* and their construction, see Aldrete 2007, 2008; Packer 1971). Intermingled with these unplanned, unstable, and impermanent constructs were some of Rome's most beautiful and architecturally sophisticated structures, such as the Pantheon and the Flavian Amphitheater, so solidly constructed that they have endured for over 2,000 years. These mighty edifices would have stunned one new to Rome with their massive scale, the number of people that they held, and their gleaming marble surfaces and facings. Our visitor would never have seen so many people congregated in one place, nor such a variety of ethnicities, with so many foreigners (identifiable by their looks, clothes, and/or hairstyles) in the mix. He or she would perhaps have experienced a feeling of personal reduction or insignificance, as merely one being in a roiling mass of humanity, and as a tiny figure surrounded by huge man-made monuments. Among the many things that soared around him, he might have seen colossal statues of Roman emperors that physically embodied their political stature in the known world, such as the famous bronze nude colossus of Nero that stood roughly 120 feet high and gave the nearby Colosseum its name, and the titanic marble statue of Constantine whose massive fragments now rest in the courtyard of the Capitoline Museum.

He would also have been struck by the opulence of the materials employed in some of those buildings. A veritable rainbow of colored stone and marble, forming the shafts of columns or arranged in handsome patterns on floors and walls, adorned temples, fora, basilicas, and baths. One could see Rome's dominance over its vast empire symbolically and literally mapped out in these valuable stones: white Pentelic marble from Attica; yellow veined Chemtou marble from Tunisia; green serpentine marble from Thebes, Egypt; red Rosso Antico marble from the Peloponnese; grey-blue marble from the island of Chios; and grey, black, and pink granites from Aswan, Egypt, to name just a few. *Opus sectile*, a type of stone marquetry employing different-colored pieces of marble, granite, and porphyry in complex patterns, would have pleased the eyes with its ornateness. The *opus sectile* floor and wall friezes of Hadrian's Pantheon, for example, contained stones reflecting several of Rome's notable conquests: from Egypt, purple porphyry; from Asia Minor, red and white Docimian pavonazzetta; from Carthage, yellow Numidian marble; and from Greece, green Lapis Lacedaemonius (on marbles and decorative stones in the Mediterranean world, see Adam 1994; Dodge and Ward-Perkins 1992).

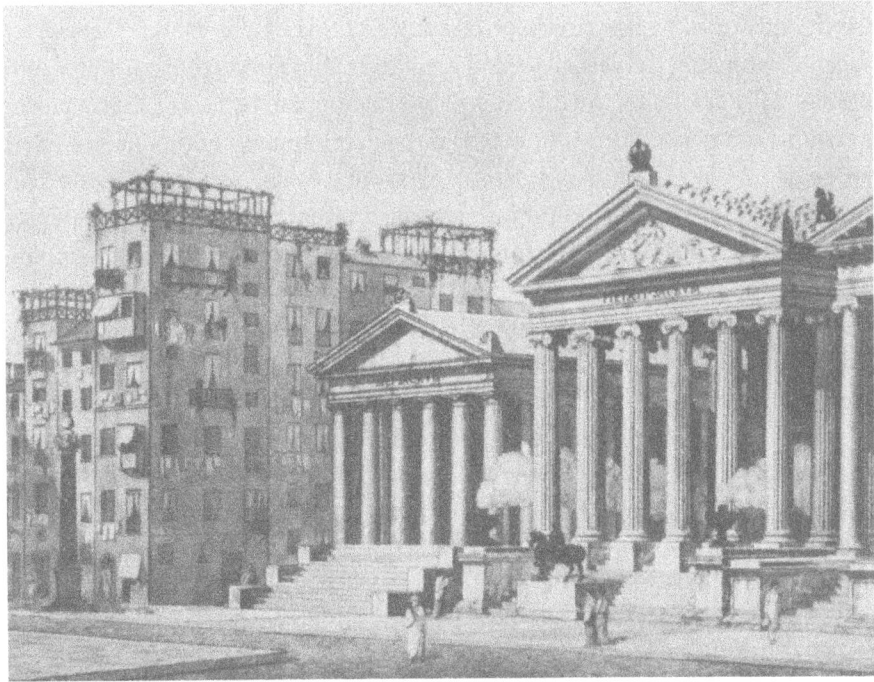

FIGURE 2.2: Reconstruction of Rome showing juxtaposition of opulence and poverty, from G. Gatteschi, Restauri della Roma Imperiale (1924).

The city would also have dazzled the eye by glittering in the Mediterranean sun. Public buildings faced with stone and marble would have gleamed; brightly painted and gilded reliefs and statuary would have throbbed with vivid color. Augustus' often-cited claim that he found Rome built of sun-dried brick and left it in marble (Suetonius *Augustus* 28) supports this vision of bright, glowing surfaces. The Temple of Jupiter Optimus Maximus on the Capitoline hill, visible from all over the city, boasted a roof and doors plated with solid gold, and would have formed a glittering focal point for the entire city. Augustus also said that he restored eighty-two temples during his sixth consulship (*Res Gestae* 20.4), which suggests the large number of structures meant to impress throughout the city (on the transformation and rebuilding of Rome under Augustus, see Favro 1996). Tacitus confirms this image when contrasting old-fashioned building styles with current ones: "Why, one might as well believe that temples are not so strongly built today because they are not put together out of coarse uncut stone and ugly-looking bricks, but shine in marble and are all agleam with gold" (*A Dialogue on Oratory* 20.7).

Abundance was an important quality that cities sought to express, and not just through buildings and proofs of material wealth. Natural resources, in particular water, were another focus of conspicuous consumption, especially at the city of Rome. By the early fourth century CE, over a dozen aqueducts were, by some estimates, delivering around a million cubic meters of fresh water into the city daily, to supply roughly 900 public and private baths and 1,500 public fountains and pools. The water flowed through the system continuously, so that people would have seen moving water all around them, even in a dense urban environment (on aqueducts and water supply in Rome and Constantinople, see Crow 2008; Hodge 2002). The sound of water splashing, gurgling, and dripping would have been one of the constant background noises of Roman cities, so ubiquitous that it probably went largely unremarked. While there were many purely functional basins and cisterns, there was also a tendency to decorate them so that the water would be even more impressively displayed. For example, in one year alone, Augustus' administrator Agrippa erected 300 statues and 400 marble pillars atop the fountains and basins of Rome. Some statues actually poured out and spewed forth water, rendering its delivery even more dynamic. All of this flowing water offered yet more sun-dappled, glittering surfaces to delight the eye. In addition, the water would have exercised a cooling effect on the air around it, especially welcome during hot Mediterranean summers. The water overflowing from fountains and sloshing onto the pavement would have further stressed the notion of luxurious abundance—while perhaps also helping to sluice away some of the muck caking the streets.

Scale and opulence thus served a propagandistic agenda, reminding Romans (and those they conquered) of the power and might of the Roman Empire as embodied in its capital city. The stones, marble, and artworks stripped from conquered territories and provinces functioned as constant visual reminders of Rome's military dominance over the world, as did the many foreign slaves who walked its streets. Overwhelming the senses of its inhabitants and visitors functioned as another sort of symbolic conquest reflecting Rome's dominion over its far-flung empire. The outrageously plentiful, constantly flowing water represented Rome's wealth and its ability to harness and control not just people and nations, but nature itself.

SMELL

The impressive sights of Rome were accompanied by equally powerful smells. The primary, omnipresent odor would have been the stench of human excrement, which would have permeated the air. By the first century BCE, Rome had reached an estimated population of around one million inhabitants, and maintained that level for several centuries. This made Rome exceptional; no other ancient Mediterranean city probably ever reached two-thirds of that size, and no other Western city hit the one million mark again until London and Paris around the beginning of the nineteenth century.[3] Rome was a densely packed city and, at its height, its populace was producing an estimated 350,000 gallons of human urine and 100,000 pounds of feces per day. While much of this may have been recycled for use in fulleries or as fertilizer and some found its way into the city's drains, a good bit also seems to have been disposed of by the most convenient method—dumping it into the street (on issues of urban waste disposal and the related topics of sanitation and disease, see Aldrete 2007; Hobson 2009; Raventós and Remolà 2000; Scheidel 2003; Scobie 1986).

Particularly for those who lived on the upper levels of apartment buildings, the idea of lugging a heavy, sloshing chamber pot full of sewage down multiple flights of stairs was much less appealing than simply emptying it out the window when no one was looking. Although this method of disposal was technically illegal, it was nonetheless rampant, as evidenced by the frequent references to such incidents in Roman law and literature (e.g., *Digest* 9.3.1; Juvenal *Satires* 3.268–78). Additionally, as there was no formalized garbage collection, this too was often thrown out of windows and lay in the streets, as did the corpses of the homeless and the destitute who could not afford a proper burial, and the carcasses of animals. As a result, for those walking through Rome's streets, the reek of decay would have incessantly filled their nostrils, their feet would have had to trudge through disgusting slop, and their eyes would have been confronted with unsavory sights and constant reminders of death.

However, for the rich, the experience of traversing the streets could be mitigated, either by covering one's nose with a perfumed cloth or by being transported in a litter carried by slaves. Juvenal vividly describes this contrast:

> When the rich man has a call of social duty, the mob makes way for him as he is borne swiftly over their heads in a huge Liburnian litter. He writes or reads or sleeps inside as he goes along, for the closed openings of the conveyance induce slumber. Yet he will arrive before us; hurry as we may, we are blocked by a surging crowd in front, and by a dense mass of people pressing in on us from behind: one man gouges his elbow into me, another pokes me with a hard sedan-pole; another bashes my head with a wooden plank. My legs are splattered with mud; soon huge feet stomp on me from every side, and a soldier grinds his hobnails on my toe.
>
> *Satires* 3.239–48

Carried above the offending sludge and surrounded by perfumed curtains, wealthy passengers could somewhat insulate themselves from the odors outside, as well as from the feeling of crowding and chaos that prevailed on Rome's busy streets. The litter became a self-contained refuge from the urban environment, which also protected one from being jostled, stepped on, and groped by one's fellow Romans.

The rich could attempt to impose a layer of pleasant scents between themselves and the dominant smells of excrement, garbage, and decomposition. Pliny describes a multitude of available oils, unguents, and blended perfumes, many famous for their high quality, among them oil of saffron, iris perfume, attar of roses, quince-blossom unguent, and blends incorporating such ingredients as lilies, gladiolus, cinnamon, bitter almonds, marjoram, pomegranate rind, balsam, myrrh, wine, and honey; there were even dried scents known as "sprinkling powders" (*Natural History* 13.2.4–13.5.25). Upon his return from Greece, Nero's triumph-like entry into Rome was accompanied by "the streets [being] sprinkled from time to time with perfume" (Suetonius *Nero* 25.2), and Nero's Golden House contained dining rooms designed so that perfume could be showered down from pipes in the ceiling upon the guests (Suetonius *Nero* 31.2). The constant heavy use of such perfumes was probably one of the most pronounced differences separating the urban sensory experience of the rich from that of the poor (on Roman perfumes, see Dalby 2002; Donato and Seefried 1989; Laurence 2010; Mattingly 1990).

A pedestrian walking through the neighborhoods of Rome would inevitably have also encountered the smells of trades being practiced, since some professions had an obvious stink. Martial insults a woman by claiming that she "smells worse than a grasping fuller's long-used crock, and that, too, just smashed in the middle of the street" or "than a hide dragged from a dog in the Transtiberim" (*Epigrams* 6.93.1–2). Fullers collected urine in jars at street corners for use at their shops, where slaves cleaned and whitened clothes by treading on them in vats of urine. The Transtiberim was a region of Rome located across the Tiber from the majority of the city, and was the home to many tanneries, which produced both unpleasant odors and biological waste (on the Transtiberim and other "marginal zones" of Rome, see Patterson 2000). A number of industries which either emitted especially noxious fumes or posed a fire danger (such as tile factories, which employed many kilns) seem to have been concentrated there, along with many foreigners, poor people, and some marginalized ethnic groups. The father of a tanner advises his son not to be bothered by the associations of his work, urging him: "Feel no disgust at a trade that must be banished to the other side of the Tiber; make no distinction between hides and unguents: the smell of gain is good whatever the thing from which it comes" (Juvenal *Satires* 14.201–5).

More appetizing smells would have come from bakeries and food for sale, either at tavern counters or from vendors walking the streets. However, the pleasant aroma of bread baking in ovens would likely have been accompanied by the loud sounds of the mills that were frequently located adjacent to the bakeries. There, millers ground grain into flour, using large, heavy, hourglass-shaped stone mills that were turned by beasts of burden such as mules, donkeys, horses, and even sometimes by slaves. This activity would have produced a lot of noise, both from the turning of the mills and from the livestock. One would have also smelled the food being served at cookshops (*popinae*), described by Horace as *uncta* ("greasy") (*Epistulae* 1.14.21), and being carried by hawkers; sausage seems to have been particularly popular as a portable snack, but there are also references to vendors of cakes, soups or pulses of legumes, and ice-water (Seneca *Naturales Quaestiones* 4.13.8).

HEARING

The large population of Rome must have produced a great deal of what today might be termed noise pollution. Seneca notes some of the annoying noises emanating from the streets surrounding his dwelling: "Among the sounds that din around me . . . I include passing carriages, a machinist in the same block, a saw-sharpener nearby, or some fellow who is demonstrating with pipes and flutes ... shouting rather than singing" (*Epistle* 56.4). The economic functioning of the city necessitated the use of draft animals and wagons to transport goods into and out of the metropolis, which generally took place at night—a regulation first established by Julius Caesar. Juvenal relates the impossibility of finding sleep when the nocturnal streets are swarming with "creaking wagons" and "shouting drovers" (3.236–8). Martial adds more details to this image of a cacophonous city:

> Neither for thought ... nor for quiet is there any place in the city for a poor man. Schoolmasters in the morning do not let you live; before daybreak, bakers; the hammers of the copper-smiths all day. On this side the money-changer idly rattles on his dirty table Nero's coins, on that the hammerer of Spanish gold-dust beats his well-worn stone with burnished mallet; and Bellona's raving priests do not rest, nor the canting shipwrecked seaman, nor the Jew taught by his mother to beg, nor the blear-eyed huckster of sulphur wares.
>
> *Epigrams* 12.57

One of the most famous and vivid descriptions of urban noises comes from the philosopher Seneca, who for a time rented lodgings above a public bath:

> Imagine, if you can, the array of noises which are so loud that I wish I was not able to hear. I can hear the bodybuilders hefting lead weights—when one is performing a hearty work-out, or at least pretending to, I hear every grunt, and when he puffs out his exhaled breath, I hear every wheeze and gasp. Or perhaps I have to endure the sounds of a lazier fellow who is content with a quick rub-down, and I hear the slap of the masseuse's open or flat palms upon his shoulder. Next, along comes a ballplayer proclaiming his point total. That's all I need. Mix in the odd loudmouth, the petty thief, the dreadful sound of the man who likes to hear his own untalented voice singing in the bath, or the eager swimmer who causes a commotion plunging into the pool with a mighty splash ... the chatty hair-plucker, who is never silent, except when he is making his victim shriek instead as he rips the hairs from his armpit. Then, too, there is the sweets-vendor hawking his varied wares, the sausage-seller, the confectioner, and all the sundry sellers of food, each one advertising his wares in a distinctive voice.
>
> *Epistle* 56.1–2

Class distinctions could make a difference in terms of noise as well as smell. Juvenal suggests that "In this city, sleep comes only to the wealthy," who could retreat into large homes up on Rome's hills or could go out to country villas to find peace and quiet (*Satires* 3.235–8).

The political rituals and public entertainments of the capital city, attended by tens or hundreds of thousands of spectators, would have contributed their share to the general noise levels. By the late empire, there may have been races or entertainments held on over 100 days per year, and the roar of the crowd emanating from these venues would have been heard all over the central city. The hard marble walls of buildings such as theaters, amphitheaters, circuses, stadia, and the public structures of Rome in general would have amplified the sounds made within them, and caused echoes to bounce back and forth about the cityscape.

Augustine elaborates upon how just the noise alone of the crowd could infect a man previously uninterested in gladiator games with a mania for them, almost against his will:

> When they arrived at the arena, the place was seething with the lust for cruelty ... Alypius shut his eyes tightly, determined to have nothing to do with these atrocities. If only he had closed his ears as well! For an incident in the fight drew a great roar from the crowd, and this thrilled him so deeply that he could not contain his curiosity ... The din had pierced his ears and forced him to open his eyes ... When he saw the blood, it was as though he had drunk a deep draught of savage passion. Instead of turning away, he fixed his eyes upon the scene and drank in all its frenzy ... he was drunk with the fascination of bloodshed. He was no longer the man who had come to the arena, but simply one of the crowd which he had joined ... He watched and cheered and grew hot with excitement, and when he left the arena, he carried away with him a diseased mind which would leave him no peace until he came back again ...
>
> *Confessions* 6.8

The great volume of the shouts made by excited crowds in the ancient world was proverbial. When, for example, it was proclaimed by a herald at the Isthmian Games in Greece that Rome planned to restore freedom to several Greek city-states, "a shout of joy arose, so incredibly loud that it reached the sea ... And that which is often said of the volume and power of the human voice was then apparent to the eye. For ravens which chanced to be flying overhead were stunned by the noise and fell down dead into the stadium"

(Plutarch *Titus Flamininus* 10.5–6; Valerius Maximus 4.8.5). An angry crowd could also allegedly harm birds with their dissent, as when a mob in the city of Rome expressed its disapproval: "At this ... the people were incensed and gave forth such a shout that a raven flying over the forum was stunned by it and fell down into the throng" (Plutarch *Pompey* 25.7). While such incidents of crowd noise literally blasting birds from the sky may be far-fetched, the popularity of this motif suggests the volume of sound that urban crowds were credited with producing.

RELIEF

The typical Roman—living in a dark and tiny apartment in a crowded *insula*, constantly battered by the mobs of people milling through the streets, and buffeted from all sides with loud sounds and strong smells—would have eagerly sought relief from the less enjoyable aspects of city life. Even if concepts of privacy, personal space, and endurable smells were less stringent than they are today, an alternative sort of environment would have been desirable. Fortunately, large ancient Greek and Roman cities usually possessed a number of public buildings and spaces that would have provided such havens.

Foremost among these were bath complexes, both large and small (on baths and bathing in the ancient world, see Fagan 1999; Yegül 1992). By the fourth century CE Rome had eleven gigantic public baths and nearly 900 smaller ones, the biggest of which, known as *thermae*, contained far more than just pools of water of varying temperature. They also featured athletic playing fields, gardens, gymnasia, food vendors, artworks, libraries, and establishments that pampered the body such as places to get massages, manicures, and haircuts. The floors were covered in handsome mosaics, nearly every surface was decorated in imported colored marbles, and skillfully carved statuary fed the eyes, while the pools of water either soothed or stimulated the body, depending on whether you plunged into the tepidarium (warm water), the calidarium (hot water), or the frigidarium (cold water). Hot air was forced beneath the floors and through the surrounding walls to heat some of the rooms, which resembled saunas with radiant heating, so that when walking across one of these floors, rather than the expected chilliness of marble on one's soles, one would have experienced the pleasant sensation of warmed marble underfoot. The largest of these complexes are estimated to have been able to accommodate 10,000 people. Baths were true social centers where people could spend an entire day; they were places you went to in order to see and be seen, to gossip, and to mingle, as well as to bathe, relax, and groom yourself.

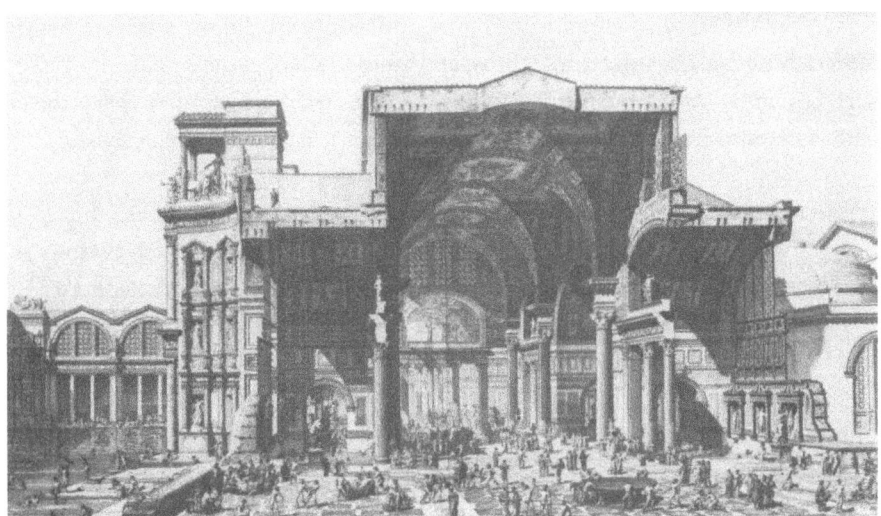

FIGURE 2.3: Reconstruction of a public bath showing ornate decor and decorative marbles, from E. Paulin, Restauration des Monuments Antique (1890).

Another important type of space supplying relief from the bustle of the city was public gardens (on urban gardens and parks, see Cima and La Rocca 1998; Farrar 1998). Rome and many other cities encompassed large expanses of land that were devoted to sumptuous urban gardens and parks. These green oases offered relief from heat, the built-up and paved-over cityscape, and the omnipresent crowding. The wealthy frequently opened their private gardens to the public or donated them to the city as a philanthropic gesture as well as to curry favor with the populace. Pompey, Julius Caesar, Agrippa, Augustus, and Lucullus all provided parks and gardens for the public's use. One of the most popular types of urban green space was the portico garden; *portici*, or covered walkways, afforded some degree of shade and shelter from the elements. Frequently encircled by colonnades, portico gardens resembled enclosed parks, often adjoining a public building such as a bath, theater, or temple, the patrons of which could retire to the nearby garden for a stroll. Other gardens were vast stretches of rolling land that contained green space, but were also adorned with fine sculptures and boasted ornate water features such as fountains, fishponds, streams, and pools. Benches positioned under trees and vine-covered, trellised arbors offered shady places to shelter from the sun and opportunities for privacy, while beds of flowers provided pleasant sights and smells even in the heart of the great city. Many ancient authors refer to walking and strolling through public gardens as being a popular pastime.

Gardens were also often a welcome addendum to dining establishments, both of fraternal organizations, clubs, and guilds, and of commercial enterprises such as inns, *tabernae*, and *cauponae*. One inn-keeper lures hot, dusty customers into her inn by tempting them with a feast for all of the senses:

> There are gardens and nooks and arbors, mixing-cups, roses, flutes, lyres, and cool bowers with shady canes. Lo! too, the pipe, which twitters sweetly within a Maenalian grotto, sounds its rustic strain in a shepherd's mouth. There is fresh wine, too, just drawn from the pitched jar, and a water-brook running noisily with hoarse murmur; there are also chaplets of violet blossoms mixed with saffron, and yellow garlands blended with crimson roses; and lilies bedewed by a virgin stream, which a nymph has brought in osier-baskets. There are little cheeses, too, dried in a basket of rushes; there are waxen plums . . . and chestnuts and sweetly blushing apples . . . blood-red mulberries with grapes in heavy clusters, and from its stalk hangs the blue-grey melon . . . rest here thy wearied frame beneath the shade of vines, and entwine thy heavy head in a garland of roses.
>
> Virgil, The Minor Poems, "Copa"

This garden aims to recreate the hallmarks of a rural idyll for its patrons, through smell (the many types of flowers growing and woven into wreaths to adorn one's head), taste (wine, cheese, and various fruits), sound (a shepherd's pipes, flutes and lyres, running water, insects' noises), vision (the emphasis on vivid colors), and touch (coolness and shade).

As the city became increasingly built up and crowded with both structures and people, urban gardens offered a necessary respite from its artificial, man-made, paved-over, mob-filled warrens. Of course, such gardens were themselves highly artificial constructs, seeking to inject idealized rural patches into an urban environment.

SENSE STRATIFICATION

Most ancient Mediterranean societies were intensely obsessed with distinctions of rank and status. In the Roman world, it made a great deal of difference, both socially and legally, whether one was a citizen or not, male or female, patrician or plebeian, a slave, a former slave, or a free-born person. Even among members of a class, formal distinctions were made, often indicated by visible differences in clothing. For example, the plain white toga was a garment reserved only for males who had citizen status, but if you were a citizen with a fortune of more than 400,000 sesterces, you wore the white toga enhanced by a thin purple stripe, and if you were of senatorial rank and wealth, you wore a white toga with a broad purple stripe. Many of your perceptions of the city would have been governed by these differences in rank and status. Thus it is possible to speak of a kind of stratification of urban sensory experience in which the sights, sounds, smells, tastes, and touches that you experienced would have been dramatically different depending upon your place within society.

Some of the most obvious differences have already been mentioned, such as the use of perfumes by the wealthy to shield them from the olfactory assault of life in the big city. Another wealth-related distinction would have been the actual feeling of one's clothing upon the body. Manufacturing garments was a time-consuming process in the ancient world, and most girls and women probably spent a great deal of their time spinning thread and weaving fabric. The more well-to-do could afford wools and linens with smooth, finer weaves, but the indigent would have had to make do with scratchy, coarser fabrics. At the extreme upper end of the wealth spectrum, exotic imported items such as silk from the East would have provided their own special sensory thrill, the very touch of them upon the skin a constant reminder of the wealth of their owner (on Roman clothing and its symbolic meanings, see Sebesta and Bonfante 2001).

Similarly, the variety of food that one ate would have been determined by wealth (on the intertwined topics of wealth and poverty in ancient Rome, see Atkins and Osborne 2006; Dalby 2002; Toner 1995). The vast majority of inhabitants around the ancient Mediterranean had to subsist on minor variations of a diet largely consisting of grains (such as wheat), olives (often ingested in the form of olive oil), and grapes (in the form of wine). This would have been occasionally supplemented by seasonally available local fruits and vegetables, perhaps some fish if near a coastline, and relatively rare bits of meat, such as goat. A popular stinky fish sauce known as *garum*, made by fermenting fish parts in olive oil, was relatively cheap and widely available, and would have provided some flavor to an otherwise relatively monotonous diet. But even within this fairly limited range of foodstuffs, status distinctions were made. Thus, wheat was viewed as more desirable than barley, which bore the social stigma of being a food typically fed to slaves, farm animals, and soldiers who were being punished for some infraction (for introductions to various aspects of food in antiquity and the average diet, see Beer 2010; Brothwell and Brothwell 1998; Garnsey 1999; Gold and Donahue 2005).

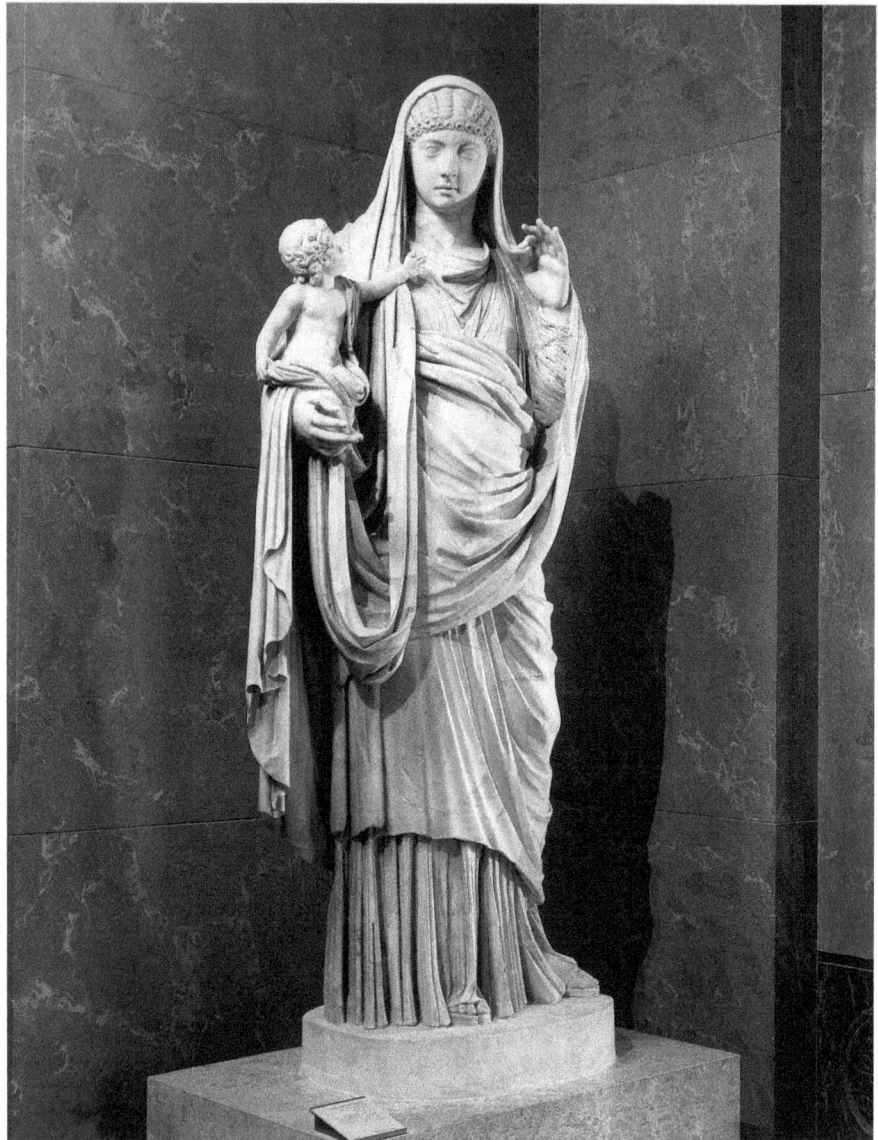

FIGURE 2.4: Marble statue of Messalina holding Britannicus. She is dressed as an upper-class Roman matron swathed in multiple layers of fabric denoting her status and modesty. Getty Images.

Wealthy Romans, on the other hand, flaunted their economic status by titillating their palates with rare delicacies. To begin with, while most Romans drank wine, there was a great deal of snobbery about various vintages and a wide range of available gradations of quality depending on type, place of origin, and age. Certain regions (and even particular fields) had reputations for producing the finest wines, and an amphora of these vintages would cost many times that of a wine of more humble provenance (on wine, see McGovern 2003; Tchernia 1986). Rich men also competed with one another through the luxuriousness and exoticism of the meals that they offered their guests, which could result in truly bizarre dishes such as pies filled with flamingo tongues or ostrich brains (on the elaborate foodstuffs available to the wealthy, see Dalby 2002; Toner 1995). In this way, the specific flavors that one experienced, and most especially the range of things that one tasted, would have been differentiated by class and status.

Another interesting sort of sensory distinction determined by wealth had to do with where one lived. Only a tiny percentage of Rome's very wealthiest would have been able to afford actual individual houses, so the overwhelming majority of the city's inhabitants lived in apartments. In many cities today, residential neighborhoods tend to be strongly geographically separated by economic levels—in other words, certain neighborhoods are mostly made up of extremely wealthy individuals while others are predominantly composed of very poor people. In ancient cities, at first glance, rich and poor were usually more intermingled, with people of a wide variety of wealth levels all living together in apartments in the same regions. There was, however, a more subtle form of stratification by wealth, one that also would have affected one's sensory impressions. Rather than being separated horizontally, ancient city dwellers were separated vertically. The apartments on the lowest floors, which tended to be larger and more luxurious, were rented by the wealthier classes. As one ascended in the building, the apartments grew progressively smaller and more crowded, with the least desirable (and shabbiest) ones on the uppermost floors or in the attic. This vertical stratification was, of course, determined by the practical consideration that, in an era before elevators, people did not want to trudge up flight after flight of stairs, making the lowest floors more desirable. Those who could afford private homes overwhelmingly chose to erect them atop Rome's small hills. These locations would have provided these elite of the elite with fresher air and more light compared to their less well-off neighbors who literally dwelt in their shadows in the valleys between the hills.

The sense experiences of some of the lowest ranking groups, such as slaves and women, would have been especially strongly affected and circumscribed by their roles in Roman society. The slave, transformed from a human being into a piece of property, was used to enhance the sensual pleasures of his or her owners, either through the work they did or as sexual objects (on Roman slaves and slavery, see Bradley 1994; Joshel 2010). Restrictions could be literal, such as being chained; Columella recommends that, for farm slaves in chains, "there should be an underground prison (*ergastulum*)," though this should be "as healthful as possible" and admit light through "many narrow windows" situated too far above the ground to be reached (*De Re Rustica* 1.6.3). Some were even made to work in chain gangs, and a sadistic master is described as delighting in the sound of floggings and "reveling in the clanking of a chain" (Juvenal *Satires* 14.18–24).

Around their necks, many slaves were made to wear collars which bore tags inscribed with their master's name and address. Such collars limited a slave's mobility by ensuring that a runaway, if captured, could be immediately returned to his owner. The sounds of slaves being flogged and tortured would have been familiar ones, and for those slaves who wore them, the clanking of a chain or the weight and touch of a slave collar around their neck probably became a part of their identity—constant reminders that their bodies belonged to another and were no longer their own.

However, the city slave often had fewer restrictions placed upon him than the rural slave, and personal or house slaves were generally allowed more freedom than those used for manual labor, farming, and mining. Thus, it is not surprising that being sent to the country was a threat leveled against urban slaves to promote good behavior (Horace *Satires* 2.7.118; Juvenal *Satires* 8.180; Plautus *Bacchides* 365). On the other hand, punishment of urban and domestic slaves could be just as brutal as that of their country cousins.

The ideal woman of antiquity expressed her chastity and fidelity to her husband through self-restraint and closing herself off from the world around her, and this would have involved an accompanying restriction of sensory stimuli.[4] In Xenophon's famous discussion of how to train a wife, she "had lived previously under diligent supervision in order that she might see and hear as little as possible," and since the gods shaped women "for indoor works and indoor concerns," she must stay indoors, sending out servants to perform errands in the world outside the house; "to the woman, it is more honorable to stay indoors than to attend to the work outside" (*Oeconomicus* 7.5–6, 7.22, 7.35, 7.30). In contrast, men were believed to have been made for outdoor tasks and activities, and were intended to move freely outside the home. The upper-class Greek women of classical Athens were swathed from head to foot, and even veiled, and figurines of aristocratic Hellenistic women portray them sheltering themselves from the sun with parasols and hats. Pale skin physically expressed a woman's sheltered existence, and cumbersome or voluminous clothing would have restricted her sensual engagement with her physical surroundings.

While urban Roman women had more freedom than those of ancient Greece, who were (at least theoretically) restricted to the home, a respectable, upper-class woman was still expected to behave with a great degree of decorum, especially under the republic. One Roman woman's tombstone reads: "I was chaste and modest; I did not know the crowd; I was faithful to my husband" (*ILS* 7472). Being out in public among the crowd meant that a woman was showing herself off to others as well as exposing herself to possible moral contagion. Early strictures against women drinking wine and public displays of affection between husbands and wives, as well as clothing styles meant to conceal a woman from chin to toes, reflected an impulse to limit her exposure to the world outside the home and its pleasures. A Roman matron's *stola*, emblematic of her chastity and modesty, reached down to the ground. A respectable married woman bound her hair with bands called *vittae*, and often used her *palla*, a type of long veil or mantle, as a head covering when out in public. The poet Ovid refers to a matron's dress as "signs of purity, thin *vittae* and long *stola* which covers the feet" (*Ars Amatoria* 1.31–2). However, such restrictions were a function of class as well as gender. Rural women of necessity spent their time laboring outside, as did those urban women who worked in the businesses and markets of the city, and they likely wore less (and less restrictive) clothing so as not to hinder their mobility.

NEGOTIATING THE CITY WITH THE SENSES

The importance of the sense of hearing in the city's political life is suggested by the many adaptations necessary due to Rome's huge population. Aristotle had pointed out that, if the population of a city-state grew too large, its orderly governance would be compromised because no herald would be capable of addressing the entire populace (*Politics* 7.4.7). Political careers were based on one's skill at public speaking, but those further back in the massive crowds that gathered before the rostra in the Forum would not have been able to hear a speaker's words. Nonverbal communication through gestures functioned as one means of dealing with this problem, thus substituting visual cues for auditory information. Another strategy was the use of heralds, who repeated and relayed messages and speeches throughout the crowd. Actors and orators alike trained their voices to achieve maximum projection, and the public spaces and entertainment venues of Rome would have been filled with shouting men competing to be heard over the constant noise of the crowd, who often supplied their own vocal commentary on what was being said (on issues of communicating at large public gatherings, see Aldrete 1999).

Crowd noise functioned as a gauge of approbation or disapproval of public figures, who coveted the people's applause and acclamations but feared their hisses and jeering. In his letters, Cicero repeatedly refers to the amount of applause bestowed upon either himself or other politicians by crowds, whether in the theater, at games, or in the streets. He comments to Atticus that "The popular feeling can be seen best in the theater and at public exhibitions," expressed through "hisses," wholehearted "cheers of the whole audience," and "tremendous uproar and outcry"; he mentions that Julius Caesar was annoyed when, upon his entrance at a gladiator show, the applause was lackluster (*Ad Atticus* 2.19). The audience knew that the noise they made could sometimes even affect governmental policy and the emperor's decisions, and took advantage of this. Thus, Romans of both the upper and lower classes would have been keenly attuned to the nature and volume of the crowd noise that they heard: whether it was positive or negative, increasing or decreasing. Whereas today, we often think of crowd noise simply as background din to be tuned out while we focus on something important in the foreground, such noise was a prominent and closely observed aspect of ancient urban life.

One of the advantages to living in a big city was the increased possibility of witnessing spectacular entertainments. In a city like Rome, some of the standard events you could observe included gladiator contests, chariot races, beast hunts, mythological re-enactments, plays, musical performances, and mime shows (on spectacles and public entertainments, see Beacham 1999; Bell 2004; Kyle 2007). People from the countryside or from villages and small cities often flocked to the larger metropolises in order to attend the great public spectacles staged there. In addition to these grand urban rituals, big-city dwellers also witnessed speeches by famous politicians, the great funeral processions of Rome's elites, the triumphs of victorious generals, religious processions, celebrity trials, the parades of clients following important men, and even fights in the streets between rival political gangs. These were all forms of public events which bystanders could both view and participate in, if they so desired.

The narrow, maze-like streets of Rome ensured that people would probably have heard urban events such as parades approaching long before they could actually see any visual evidence of them, and such noise would have produced anticipation—people craning their necks to see above those around them, and rumors circulating as to what was coming and how soon. Similarly, in the vast expanse of the quarter-mile long, dust-obscured Circus Maximus, attendees would often have perceived these events primarily through the sense of hearing rather than sight. When audiences numbering in the tens or even hundreds of thousands were gathered together to observe great spectacles such as these, the roar of the crowd would have echoed far beyond the Colosseum and the Circus Maximus, so that even those not present would have known that something exciting (and likely bloody) had occurred.

Experienced urban listeners would have been able to interpret and make subtle distinctions among different types of applause, cheers, shouts, and chants, in order to discern details about what was transpiring even when they could not see the spectacle directly. Certain formulaic chants and rhythms of applause appear to have been specific to particular cultures, and even to individual cities, and thus these aural clues would have conveyed clear meanings to locals, but would have puzzled outsiders. Evidence for the specificity of these formulas can be found in an amusing incident during the reign of Nero when the Quinquennial Games were being held at Rome and large numbers of people from the countryside had flocked to the city to observe them. At the games, the complex rhythmic forms of applause habitually employed by the urban populace of Rome were totally disrupted by the crude clapping and stomping of the rustics, who were unfamiliar with the distinctive formulas used at Rome (Tacitus *Annals* 16.5).[5]

Being able to negotiate the city by sound was especially important in Rome, with its narrow, twisting streets and up-and-down topography, which would have severely limited lines of sight. You could rarely see very far in the city, so the perception of being in a dense, jumbled maze would have been intensified. Conversely, when you encountered one of the large open spaces of the city, such as some of the great parks and gardens, the Circus Maximus or the Colosseum, the effect would have been made all the more impressive by the contrast with the normally cramped urban experience.

While many ancient cities shared the organic, narrow, winding street pattern of Rome, this would have contrasted sharply with some Greek and Hellenistic cities and even with other Roman ones (on ancient urban planning, see Favro 1996; Owens 1991; Ward-Perkins 1974). Greek cities, especially those founded as colonies, were often laid out on a Hippodamian grid plan, with intersecting right-angle streets meeting at regularly spaced intervals. A number of cities founded by the Romans had their origins as legionary camps whose roads were also laid out in a grid. The most impressive city of this planned type was probably Alexandria in Egypt, founded by Alexander the Great and immodestly named after himself. Alexander founded several dozen cities scattered all over the areas he conquered, some as far away as modern Afghanistan, but all were erected on the model of an ideal Greek city, complete with Greek-style temples, gymnasia, stoas, and structures.

At Alexandria, not only were the main avenues straight, but they were unusually wide as well, with the two main intersecting avenues said to have been nearly 200 feet wide. One asset of having straight, broad roadways in cities such as Alexandria was that this enabled their rulers to hold truly impressive parades. This perhaps reached a peak during the Hellenistic era, when rival kings were fiercely competing with one another in a variety of ways for prestige and power. Their parades were planned with distinct features designed to dazzle and engage each one of the five senses. As an illustration that sensory extravaganzas in the ancient world were by no means unique to Rome, this chapter will conclude with a description of one such parade, staged in the third century BCE by the ruler Ptolemy II Philadelphus at the stadium of Alexandria.

It began with dozens of people with their bodies painted and dressed up in finery pretending to be mythological figures, such as satyrs bearing golden torches and Victories with golden wings. Accompanying them were several hundred boys bearing censers of incense and basins containing exotic perfumes and spices, including vats of oil of frankincense, myrrh, and saffron. At similar parades, the spectators could anoint themselves with the fragrant oils, and this was probably the case here as well. The procession featured a number of ornate wagons or carts bearing huge statues or entire tableaus of figures, which would have resembled the floats found in modern parades. One of these, for example, was a cart over twenty feet long pulled by 180 men which contained a 15-foot high statue of the god Dionysus dressed in purple and gold, pouring out a libation from a golden goblet into a 150-gallon golden wine bowl and surrounded by basins of fragrant casia and saffron, while over him soared a trellis covered in ivy, grape vines, and fruit, and from which hung wreaths, ribbons, and masks. On other floats, there were animated statues that could stand up, pour out libations and wave their arms, or oversized objects such as a 90-foot-long spear made of silver, a 30-foot high statue of an eagle, and a solid-gold horn 40 feet in length. Exotic sights included 300 harpists playing in unison, 600 elephant tusks, 24 chariots drawn by elephants, and a veritable menagerie of animals, among them 2,400 dogs, 2,000 color-matched oxen, dozens of teams of ostriches, antelopes, deer, goats pulling chariots, hundreds of parrots, peacocks and other birds, 350 sheep, twenty-six Indian zebus, fourteen leopards, twenty-four lions, a giraffe, a rhinoceros, and an albino bear.

For the drinking pleasure of the crowd, thousands of boys carried flagons of wine which were distributed to the onlookers, while, to further stimulate their senses, hundreds of camels were each laden with 300-pound containers of spices, including frankincense, myrrh, saffron, casia, cinnamon, and orris. One remarkable wagon carried a mock-up of a cave out of which were released

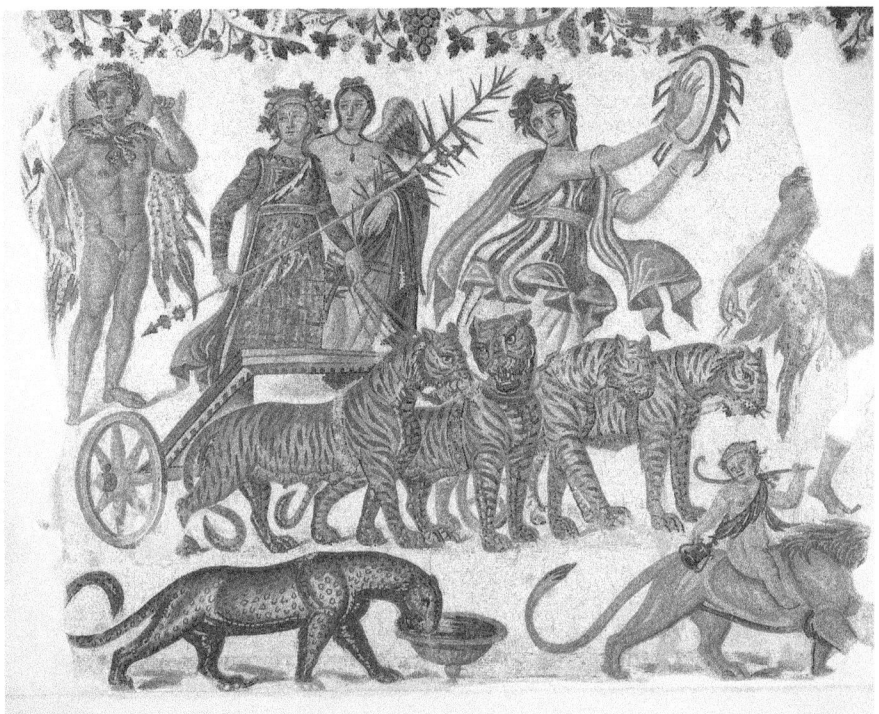

FIGURE 2.5: Mosaic of the Triumph of Bacchus (Dionysus). Getty Images.

flocks of pigeons and doves conveniently equipped with nooses tied to their feet so that the spectators could grab them as they flew by. From the same cavern also gushed forth two fountains, one of milk and one of wine. Another wagon bore a 36-foot long wine press in which sixty men dressed as satyrs trod grapes so that the juice flowed out and coated the roadway, while from another cart a colossal wine-skin stitched together from leopard skins and with a capacity of 30,000 gallons spewed wine directly into the mouths of eager spectators. Finally, there was a 180-foot phallus painted in various colors and wrapped in golden ribbons at whose tip was a 9-foot golden star. After all this, the subsequent military parade of 80,000 soldiers almost seemed an afterthought (Athenaeus *Deipnosophists* 5.197–203). From the rumble of the carts as they passed to the exoticism of the bizarre sights, from the overwhelming opulence of the mingling fragrances to the rich flavor of and (literal) intoxication from the wine, this procession was a true extravaganza for all the senses, and one that the modern world would be hard-pressed to match.

CHAPTER THREE

The Senses in the Marketplace: The Luxury Market and Eastern Trade in Imperial Rome

ANDREW WALLACE-HADRILL

In 16 CE, two years into the reign of Tiberius, a lively debate arose in the senate about the growth of luxury (Tacitus *Annals* 2.33). A former consul, Q. Haterius, protested against the use of solid gold drinking cups and the wearing of Chinese silks by men. The counterargument was made that with the growth of empire, the growth of private wealth was inevitable, and Romans could scarcely be expected to live like their ancestors. The emperor, who was famous for setting an example of a parsimonious lifestyle, reassuringly added that this was no time for censorial action, but that when action was needed, he would not hold back. Within a few years, his reassurances sounded hollow. The debate bubbled up again in the senate in 22 CE. Prices in the market were rising beyond control (Tacitus *Annals* 3.52f.). The aediles, who traditionally had responsibility for the market and its prices, complained that the regulations of the legislation against luxury were being ignored, and the prices of forbidden goods were rising by the day: serious measures were required, and they invited the emperor to take action. To their invitation, Tiberius gave a spectacularly evasive reply. He wrote, rather than addressing the senate in person, to spare the blushes, he claimed, of the individuals who were offenders. He applauded the energy of the aediles, and urged them to do what they could. But imperial intervention was scarcely appropriate. In any case, luxury spread far beyond the food market, to housing, slaves, precious metals, works of art, and the fashion among women for gemstones which resulted in a vast transfer of resources to foreign countries. The emperor had bigger concerns to trouble himself about, and the matters of which the aediles complained were by comparison a trifle. He had to ensure a food supply for the city of Rome, which could no longer be satisfied by domestic produce. That, not luxury, was what threatened to bring the republic down.

This imperial letter, as Tacitus grasped, marked a sea-change in official policy. For two centuries the senate had been producing ever more complex legislation to control the consumption of what were regarded as luxurious foodstuffs. Tiberius' response was the final admission of defeat. But at the same time, it put the debate about luxury back into context. On the one hand, it was futile to worry about luxury food prices, and ignore the flourishing market in silks and gemstones. On the other, the food prices that mattered were those of staples, above all wheat. And since Rome had become dependent on imported wheat, it was no good complaining about imports.

Anybody who knew about the trade from Alexandria would understand how intimate were the links between staples and luxuries. The Alexandrian grain ships were what stood between a bloated city of perhaps a million souls and starvation, rocketing prices, and the riots that could bring down a government. Emperors did all they could to promote this trade, both through their control of the Egyptian economy, and through offering generous incentives to shippers. But the same Alexandria was the principal gateway for luxuries into the Mediterranean. Add a few bales of silk and a few boxes of gemstones to your heavy tonnage of wheat, and your profits could increase spectacularly. Did Tiberius really want to choke off the corn shippers by killing the market in luxuries? Tiberius, who so faithfully followed the example of Augustus, will have been aware of the lengths to which his predecessor had gone to stimulate the luxury trade.

Effectively, the conquest of Egypt by the future Augustus at the start of his reign opened up a trade route to the Orient, and thereby changed the tastes, smells, sights, and sensations of the Mediterranean world. Silks from China, incenses from Arabia, spices from India, had been reaching the Mediterranean for a long time, but it was a small trickle, made difficult by the passage through areas like Mesopotamia, the Near East, and Egypt, over which Rome had no

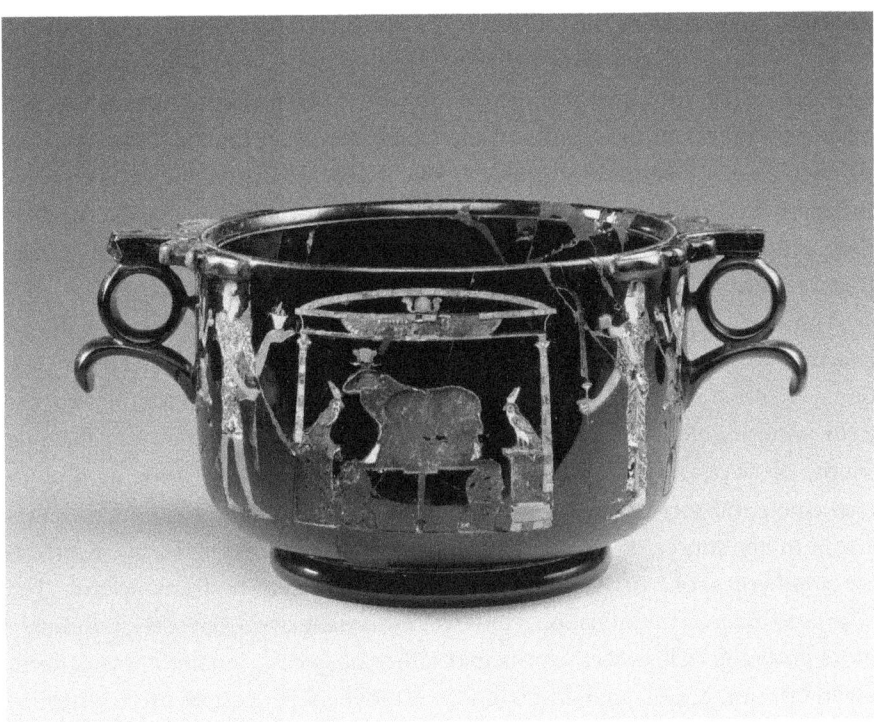

FIGURE 3.1: Egyptian style black obsidian bowl with white and pink coral inlays, lapis lazuli, malachite and gold, from Villa San Marco, Stabiae. Getty Images.

control. The conquest of Egypt not only opened up Alexandria as the great door of the Orient on the Mediterranean, but it opened up new direct shipping lanes to Arabia, East Africa, and India. The route was via two ports on the Red Sea, Myos Hormos and Berenike, both founded by the Ptolemies. The barren Red Sea coast was no welcoming one for ports, and to reach them and transfer goods to the Nile involved a trek of many days on camel across the desert. But Augustus swiftly grasped their importance, sending his general Aelius Gallus (the adoptive father of Tiberius' praetorian prefect Sejanus) on campaign into the Sudan and Arabia. Recent archaeological exploration of Berenike (conducted under adverse, waterless circumstances) has confirmed the Augustan boom of a port which played a minor role under the Ptolemies.

About the copious trade which passed through these ports, making its unmistakable impact on the Roman world of senses, we are surprisingly well informed. The *Periplus Maris Erythraei* is a manual of voyages from these Red Sea ports, written probably in the mid to late first century CE. It offers detailed accounts of the ports along the east African coast down to Rhapta, opposite

Zanzibar; of those along the Arabian gulf to Kane, the great port for frankincense; and of the routes to India, following the monsoon winds, blustery south-westerlies from July onwards, gentler north-easterlies for the return journey from November onwards, and leading to the two great trading areas of India, Barbarikon and Barygaza on the north-west coast, Muziris and Nelkynda on the south-west tip. Our manual explains in detail not only what exports each of these ports had to offer, but what sorts of imports they were interested in. The traders never sailed with empty hulls, but exchanged as they went.

The traders had a sharp eye for quality. Some commodities could be procured in several of the ports, but each area had its specialities. The voyage down to Rhapta was relatively risk-free, if time-consuming (waiting for the right winds could drag the round trip on to two years), but it was the best source of elephant tusks for ivory, rhinoceros horn (prized then as now in medicine), and tortoiseshell from the turtles of the Indian Ocean. Africa was also a minor source of incense and aromatics, especially ginger, but Kane on the southern shore of Arabia was the proper source of frankincense. The voyage to India on the monsoon winds was more dangerous, but correspondingly more profitable. This was the principal source of spices, cinnamon, casia, nard, malabathrum, costus, myrrh, lykion, but above all pepper; of precious gems, sapphires, diamonds, agate, onyx, carnelian, but especially pearls; and of fine textiles, Indian cottons, and finely-woven muslins as well as Chinese silks.

All these commodities (and many besides) are found also listed in Pliny's encyclopedia, the *Naturalis Historia*, in which (with suitable moralizing disapproval) he offers the anatomy of Roman luxury and the indulgence of the senses. He also with some frequency provides market prices, presumably based on the *macellum* in Rome, and thereby illustrates the concerns of the Tiberian aediles about market prices. Pepper is a good example. Pliny has little time for pepper. "That its use is so popular is remarkable: other fruit have pleasant tastes, or pleasant appearance, this has only its bitterness to recommend it, and for that it is sought from the Indies!" (Pliny *NH* 12.29). Nevertheless, it is a costly item, and as with so much else he catalogues, its price depends on quality and variety. The long pepper from northern India, which is hottest, fetches 15 *denarii* the pound, whereas the white and black peppers from south India fetch 7 and 4 *denarii* respectively. This may have seemed like a waste of money to Pliny, but the popularity of pepper, as he concedes, was vast. Particularly black pepper, the cheapest, became a standard item in Roman cuisine, and not only in dishes, but drinks like spiced wines, let alone in medicines. Its use must have reached a high degree of social diffusion: it is met in a document from the Roman garrison at Vindolanda, and is encountered in the sewer at Herculaneum

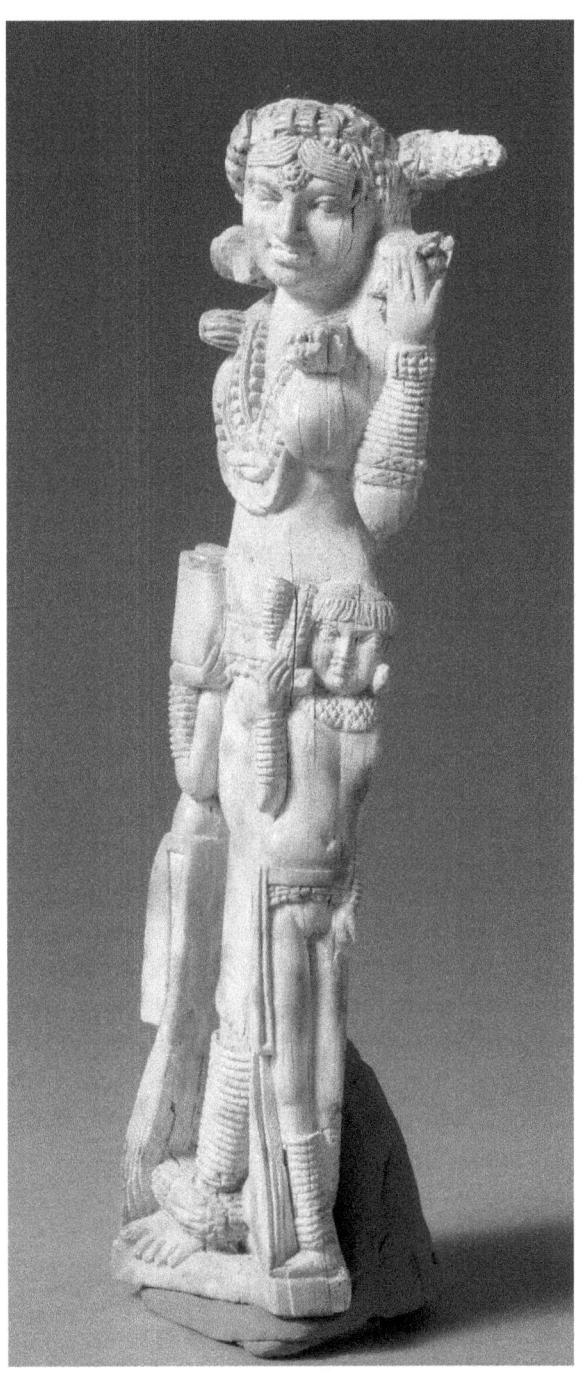

FIGURE 3.2: Indian ivory statue found at Pompeii, possibly of the goddess Lakshmi. Getty Images.

beneath a modest block of shops and flats. It reached Rome in very considerable quantities, stored in a vast warehouse constructed for the purpose under Domitian, the *Horrea Piperataria*, still partially preserved beneath the Basilica of Constantine. The Roman state took a direct interest in the pepper supply, and when Alaric held the city to ransom in 408 CE, part of the deal was 3,000 lbs of pepper—an amount that sounds impressive, yet at Pliny's prices, worth as little as 12,000 *denarii*, no prince's ransom. Pepper, like so many of the other commodities traded through the Red Sea ports, has been found at Berenike, not as elsewhere in small traces, but in a jar containing 7.5 kg stored in a temple.

Pepper was thus, in contrast to the rarer spices and incenses, a large bulk, low value luxury. The great merchantmen which braved the monsoon winds, with loads of 75 to 1,000 tons, needed bulk to make weight. They could scarcely fill up with gemstones and light muslins. They were greedy for pepper, and met a warm welcome at the port of Muziris which supplied them. The trade can be seen from the other side through a Tamil poet: "the city where the beautiful vessels, the masterpieces of the Yavanas [Westerners] stir white foam on the Periyar, river of Kerala, arriving with gold and departing with pepper—when that Muçiri, brimming with prosperity, was besieged by the din of war." That part at least of the exchange was gold and silver coin is abundantly confirmed by the large quantities of early imperial *aurei* and *denarii* found in south India—notably more so there than in the north, and with a peak under no less than Tiberius, and a sharp falling off after Nero's reduction of the purity of those coinages. The Romans were admired in the east for their honesty, on the grounds that their coinages were of consistent weight and purity from emperor to emperor.

Tiberius' concerns about the drainage of resources created by the luxury market is echoed by the figures which Pliny indignantly offers for the annual currency loss to the East, apparently 100 million sesterces, and specifically 50 million to India. The figures preserved in the manuscripts are unreliable, and if the "losses" ran at the rate suggested by Pliny, it was a mere trifle. The value of the Eastern trade must have been several orders of magnitude higher. Our best evidence comes from a papyrus recording a loan against a shipment of goods from Muziris. The quantities given are precise, with weights, values, and amount deducted in tax. The consignment consisted of sixty boxes of nard, and a large quantity of elephant trunks, both whole and partial. The total weight was 3.5 tons, and the value just short of 7 million sesterces, but as that was after the deduction of the *tetarte*, the 25 percent tax imposed on luxury goods by the Roman authorities, it brings the total value closer to 10 million.

A relatively small 75-ton ship could carry over twenty such consignments, and double the value of Pliny's supposed figure for the cost of Eastern trade. So either Pliny's figures are a vast understatement, or they are based on very partial information, excluding for instance the numerous goods which, as our Red Sea trader makes plain, were shipped outwards in exchange. Some modern scholars have followed Pliny's moralizing in translating this into a balance of payments deficit, though as the Athenians blessed with Laurion and minting coinage for an empire discovered, when the state both owns the mines and monopolizes the currency, it can mint coinage without loss or even fear of inflation. The trade was vastly profitable to Rome, not least as a source of tax. The geographer Strabo reckoned that 120 ships a year sailed out of Myos Hormos under Augustus. Berenike rapidly became larger than Myos Hormos, and it is clear that trade grew in the first century CE, so we must be looking at at least 300 shipments a year, each with a value in the tens or hundreds of millions, with a total trade evidently worth billions. Small wonder that Tiberius, for all his parsimony, felt he had better things to do than discourage the luxury trade.

SMELLS AND TASTES

What was its impact, not so much on the Roman economy, as on the world of Roman senses? It is easier to feel than to quantify. Walk around not just the Roman marketplace, but Roman life, with the taste-buds alert, the nose twitching, the eye out for sparkle, the touch sensitive to the feel of fabric. The Eastern trade impacted on what they ate and drank, on the medicines they were dosed with, the smells of their rituals, the great sacrifices at festivals, or the quiet domestic offerings, the jewels and perfume they wore, the oils they anointed themselves with in the baths, and the fine dresses they put on for dinner parties. The "luxury" label makes us initially think of a lucky elite, better fed, better clothed, and better smelling than the rest, and maybe this was true to an extent. The smells of the countryside must always have been different from those of the town (unless you found yourself in a luxury villa). The officer who presented himself to Vespasian smelling of perfume received a sharp rebuke: the emperor would rather he smelt of garlic like a peasant (Suetonius *Vespasian* 8.2). But on the other hand, we should not underestimate the degree to which luxuries were penetrating the more middling ranks, especially in urban contexts, and the degree to which luxury was "aspirational," desirable to those who like Vespasian's officer wished to rise in the world.

An interesting test case is offered by the recipe book that goes under the name of Apicius. It is sometimes taken as a book for the rich, not least because of its association with Apicius, the by-word for gourmandize under Tiberius and the early Julio-Claudians. But it is evident that the book is a later compilation, with recipes attributed to the emperors Vitellius, Trajan, and Commodus, and it is likely that even if some recipes go back to the early first century CE, even to the hand of Apicius, we are looking at a cumulative compilation. Some recipes may indeed serve the luxurious tastes of the rich. Among the recipes for fowl are a couple for flamingo, an import, naturally, from Africa, which must have been rare and expensive, even when Caligula insisted on its use in sacrifices to the imperial cult. But these are exceptions alongside the numerous recipes for duck, woodpigeon, and crane, all locally sourced, let alone the chicken that dominates the section on fowl. Fish could be a highly priced speciality, especially if of exceptional size, like the mullet which was donated to Tiberius, though the parsimonious emperor had it sold on in the market and commented that there were gluttons like Apicius prepared to blow a fortune on such a fish (Seneca *Letters* 95.42). But the fish which the cookbook mentions are the mullet, perch, gilthead bream, dentex, mackerel, scorpion fish, tuna, and eel, which abound in the Mediterranean and are typical of present-day Italian cuisine. The section on meat and game has recipes for wild boar, a standby for high Roman cuisine, venison and wild goat, alongside beef, lamb, pork, and hare: all of these are locally sourced and standard in Italian cuisine. Only the solitary recipe for stuffed dormouse takes us into a less familiar world, and then the frequency with which *gliraria* are found in the Vesuvian cities for fattening up dormice suggests this more *outré* taste could be met by local supply. The entire book dedicated to vegetable dishes suggests nothing beyond the budget of a large number of Romans.

If we take Apicius, rather than the satirists who constantly made fun of culinary excess, as our guide, we may ask where the world of exotic luxury impinged on Roman taste buds. The answer must surely lie in the sauces, the spices, herbs and condiments, that gave Roman cuisine its characteristic flavors. It is here that the exotic spices that led merchants to brave the monsoons play their distinctive role. Many of the spices which the *Periplus* sources to India, and which Pliny disapprovingly records prices for, find their place in "Apicius." There are ginger and cardamom, spikenard, cumin, malabathrum, costus and the spice called folium, and above all black pepper, all Eastern imports. There is also *silphium* or *laser*, originally sourced from Cyrenaica and regarded as a precious commodity (Caesar found the Roman treasury had a good supply of it); but this seems to have become extinct in the mid-first century CE, and was substituted by asafoetida or Devil's Dung, the acridly pungent resin of an umbellifer which grew in Afghanistan, where Alexander's troops discovered it. All of these required the luxury trade to supply them.

But though Apicius uses Eastern spices, they are hardly the predominant taste of his cuisine. Spikenard, cardamom, the prized malabathrum and costus, feature in two, three, four, and five recipes respectively. Cumin is a good deal commoner (fifty-five recipes), but it is only black pepper that features again and again in over a hundred recipes. Cinnamon and cloves are absent. The commonest herbs and flavors are those standard in Italy: coriander, lovage, parsley, rue, oregano, celery, onion, pine nuts, and onion. The only notable absentee by contrast with modern Italian cuisine is garlic, which evidently retained its reputation as a peasant taste. The dominant taste is not that of the spices of the Orient, with the egregious exception of pepper, but of fermented fish sauce, *garum* or *liquamen*, the production of which, especially in south Italy, North Africa, and Spain, was on an industrial scale. What makes it hardest for us to imagine the dominant taste of Roman cooking is the lack of modern production of fish sauce (unless possibly the sauces of Thailand and Vietnam are indeed similar), and lack of clarity as to how it was made, from fish blood, blood and guts or a mixture of these and small fry, layered with salt and left to ferment. Devil's Dung is the other ingredient that strains our imagination. These, with oil, vinegar and honey, find their ways into dish after dish. India supplied the ubiquitous pepper, appreciated by everyone except Pliny.

For the smells and the tastes of the East to dominate, we need to move into different spheres. In medicine they were regarded as essential. The first century CE *Materia Medica* by Dioscurides enumerates in detail the powers of herbs and spices in pharmacology. Pepper and ginger, cinnamon and casia, and the full range of rarer Indian spices are listed. Other medical texts too, like the early first century CE Celsus *On Medicine*, deploy these spices. But then, as everyone from the Elder Cato knew, doctors were out to fleece their customers, or, more kindly put, medical drugs were frequently hard to source and expensive. How many could afford the sort of treatments they offered is open to question, but the point is that medicine is another significant area to which Eastern imports added their smells and flavors.

So too with ritual. Much of the business of sacrifice depended on the richness of the land, whether the classic pigs, sheep, and cattle, or the more modest offering of spelt cakes, honey, and eggs. Domestic offerings excavated in Pompeii include nuts, fruit, pinecones, and the inedible extremities of chickens. But while all of these could be locally sourced, what sacrifice was complete without the smell of incense, the frankincense, *tus*, which the southern Arabs managed to restrict to the port of Kane, along with myrrh, nard and the like? The olfactory sensations of a Catholic mass are the direct descendants of Roman sacrificial practice.

Funerals were a specific ritual that demanded incense. The richness of the incenses burnt to disguise the stench of death was also an important indicator of status. Here the nards and frankincense imported from Arabia and India came into their own. Statius speaks of Atedius Melior as spending an entire fortune on the scents for the funeral of his favorite Glaucias: the flowers of Cilicia, the grass of India, the liquids of Arabia, Pharos, and Palestine (*Silvae* 2.1.160f.). Poetry may not be able to evoke the pot-pourri of scents, but it can catalog the geographical range on which it depended. That vast sums of money could be involved is likely enough. Nero burnt so much cinnamon or casia at the funeral of his wife Poppaea, according to Pliny (*NH* 12.83), as to consume the equivalent of an entire year's produce. But even after death these unguents remained vital: at the ritual visits to the grave on the Parentalia or Rosalia, the stench of death still needed to be masked by offerings of unguents, poured down the tubes into the grave, and excavation shows burial sites to be littered with glass unguent bottles.

The ritual use of incenses linked closely to perfumes. Ovid in his *Medicamina Faciei Femineae* (the *Medicaments of the Female Face* 83ff) wickedly suggests that though frankincense was useful for keeping the gods happy, it was as well to keep some aside for personal use: mix *tus* with nitre, add cumin bark and a cube of myrrh, a handful of dry rose leaves and sal ammoniac, and apply to the skin.

The tastes and smells of early imperial Rome were a blend. The home-grown dominated; but the flavors made possible by the Red Sea trade made an important contribution. One may be struck, not so much by the luxury, as the integration of these tastes and smells into the local ones: just as pepper and cumin sit indifferently alongside marjoram and thyme in the modern spice rack, so they blended in with the tastes of the Mediterranean, olive oil, wine, and the inescapable fish sauce. But one point we may note about this cuisine, a point also true of medical concoctions, was the love for mixing multiple tastes, and throwing in a bit of everything. Apicius rarely recommends less than half a dozen flavors. Modern Italian cooking, which urges simplicity of taste combinations, in this sense is closer to classical Greek cuisine, to judge by Archestratus' pleading for the same principle, and his disapproval of the pot-pourri of tastes favored by the Italians.

SIGHT AND TOUCH

From tastes and smells to sight and touch, trade not only across the Mediterranean but with a larger world outside enhanced variety and pleasure. The same Taprobane (Sri Lanka/Ceylon) that was the best source for black pepper and cinnamon was the prime supplier of gemstones and pearls. Our Red Sea trader identified the southern Indian ports as a source for pearls, diamonds, sapphires, and all types of transparent gemstones. These included, as Pliny could spell out in detail, onyx, rock crystal, beryl, carnelian, amethyst, aquamarine, emerald, garnet, and agate, as well as the double-layered sardonyx that lent itself to cameos. These were prized items, incised in Alexandria or closer to home and set in golden rings, or strung with beads in necklaces. Gems were already prized in Ptolemaic Egypt, and, as a recently published papyrus has revealed, the epigrammatist Posidippus produced a sequence of epigrams on each gem. But again the imperial take-over of Egypt allowed a quantum leap in the market for gems. Gold rings set with intaglios, most commonly of carnelian, are found in each of the Vesuvian sites, including the rural ones, and are typically associated with skeletons who clung to them for their transportable value. In Herculaneum, the workshop of a *gemmarius* had produced a dozen such intaglios, not yet in settings, while half a dozen more had been carried down to the sewer.

Again the question arises of the social spectrum of those who possessed such gems. Pliny makes clear the range. These could be amongst the most valuable of possessions. When one Nonius Struma was proscribed by Antony as triumvir, he fled with his one treasured possession, a ring with a beryl said to be worth 2 million sesterces: the ring was his undoing (*NH* 37.82). Myrrhine (probably agate) and rock crystal were cut into drinking vessels and wine dippers of vast cost: Petronius, author of the *Satirica*, broke a myrrhine dipper worth 300,000 sesterces before his suicide to stop Nero laying hands on it, while Nero upon his own suicide smashed two rock-crystal cups (*NH* 37.20, 29).

But the highest values were attached to pearls, *margaritae* or *uniones*. Pliny waxes indignant at the fortunes spent on pearls: Lollia Paulina, wife of the emperor Gaius, appeared at a banquet draped with a rope of pearls and emeralds said to be worth 40 million, while Cleopatra famously squandered 10 million by dissolving a single pearl in vinegar, the twin of which was dedicated to Venus Genetrix in Rome (*NH* 9.106–22). But despite this giddying sum for a single pearl, there were smaller ones at a fraction of the cost: to such an extent that Pliny complains that the fashion for twin-pearl earrings called "castanets" had spread so far that even the poor, *pauperes*, craved them (*NH* 9.114). That finds some confirmation in the Vesuvian sites, where earrings with two pearls suspended from a golden bar are a regular type found in dozens of examples. One may argue over how poor the *pauperes* might be, but there can be little doubt that golden rings with incised gems and pearl earrings were common among people far below the level of the elite (see Fig. 3.4 for an example of gold pins and pearls from Pompeii).

Not all roads for luxury goods led from India. There was one northern route of importance which led from the Baltic, and supplied the Roman world

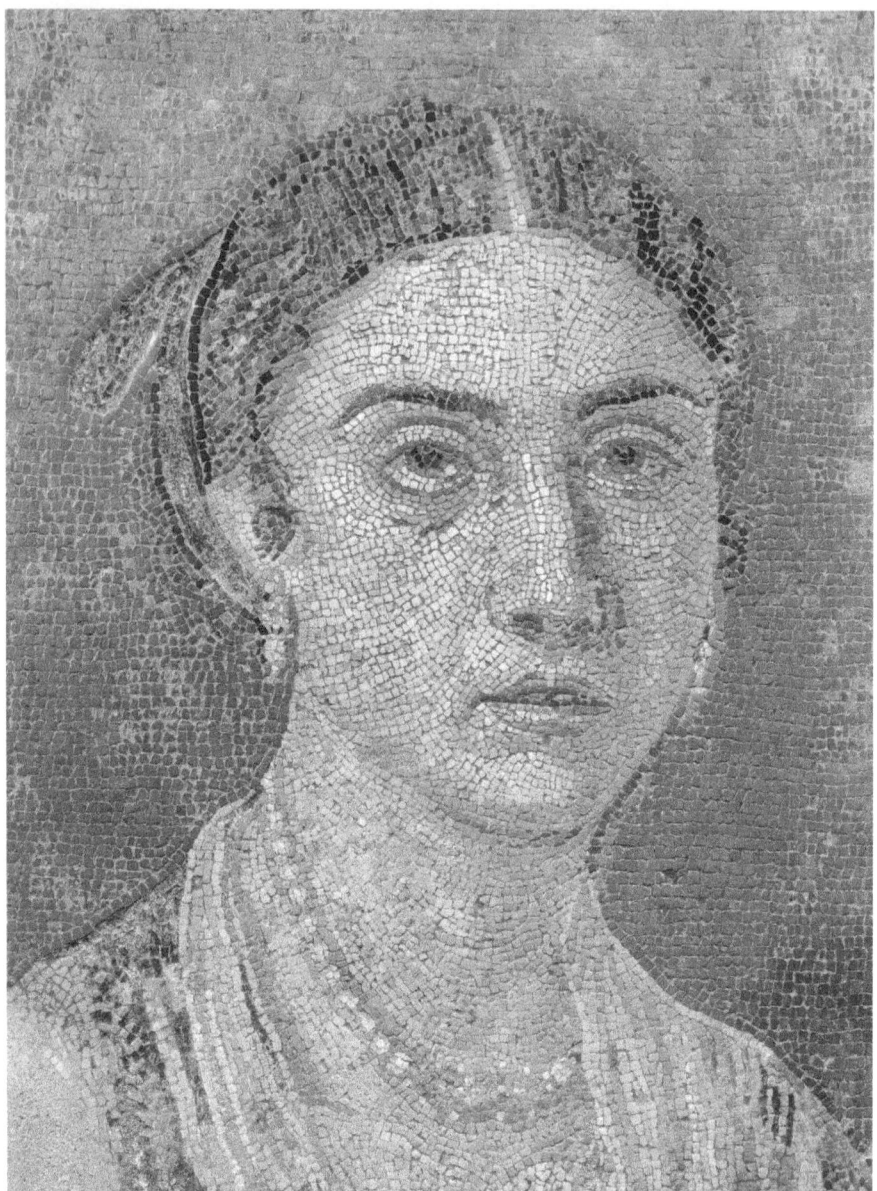

FIGURE 3.3: Mosaic from Pompeii showing a woman wearing a pearl necklace and earrings. Getty Images.

with amber. Pliny ranks amber as behind only myrrhine-ware and rock-crystal among luxuries (*NH* 37.30). He is well aware of its source on the Baltic, and its nature as a crystallized resin—he has no time for the story that it is made of lynx's urine. And he knows the role of the Veneti in bringing amber to the

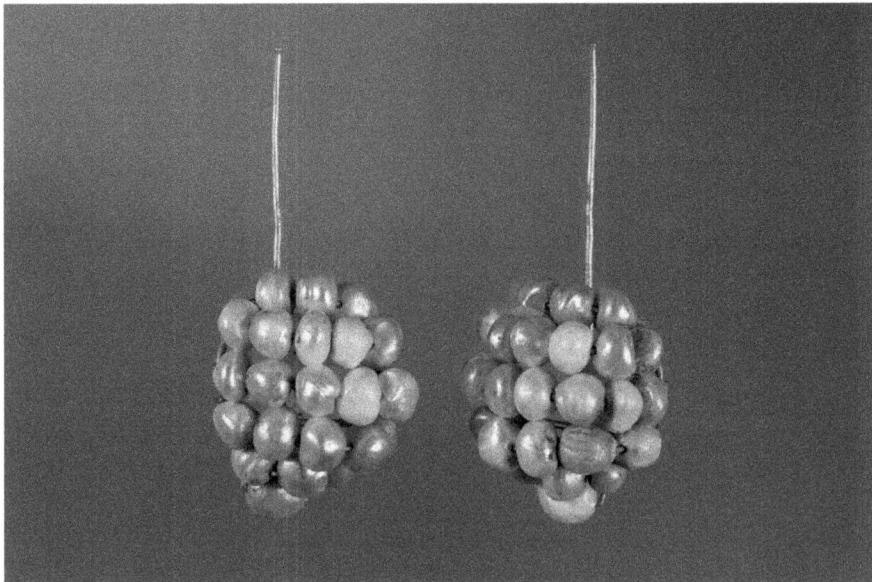

FIGURE 3.4: Pair of gold pins and pearls from Pompeii. Getty Images.

Adriatic. The excavations of Aquileia, just round the coast from Venice, have produced copious amounts of amber, which was worked there into jewelry and objects, along with a considerable glass production, making Aquileia the Murano of antiquity. There must have been other luxury goods too that traveled down the amber road from the Baltic. One might think of Pliny's story of auxiliary officers in Germany detaching whole cohorts to hunt white geese, for the sake of the downy feathers for soft pillows (NH 10.54).

Goose-feather pillows were not the only soft touch in Roman luxury, and here we think above all of silks. As we have seen, Chinese silks reached Rome with spices and gems along the Red Sea route. But there were overland routes across Asia of enormous importance which made the desert cities of Palmyra and Petra flourish in the early empire. Despite its fame and romantic appeal, the "Silk Road" was by no means so well established and well-traveled as its fame suggests. Rather than a single, well-defined and well-beaten track, it was a series of links, with goods constantly changing hands, and various routes traversing the daunting obstacles of the Lop and Gobi deserts, and the mountain ranges of the Pamirs and Hindu Kush. It was an extreme rarity for a Roman to reach China in person, or for a Chinese traveler to reach Rome, and trade depended on a chain of intermediaries long enough for mutual knowledge and understanding to fail to penetrate. Indeed the Romans were aware of the Chinese, whom they called Seres, and Augustus claimed to have received embassies from China. But Roman geographical knowledge of the route, let alone China itself, was extremely sketchy.

Reciprocally, the Chinese were aware of Rome, but only sketchily. The Han dynasty (206 BCE–220 CE) was interested in exchange with the West, but without establishing direct or reliable contact. A valuable record of their knowledge is preserved in the *Chronicle of the Western Regions* from the Hou Hanshu, compiled in the second century CE. The Roman Empire, Da Qin, is seen in a positive, but not wholly accurate light. Their land is seen as a rich one, producing "plenty of gold and silver, and of rare and precious things." But the list that follows is not one of products of the Roman Empire, but precisely the goods which Roman traders *pursued*: luminous jade, bright moon pearls, Haiji rhinoceros, coral, yellow amber, opaque glass, whitish chalcedony, red cinnabar, green gemstones, gold-thread embroideries, and delicate polychrome silks painted with gold. It makes a fine shopping list for a Roman, and of course doubtless all these goods were indeed available in Rome.

More curiously, the *Chronicle of the Western Regions* attributes silk production to Rome. "They also have a fine cloth which some people say is made from the down of 'water sheep,' but which is made, in fact, from the cocoons of wild silkworms." This, by a strange mirror reflection, could be Pliny talking about China, not the reverse. The *Chronicle* has a high opinion of the honesty of Roman traders, who "do not have two prices." But it acknowledges the difficulty of communication: "the king of this country [Rome] always wanted to send envoys to Han, but the Parthians, wishing to control the trade in multi-colored Chinese silks, blocked the route to prevent the Romans getting through." Whether or not there was active Parthian obstructionism, the route was evidently an insuperable barrier, though the *Chronicle* claims that one embassy made its way through in the year 166 CE, in the reign of the Roman emperor An-tun—Marcus Aurelius Antoninus. The embassy offered gifts of elephant tusks, rhinoceros horn and tortoiseshell, but the Chinese were deeply unimpressed: "The tribute brought was neither precious nor rare, therefore raising suspicions that the accounts might have been exaggerated." If there is any truth in this, the luxuries offered were the typical products of East Africa. It might have been a trader who loaded up at Rhapta, and was blown off course to find himself in the South China Sea.

Chinese silk certainly reached Rome, but through intermediaries rather than directly, whether overland on the "Silk Road," or more easily by sea via India. But, reflecting the tenuous links of communication, Chinese silks were actually transformed before they reached the Roman market. There is no sign of Chinese designs reaching Rome, and this is because, as Pliny bitterly complains, demonstrating a strange ignorance of the silkworm and the mulberry tree:

> the people called the Seres are famous for the woollen substance obtained from their forests; after a soaking in water they comb off the white down of the leaves, and so supply our women with the double task of unravelling the threads and weaving them together again. So manifold is the labour employed, and so distant is the region of the globe drawn upon, to enable the Roman matron to flaunt transparent raiment in public.
>
> NH 6.54

From this weird amalgam of ignorance and prejudice, it emerges that Chinese woven silks were elaborately unpicked and rewoven, presumably in order to enhance the quality of silk which Romans most appreciated, its translucency. Pliny may exaggerate the labors of the weavers if, as seems likely, the majority of Chinese silk was imported in skeins. In any case, by the time it is found in the Roman empire, silk is not typified by Chinese patterns.

Chinese silk was more prestigious than the local Mediterranean equivalent, from the island of Cos, but this too was regarded as a scandalous luxury. Pliny said that it was one Pamphile who had the glory of inventing a fabric that would leave women naked (*NH* 11.76). For Propertius, wearing Coan fabric made you a loose woman (4.2.23). The sight of his beloved was enough to make him want to write his whole volume of poetry on Coan silk (2.1.5). Propertius took the anti-luxury line that nature was the highest beauty, and no artifice could improve it: no need to wrap her slender curves in Coan cloth, or drench the hair with the myrrh of the Orontes (1.2.1ff.)

The protests of Tiberius and Pliny against the wearing of diaphanous silks by respectable married women are both on grounds of indecency and expense. Seneca elaborates both points:

> I see silk dresses, if dresses they can be called when they have no substance with which to protect either the body or the reputation, though they let her swear blind she is not naked. These dresses are brought in from trade with unknown peoples for vast sums, just so our married women can flaunt in public even more than they reveal to their lovers in the bedroom.
>
> Seneca *On Benefits* 7.9.5

As on other luxuries, emperor, philosopher, and encyclopedist sing from the same hymn sheet, protesting a tad too loudly. More realistically, Martial

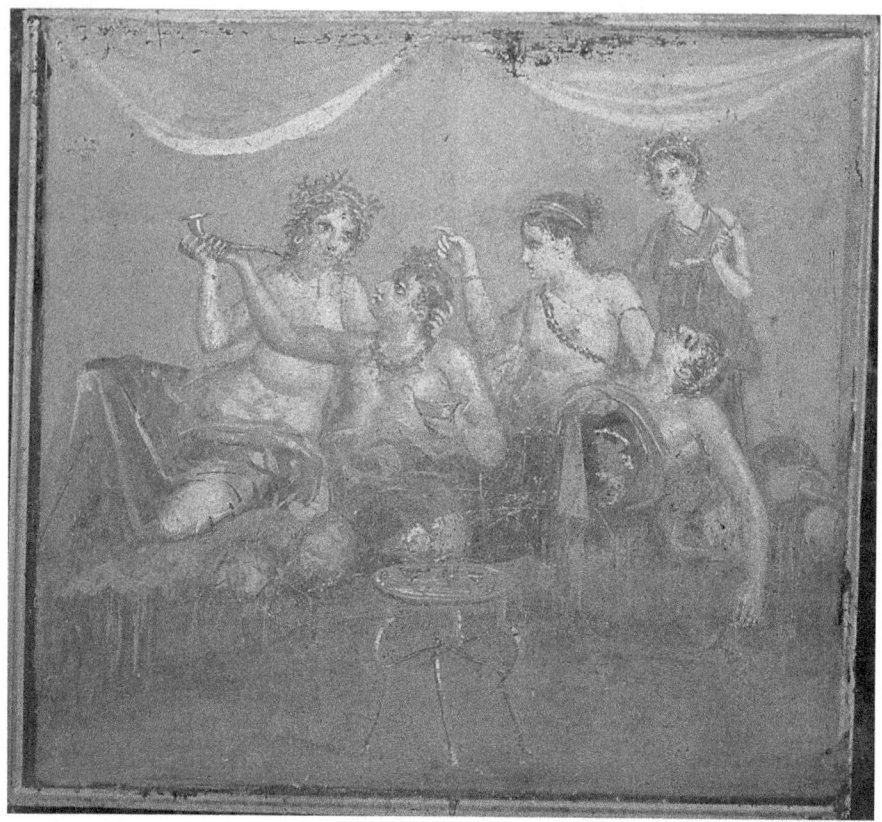

FIGURE 3.5: Fresco with banquet scene from the *Casa dei Casti Amanti* showing woman wearing see-through silk. Photo by Michael Harvey, courtesy Soprintendenza Archeologica di Pompei, Ercolano e Stabia.

warns not to be tricked by a girlfriend into a shopping trip to the Vicus Tuscus, where she can beg for a pound of nard, choice emeralds and silk dresses (*Epigrams* 11.27). If they represented a female fashion item, the fashion must have been one for the really rich, as Galen indicates.

The route to China was too long and difficult for silk to become a standard item like pepper or pearl earrings. On the other hand, one wonders how many could endure the Italian summer heat wrapped in wool. There was a lighter evening dress for dinner parties, the *synthesis*, and here the trade in Indian cottons and muslins might have provided a more endurable alternative to heavy wool. Martial describes a dinner guest, one Zoilus, changing his sweaty *synthesis* eleven times in a single dinner: he was not impressed (5.79). Pliny knew about "wool-trees" (*laniferae*, corresponding to the Greek term "erioxylon") growing on the islands of the Bahrein group in the Persian gulf (*NH* 12.37), and in Ethiopia on the borders of Egypt (13.90). Moreover, cotton was grown in Egypt itself, as later Egyptian papyri and ostraca reveal, backed up by finds of cotton seeds and bolls associated with spindle-whorls. Both Indian and Egyptian cottons are found at Berenike, and it is possible to distinguish them by the different traditions of spinning the yarn (an activity more than proverbial): the Egyptian spun anti-clockwise in an S-pattern, the Indian clockwise in a Z-pattern. But despite the availability and seeming potential of cotton, it seems to have remained a rarity across the empire, with only isolated finds in Italy, Germany, Hungary, and Spain (Palmyra, the gate to the East, is another story).

Instead the market was captured by silks, and for all the moral objections so hysterically raised in the first century CE, silk established a firm place as a sign of elite status, and is frequently met in elite burials into late antiquity. The ideal combination of luxury was silk interwoven with wool, dyed with the purple of the *murex*, in itself an important luxury, and with threads of pure gold. Such garments mark the richest burials, from Trier, where the great cemetery of St. Maximin provides numerous examples, to various sites in Britain.

Fabrics and textiles are at best patchily served by the archaeological record because of their delicacy. To judge from the representation of fabrics in wall paintings, dresses were characterized by bright colors not so much in complex patterns, but in the superimposition of brightly colored pieces. The world of colors is preserved for us far better in architecture, and it is on Roman walls and floors that we can grasp the rich and varied palette made possible by Roman imperial power. Just as Roman food came to incorporate a rich variety of tastes from across the Mediterranean with exotic imports, so the surfaces of Roman rooms glittered with hues that depended on wide geographic control and contacts.

Brightness and variety of color typifies the imperial period, which by opening up trade gave access to a greater range than had been traditional in the Mediterranean, with the significant exception of Alexandria. Polychrome marble flooring, known as *opus sectile*, becomes a key marker of luxury in the early empire. Again, it is Augustus' conquest of Egypt that marks a turning point, not only opening up access to the prized purple porphyry and pinkish flecked granite, but also spreading technologies long used for quarrying, cutting, and transporting these hard rocks. The exploration of the Roman quarries at Mons Porphyrites and Mons Claudianus can only increase our respect for the technological skills in quarrying enormous weights of granite from these inhospitable mountains, and transporting the stones across the equally inhospitable desert before it reached the Nile and the relative ease of water transport.

It is in the early imperial period that a series of quarries across the eastern Mediterranean are absorbed into imperial control and management: from Simitthus (Chemtou) in Numidia the prized yellow/orange of *numidicum* (Giallo antico); from Mt. Taenaros in the Peloponnese the red *taenareum* (*rosso antico*) and the green serpentine of Sparta (*lacedaemonium*); from Carystos on Euboea's southern tip, the green and white onion veins of *carystium* (*cipollino*); from Chios in the Aegean the pastel breccia of pinks, purples, and grays, *chium* (portasanta); from Docimium in central Phrygia the purpled salami cuts of *phrygium* (pavonazetto); from Bithynia the coral breccia, of reds, pinks, and whites in a coral matrix—and this is to name only the commonest of a varied supply. Each of these stones is in itself rich in color, and in their most prestigious forms they provided monolith columns and large architectural elements, largely restricted to public buildings (and hence the imperial interest in controlling the trade). But the use of colored marbles spread far into the private sphere in the form of veneers (a fashion attributed to the luxurious Mamurra, an engineer of Caesar sometimes identified with Vitruvius), and here the taste was to mix as many different marbles as possible in a counterpane of pattern. Cutting marble produced progressively smaller offcuts. Small chips could be used to give life to a mosaic floor, woven into patterns with other cheaper stones. And there was always a market for recycling, so that we find shop-counters in Pompeii set with odds and ends of colored marbles.

This taste for bright color mixes is seen equally in wall decoration. The painters of classical Athens, claims Pliny, were content with just four natural earth colors, the white of Melinum, the ochre of Attica, the red of Sinope ("sinopia" is still used of the red used to sketch out a fresco design), and soot black; he contrasts the rich hues of contemporary Roman painting, which he says include purples and Indian indigo, which he wrongly believes to include snake and elephant blood (*NH* 35.50), produced by the crushing of the snake by a dying elephant so that their bloods comingle (*NH* 33.116). Pliny lists no fewer than thirty-five different pigments, of which modern chemical analysis has been able to identify twenty-eight in the wall paintings of Pompeii. Most are sourced from a variety of locations around the Mediterranean. But the brightest and most prized colors were harder to source, and Pliny specifies that for these the client had to pay extra, presumably at a mark-up on market price. The fancy colors were minium, Arminium, cinnabar, chrysocolla, Indicum and purpurissum (*NH* 35.30). Of these, minium and cinnabar seem to overlap, the vermillion of mercury sulphite, a byproduct of mining precious metals. Arminium was a dark blue, originally from Armenia, with a correspondingly exorbitant price (300 sesterces the pound), but the discovery of a Spanish version brought the price down to 6 *denarii* the pound, even so a high price (*NH* 35.47). Chrysocolla is identified as malachite, an expensive product of the Red Sea trade. Indicum is the supposedly snake-blood import from India, while purpurissum takes its purple from the murex, a color special enough to become an imperial privilege.

Where there is luxury and expense, there is also the drive to find cheaper versions. The classic example is Egyptian blue. A friend of Cicero's, Vestorius, made a fortune by importing from Alexandria to Puteoli the "Egyptian blue" called *caeruleum*. But, as Vitruvius explains (VII.11), he went a step further, and having determined the simple recipe, based on sand crushed with sodium nitrate with copper shavings fired in the furnace, produced it at Puteoli itself. The price remained high, given by Pliny (*NH* 33.162) as 11 *denarii* the pound; archaeology can demonstrate its extensive use in decorating the walls of Pompeii and Herculaneum, and *amphorae* from a wreck outside Marseilles suggest that the importer took to a flourishing export business.

Wall painting is where the astonishing color range of Roman pigments is most visible to us, but of course pigments were not limited to painting: as well as fabrics, they were used in architectural decoration, cosmetics, make-up, ointments, and medicines in general: the pages of Dioscurides reveal how close the overlap was between medicine and the world of luxury. Consider Ovid's advice to women on self-presentation: the effect is full of color (*Ars Amatoria* 3.161ff.). Women should not hesitate to dye their hair with "German herbs." We hear elsewhere of the use of various dyes to give black hair (Pliny suggested leeches rotted for forty days in wine, while Dioscurides suggested kermes rotted in water), red hair (the juice of young walnuts, suggested Pliny), or how to dye blond by the use of *sapo*, goat's fat mixed with beechwood ash. Wigs became commoner and more elaborate among the rich, and the hair of German captives was valued for its blond color. Then there is dress. No need, suggests Ovid, to blow a fortune on Tyrian purple, for a host of colors can dye wool at lower cost: sky-blue, sea-blue, crocus yellow, myrtle green, amethyst purple, and pale rose. He points to the effect of a meadow full of flowers, and that is indeed the effect of the bright colors represented (for example) in the house of the Chaste Lovers at Pompeii. Then there is make-up, and here the essential colors are white and red: white from white clay, safer than the white lead of *cerussa* that was poisonous, and ruddle red, cheaper than the pricey cinnabar used for decoration. Eyebrows could be subtly picked out with ashes or crocus yellow. A girl's dressing table will be covered with little pots, *pyxides*; but beware of letting your lover see them for the secrets of make-up are best concealed, and the contents might disgust. The contents of crocodile intestines were used for rouge, but best not to know about it.

How many of these scents and colors reached the poor of the empire? The agricultural worker may have continued to smell of sweat and garlic, untouched by the Eastern luxuries of the rich. But within the context of the city, the situation was more nuanced. What of the smells of the greasy *popina* for which Horace's farm bailiff yearned? The early emperors wanted to close down such cookshops: it is unlikely to have been on health and safety grounds, more likely that they were felt to offer the poor excessive temptation, as well as incitement to gamble and brawl. The emperor Claudius may have let the cat out of the bag in remarking to the senate, "Who can live without a snack, *offula*?" (Suetonius *Claudius* 40.1). The food was surely laced with *garum* and *asafoetida* as "Apicius" would have recommended for the rich; and it is dangerous to assume that no spices or pepper reached the diet of the urban poor.

Then we must allow for the impact of the public baths, with which Roman cities were so generously provided. Even if they did not rise to modern standards of hygiene, the habit of regular washing was constructed as a universal amenity, at least for the free. The glass ampoules of oil with which they scraped down doubtless had downmarket versions with cheap oil and cheap scents: not everyone would emerge smelling of frankincense and malabathrum. But given the power of social pressures, they are more likely to have emerged smelling of cheap, downmarket perfumes than of human sweat. Humans smell too of what they eat: we may suspect a barbarian could recognize a Roman by his or her breath. Sacrifices and festivals played an important role in diffusing culture: the smell of the incense and the flavors of the cooking of a public feast may have engendered more homogeneity than we expect.

CONCLUSION

The Roman art of seduction was an assault on the senses, with colors and scents and sensuous fabrics; and the Roman marketplace, supported by a trade network that spread across the empire and beyond, abundantly supplied it. Tiberius was right to hesitate to impose controls on the luxuries available in the market. They both rode on the back of the market in staples, and played a crucial role in stimulating Mediterranean trade. It is doubtless right to think of the great ports of Puteoli on the Bay of Naples and Portus, the port of Rome, on the mouth of the Tiber, as primarily aimed at ensuring a supply of grain, oil, and wine to the overcrowded population of the metropolis. But on the back of this trade came an astonishing variety of non-staple products: spices from Arabia and India that transformed the expectations of Roman taste-buds; aromatics and perfumes that transformed the smell of religious ritual and personal hygiene; silks, cottons, and fabric that transformed the way Romans dressed or covered their furnishings; gemstones, from pearls to glass beads, that became potent status symbols, women's "lictors," objects of such value as to be grasped by the victims fleeing from the wrath of Vesuvius; pigments that transformed the colors of their clothes, decorated walls and cosmetics; colored marbles that meant both public spaces and private were not just gleaming white, as Hollywood has imagined them, but a rainbow of bright and subtle hues.

Luxury was consistently identified by the Romans with the Orient, and with some reason: the brightest gems, the finest spices and perfumes, the softest silks, depended on a vast trade with the East, with Arabia, East Africa, India, and at a distant remove with China, which the conquest of Egypt in 30 BCE opened up in a spectacular fashion. Alexandria was seen as a font of corruption: an enormous proportion of this trade must have passed through its docks. But for all that, the quantity of merchandise attributable to internal trade within the Mediterranean must have been of a different order of magnitude. The Roman imperial world of senses was characterized by its variety and mixture: when a Roman dish or a Roman wall painting was likely to have some ingredients from beyond the empire, a hint of Oriental spice, but this was a mere extra to what could be sourced more locally.

While Tiberius may have despaired of controlling the trade in luxuries, that does not mean that the Roman approach was completely *laissez-faire*. The aediles evidently did continue to monitor prices in the marketplace. The Elder Pliny has an enormous amount of information about the prices of these luxury goods, though on the whole he only cites them to express outrage. It is hard to imagine that he went down to the *macellum* to monitor prices himself. His knowledge reflects the knowledge generated by Roman officials, the aediles and their agents. Two centuries later, when Diocletian produced his great Price Edict, setting maximum prices, it is clear that the government still had intimate knowledge of the vast range of differentiation in luxury prices. However effective that Edict may or may not have been, it is striking that it was not felt to be enough to regulate the prices of staples, but of the full range of commodities.

CHAPTER FOUR

The Senses in Religion: Piety, Critique, Competition

SUSAN ASHBROOK HARVEY

What can we learn by studying the senses in ancient religion? In this chapter, I will argue three points: (1) religion in antiquity was a fully and complexly embodied endeavor, for which the senses were not simply intrinsic but also functionally significant; (2) sensory awareness played a crucial role in ancient religious critique and in configuring religious reforms; and (3) sensory perception and experience were utilized for purposes of competition between religions. In all three areas, sensory engagement elicited and marked divine presence or absence, danger or deviance, truth or falsehood. While there is surely more, I suggest that attention to the senses yields a far richer, more nuanced understanding of ancient religion than is otherwise possible.

I will focus on religion in the Roman Empire between the first and sixth centuries CE. The geographical extent of the empire during this era as well as the logistics of infrastructure facilitated continual interaction between peoples, cultures, and religious practices. In such a context, influence, exchange, and critique flourished, whether of one's own practices or those of others. At the same time, religion during this period demonstrated profoundly shared sensibilities across different traditions, whether Greek, Roman, Jewish,

Christian, or others. Hence one can speak of "religion" in the singular, even while discussing its various forms (Rives 2007: 13–53). Further, all forms engaged much older traditions, whether ritually through worship practices, narratively through sacred stories, or in social memory, through festivals, memorials, shrines and other markers, thereby fostering a deep sense of historical continuum. Cultural memory was both inscribed and sustained through religious traditions. The Roman era incorporated a long past, even as it turned towards new directions.

RELIGION IN A SENSING BODY

Religion was a pervasive and varied presence in the ancient Mediterranean world. As the second-century Greek philosopher Artemidorus remarked, "no nation is without gods ... different people honor different gods, but they all have recourse to the same thing" (*Dreams* 1.8, cited in Rives 2007: 86). Ancient religions were fundamentally relational systems, first between the human and divine realms, and then within human social order. Religion comprised the practices and structures by which people established and maintained human-divine relations; and by which they accordingly defined themselves within families, communities, and states, by gender, class or rank, age, and ethnicity. In similar terms, religious practices defined and integrated the spaces of peoples' lives, whether domestic or civic; and they articulated roles that intersected various social and political locations.

A shared treasure chest of ritual tools provided the practices that enabled such relationality, enacting it across social and political landscapes (Beard *et al.* 1998; Bremmer 1994; Burkert 1985; Rives 2007). These practices engaged a rich sensorium, whether in the simplest individual act or in the grandest public spectacle.

Sacrifice was the basic marker of human initiative towards the divine. It could be a few grains of pungent incense or a honey cake offered at the prayer niche of a domestic room, or an aromatic libation of wine, oil, milk, or honey poured out by the pious householder. Again, sacrifice could be the elaborate festival of a civic community or imperial celebration, where incense, grains, and animal offerings were consumed by fire, yielding fragrant smoke, "divine and holy," visibly ascending heavenward (Lucian *Sacrifice* 13; Harmon 1968, 3: 189). Flowers, aromatic plants, sacred oils and perfumes adorned the offerings, statues, altars, sacred buildings, and persons conducting the ceremonies, along with shining garments, embroidered silks, elaborate tapestries, brightly painted colors, gold or silver trim, and jeweled utensils. Prayers, hymns, musical

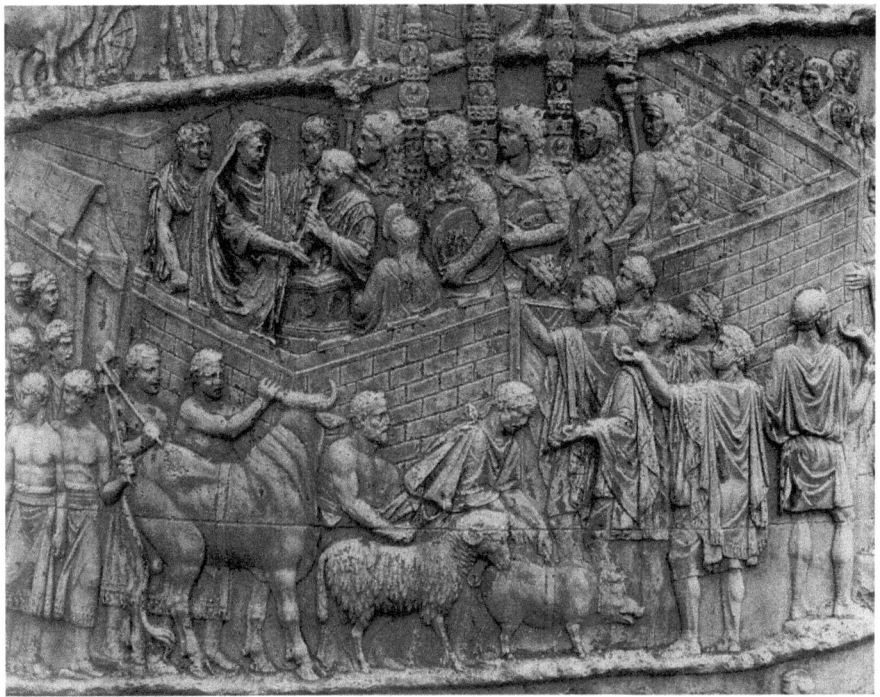

FIGURE 4.1: Detail from the Column of Trajan showing the emperor wearing the veil of the Pontifex Maximus and performing libations at the altar. In the foreground a lustral procession with musical fanfare prepares to enter for sacrifice. Photo: Filippo Coarelli, *The Column of Trajan*, trans. C. Rockwell (Rome: Editore Colombo, 2000), vol. 1, p. 99, pl. 55.

instruments and choreography accompanied the ritual procession and process. Holy taste followed in the foods that resulted: whether the festival celebration cooked from the sacrificed meat, or the good harvest resulting from the right relation between person and god(s). The sensory qualities of each component, whether in a poor household or a grand temple, conveyed human initiative towards the divine, and the blessing of divine presence in responsive return. A dialogic, interactive human-divine relationship was presumed, sought, and affirmed throughout the ancient world (Ullucci 2012: 23–30).

Hence in Ovid's *Fasti*, a lyrical catalog of religious rites and celebrations following the calendar year, the poet describes parallel ritual structures for the household and for the city of Rome itself (Nagle 1995). Though wonderfully varied in the specifics he cites, Ovid portrays a consistent pattern of personal and communal offerings to acknowledge and honor divine presence. For New Year's Day, sweet scents should be sprinkled on the hearth just as in the gleaming fires of the great temples (1.71–88). Fragrant wreaths should be hung on doors, animals garlanded, special clothes brought out for the special days. On February 21, small plates dedicated to ancestral spirits should have arrangements of "wreaths, a sprinkling of grain and a bit of salt, bread soaked in wine and violets scattered about" (2.533–9; Nagle 1995: 71–2), followed the next day by incense and plates of food for the household deities (2.631–8). Depending on the festival or the occasion, he mentions cinnamon incense, honey-drenched libation cakes or mixtures of spelt, salt, and incense; or myrtle, mint, and roses. Ovid enumerates special fumigants for cleansing; and occasions when special dishes are needed, such as roasted cow, millet cakes with milk, or a stew of bacon, beans, and barley. Celebrations might call for white robes (for Ceres, 4.619–20), others for multi-colored dress (for Flora, 5.193–377), still another for long robes and masks (for Minerva, 6.650–710). Incense, garlands, baskets of flowers, and fragrant woods repeatedly and continuously accompany the rites he mentions, whether in the household, in field or stable, or in elaborate temple ritual. Indeed, lists of ritual objects needed for various festivals survive to us in documentary papyri, and inscriptions enumerate many types of dedicated offerings. Colors, fragrances, textures, and variety characterize these lists (Beard *et al.* 1998, 2: 60–77 for calendars, 148–65 for sacrifice).

Sensory attention kept one mindful of the divine amidst daily activity. Vivid images of gods or goddesses were woven into curtains, carved into household vessels, incised into rings, belts, hairpins, and other personal accessories, providing tactile and visual engagement. Deities were depicted in colorful statues, sculptures, reliefs, and paintings that graced civic landscapes, rural shrines, and domestic buildings.

Sweet fragrances of incense, flowers, aromatic woods and plants were continually encountered throughout one's day; invariably, they were held to be evocative of divine presence. Scents were particularly important for their capacity to add religious resonance to an action or encounter. Their inclusion in religious ritual was ubiquitous. In every instance, what granted efficacy to the smells, whether pungent or sweet, were the olfactory meanings drawn from other contexts, particularly those of medicine and hygiene. Aromatic products were commonly used as cleaning agents and as key ingredients for medical treatments of all kinds; they were everywhere employed in burial rites. Cleaning was done by a sequence of washing, fumigating and perfuming. While this was the common method for housework, the same process was used for religious rites of initiation, purification, and consecration—whether of persons, objects, or places. Because aromatics were known to be effective cleaning agents and powerful medicines, they were also understood to be functional elements in religious ritual (Caseau 2001; Harvey 2006).

Consequently, stench or ill-odor in the form of working fumigants could be appropriate for rites of purification. While religious purity in its oldest forms was a matter of ritual state rather than moral condition, by Roman times the two concepts were largely combined. Ovid describes the pastoral rites of Pales that required a fumigant from the Vestal Virgins made from "horse's blood and calf's ash," as well as "purification" of the sheep flocks with "the smoke of burning sulphur" (4.723–82; Nagle 1995: 124–5). These ingredients were familiar to his contemporaries as active disinfectants. In the rites Ovid enumerated for the occasion, celebrated on April 21, these harsh smells were intertwined with a larger olfactory palette. Ovid mentions additional adornments of fragrant plants on the sheepfolds and garlands of flowers wreathing the doors; burning fires of olive, pine, Sabine juniper, and laurel wood; millet cakes, milk, and grape must; the use of water. In this instance, the harsh stench of some ritual components would have indicated strong cleaning, inducing ritual purity, and indeed its moral counterpart. But the broader olfactory mix contextualized the harshness, rendering it effectively hygienic, and more: blessedly health-giving and fruitful.

The densely textured sensory qualities of such patterned activities distinguished religious ritual from other actions, and were crucial to their perceived efficacy. Another example of the sensory details of religious ritual, and especially of the daily tasks that bound household piety to grander sacrificial structures, is strongly evident in the archaeological remains of Second Temple Judaism, for example, prior to the destruction of the Jerusalem Temple in 70 CE (Magness 2011). The material evidence demonstrates the various ways that personal household practices operated: for the preparation and consumption of food (or abstinence from it), for ritual bathing, Sabbath observances, special clothing needs, toilet habits, burial customs. Religion functioned at the level of deep daily habits and structures.

Religion, then, consisted of multiple (sensorily marked) acts every day, performed individually and with others. For this reason the early Christian intellectual Tertullian vehemently opposed "mixed" marriages, where only one partner was Christian (notably in "To His Wife," 2.3–8; Le Saint 1951: 23–36). His concern was precisely the ordinary religious practices of daily life: the personal gestures of prayer or blessing, the times of fasting or ritual food, the lighting of the hearth or the placement of wreaths. Even mundane acts carried religious significance: "we make the sign of the cross on our foreheads at every turn, at our going in or coming out of the house, while dressing, while putting on our shoes, when we are taking a bath, before and after meals, when we light the lamps, when we go to bed or sit down, and in all the ordinary actions of daily life" ("The Chaplet," 3.4; Arbesmann *et al.* 1959: 237). One saw, heard, touched, smelled, and tasted by numerous daily routines a continually present relationship between humans and their god(s). The senses enabled the body to experience human–divine relation, to express that relation, to know and to negotiate its contours.

Underlying this perspective was a cosmology in which human and divine domains intersected. However separate, these domains were constantly permeable. Hence religious practices molded sensory awareness and continuously engaged it, promoting a fundamental religious epistemology: the divine could be perceived, and thereby experienced. Religious instruction cultivated such attunement, while religious rituals utilized such sensibilities. Indeed, where sight was often the most valued sense from the view of philosophy, yet religious practices engaged the other senses in even more significant terms since these made every encounter tangible, and every practice greater than its appearance. One could *sense* more than one could do. Insofar as bodily experience was known through the senses, the senses provided vividly real knowledge of the divine. A dialogic exchange between human and divine realities resulted.

Because the ancient person expected such interaction, it was constantly available. Divinatory practices were common (Beard *et al.* 1998, 2: 166–93). Augurs interpreted the flights of birds and read the entrails of sacrificial animals as signs conveying divine purpose or intention. Oracles were frequently consulted, and some, like that of Apollo at Delphi, were held in grave esteem, with pilgrims from near and far (Elsner and Rutherford 2005). Incubation at healing shrines such as those of Epidauros or Claros produced dreams and visions in which gods or other divine beings gave instructions or prescribed cures. The natural world could bespeak divine favor or anger. Thus the great fourth-century orator Libanius asserted that one could know the blessings of the gods upon his beloved city of Antioch, by "the evidence of our senses" ("Antiochikos" 115; Norman 2000: 28). Libanius himself consulted Asclepius as well as soothsayers about his various maladies (*Autobio.* 143; *Ep.* 146); similarly, he sensed the tragic death of the emperor Julian before the arrival of messengers, when destructive earthquakes struck the region (*Autobio.* 134).

The natural world was the constant interface between the human and the divine realms, communicating from one domain to the other. The second-century Latin orator and writer Apuleius described how travelers expressed the pervasive awareness of divine presence as imminent and felt through attunement to the natural world:

It is the custom of pious travelers, whenever they come across a sacred grove or holy place along their way, to make a vow, offer fruit, and sit for awhile . . . [one might encounter] an altar wreathed with flowers, a cave shaded by leafy boughs, an oak weighed down with horns, a beech crowned with pelts, a little hill sanctified by an enclosure, a tree-trunk hewn into an effigy, a turf altar moistened with libations, a stone smeared with unguent.

Bouquet (Florida) 1, cited in Rives 2007: 90

The trajectory of Christianity during the Roman era highlights the issues with particular force. Earliest Christian literature showed little interest in the senses *per se*. But during the fourth century, Christianity gained legal protections and imperial favor under the reigns of Constantine and his sons. In wholly unexpected quantities, wealth, prestige, and converts flooded Christian communities. Liturgy expanded, as did all forms of public or domestic expression available to Christians. Christian texts not only enumerate these changes, but also draw attention to their sensory qualities.

For example, catechetical homilies instructed the newly converted specifically on the sensory aspects of liturgy. Cyril of Jerusalem, for one, explained that incense both called for and heralded divine presence; further, that perfumed holy oil anointed the newly baptized, distinguishing them from the catechumens (anointed with unscented oil) in order to grasp already the fragrance of Paradise wafting towards them (*Procat.* 1). Moreover, he urged the neophytes not to be disappointed if the holy oblation seemed to taste like ordinary bread and wine: the properly initiated would recognize Christ's flesh and blood instead (*Cat.* 4).

Christian teachings on the incarnation and physical resurrection of Christ set the body into high relief. Physicality itself became significant: whether by the dramatic explosion of the monastic movement and its increasingly harsh ascetic forms; or by the sudden interest in the idea of the Holy Land, and its attendant—and equally dramatic—development of pilgrimage, the cult of relics, and healing shrines. John Chrysostom urged his congregation to embrace the blessings of martyrs' tombs, especially the holy oil poured over their bones and collected for veneration: "Embrace the coffin, nail yourself to the chest . . . Take holy oil and anoint your whole body—your tongue, your lips, your neck, your eyes . . . For through its pleasant smell the oil reminds you of the martyrs' contests, and bridles and restrains all wantonness in considerable patience, and overcomes the diseases of the soul" ("A Homily on Martyrs"; Mayer and Allen 2000: 96).

Thus the sensations of holy encounter should continue to instruct the faithful even after leaving the sacred site, lingering in one's consciousness as a sensory accompaniment through one's daily activities. The pilgrim Paula had licked the ground at the very spot in Bethlehem where Christ was born (Jerome *Ep.* 108): divine incarnation rendered the physical itself an ever-flowing stream of divine encounter.

Not only were the sensory experiences highlighted as such, but further, Christian authors considered the significance of what those experiences were. In homilies and hymns, Christian leaders noted how sense perception affected one's body, and more importantly, its resulting impact on one's religious understanding. Just so did the fourth-century hymn writer Ephrem the Syrian sing the wonders of bodily experience:

> Let us see those things [God] does for us every day!
> How many tastes for the mouth! How many beauties for the eye!
> How many melodies for the ear! How many scents for the nostrils!
> Who is sufficient in comparison to the goodness of these little things?
> *Hymns on Virginity* 31.16; McVey 1989: 401

Most often, Christian authors showed an interest in the epistemological result: how the sensory encounter yielded greater knowledge of God, or what kind of knowledge was gained. Basil of Caesarea, like other Christian leaders, exhorted his congregation to study the beauty of creation as a means of grasping the infinitely greater beauty of the Creator (*Hexaemeron* Hom. 1).

The ancients themselves sometimes distinguished the sensory and the physical as distinct, separable domains. Christians such as Origen of Alexandria and Gregory of Nyssa, for example, building on earlier philosophical inquiry, would develop an elaborate system of "spiritual" as opposed to "carnal" senses, in the effort to articulate more clearly how the senses could engage the divine. Yet these spiritual senses for these authors were more properly the physical senses sacramentally transformed, rendered permeable and open to direct perception of the divine, beyond and in addition to what the limited physical realm could allow (Harvey 2006: 169–80).

In fact, late antiquity brought new attention to sensory experience throughout religious contexts. This was the era of Neoplatonism's interest in theurgy: the conviction that matter itself might convey, mark, or mediate divine presence (Miller 2010; Shaw 1995). In the "material turn" of the time, matter's capacity for divine penetration became a theme across religious spheres. For example, complex Manichaean food rituals worked not to destroy the body but to transform it: to change matter physiologically from the vehicle of dark or evil, to a receptacle for the saving particles of light (BeDuhn 2000).

Jewish piety of the same period also flourished with sensory richness, despite the devastating loss of the Jerusalem Temple and its extensive sacrificial system in 70 CE. Cultivation of a sensory appreciation can be seen in the archaeological remains of synagogues decorated with exuberant wall paintings and lavish floor mosaics of biblical stories (Elsner 2003; Levine 2005; Levine and Weiss 2000); in the appearance of votive offerings and dedicatory inscriptions (Satlow 2005); and in rabbinic reflection deeply attentive to the senses as mediators of righteous devotion (Green 2011).

The intensification of Christian asceticism, even in its harshest forms, must be seen as part of the same general orientation. Greek and Roman philosophical asceticism had advocated a benign neglect of the body, in order to focus on the higher realms of the intellect. The extremes of Christian asceticism emerge during the fourth and fifth centuries, coinciding with the changed interest Christian leaders showed in valuing the physical realm and bodily experience. The desert-dweller in a cave, the stylite on a pillar, the monastic crippled under weighty irons, all deliberately engaged a physicality of ascetic discipline wherein its sensory qualities were inescapable—both for the practitioner and

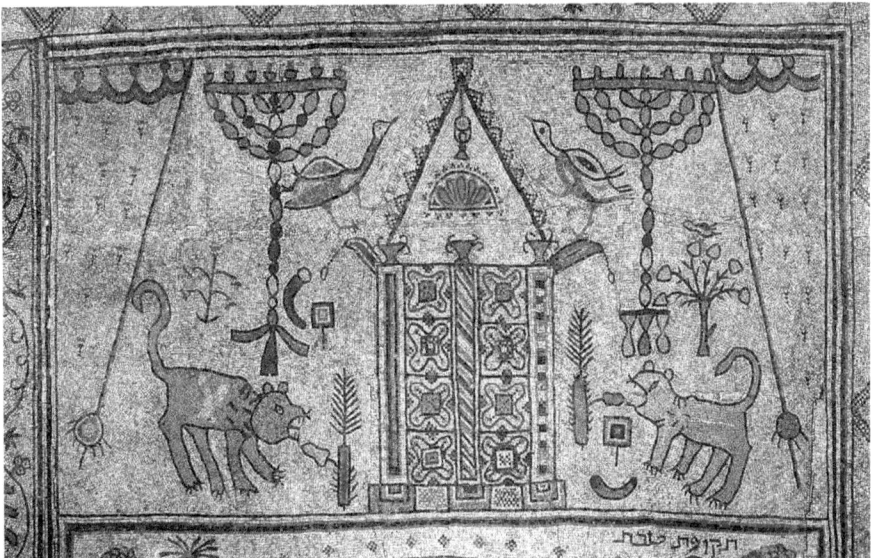

FIGURE 4.2: Floor mosaic from the Beth Alpha synagogue showing instruments of sacred ritual, including the sacred lulav (palm branch), etrog (citron), shofar (ram's horn), and incense shovel. Copyright: Zev Radovan.

for the observer. Critics (including ascetics!) complained about the odor of unwashed monks, and the smell of fasting breath. The coarse cloth of monastic habits continually chafed the skin; bare feet bled constantly. Sensory discomfort contributed to the ascetic's discipline, sometimes with penitential intent. But for Christians, asceticism was never a simple matter of self-mortification or even of renunciation. Rather, it was also an effort at transformation, rendering the physical body anew, towards its angelic, radiant and resurrected state to come (Brown [1988] 2008; Harvey 1998, 2006: esp. 201–21; Shaw 1995).

Finally, religion in late antiquity shared a palpable conviction that the afterlife, in whatever form, was a sensorily vibrant existence. From the elaborate underworld geography of Virgil's *Aeneid*, Book VI, or the otherworld journeys of I Enoch or the *Acts of Thomas*; the lush Paradise of the Manichean Psalms, the visions of martyrs, or the longing of burial inscriptions, the ancient Mediterranean shared widespread agreement that whatever kind of existence the afterlife would bring, it would surely, and necessarily, be known in and through the sensory experience of bodies, however much transformed.

SENSING CRITIQUE

In literary sources, genre and rhetorical mode determined representation of religion. Hymnography and panegyric, for example, contained exquisitely exalted portrayals of human-divine relation. In turn, comedy and satire in any form easily skewered religious practices, often by inflated caricature of sensory experience. Nonetheless, there were serious issues of religious critique debated by ancient authors (Beard *et al.* 1998, 2: 349–64). Religion was omnipresent in the ancient world, and so, too, was concern for its proper observance (Knust and Várhelyi 2011). Attention to the senses highlighted the issues.

During the Roman era, religious critique commonly pitted sensory richness against true piety. The poet Ovid expressed a cynical reserve towards the extravagance that characterized Roman religion in the wake of the empire's new trade routes, luxury goods, and markets. He lamented for a past golden era of simpler hearts and simpler worship; a time when a little grain and some salt, offered with devotion, sufficed for the gods' good will. "That was before strange ships had sailed the watery seas / transporting tears that the myrrh tree wept; / before Syria sent us frankincense, and India, balsam, / before anyone knew what saffron looked like" (*Fasti* 1.337–42; Nagle 1995: 46). The first-century Jewish philosopher Philo agreed. Prior to the destruction of the Jerusalem Temple, he complained bitterly about those who provided expensive, ostentatious sacrifices, but with "impure" hearts: "Even the least morsel of incense offered by a man of religion is more precious in the sight of God than thousands of cattle sacrificed by men of little worth" (Spec. 1. 275; Colson 1984, 7: 259).

Skepticism towards religious ceremonial was not new for the Mediterranean world. Such sentiments recurred throughout the Hebrew Bible (e.g., Ps 50 [LXX 49]; Ps 51 [LXX 50]; Amos 5: 21–4; Hos 6:6; Jer 7: 21–4). Known to early Christians through the Septuagint (Greek translation), they were often cited by Christians in critique against the sacrificial traditions of both Jews and pagans. But these biblical passages did not reject sacrifice as the basic practice by which human-divine relation was performed and maintained. Instead, because they identified a wrong kind of sacrifice, they directed the audience towards a "true" sacrifice that would effect a "right" relation with God. Jesus' denouncement of the merchants at the Jerusalem Temple had been a similar, and traditional, performance (Mt 21: 12–13; Mk 11: 15–17; Lk 19: 45–6; Jn 2: 13–17). Again, the Jewish sectarian communities of Qumran rejected the Jerusalem Temple and its priesthood as irrevocably corrupt. They presented an alternative sacrifice, in language easily recognizable to philosophers: "And prayer rightly offered shall be as an acceptable fragrance of righteousness, and perfection of way as a delectable freewill offering" (I QS 9: 4–5; Green 1997; Vermes 1997: 110).

For Greek and Roman philosophers had long debated how best to worship the gods. For them, religious critique was part of the fierce rivalry between philosophical schools (Ullucci 2012). The premise of such critiques was not that sacrifice—the premier ritual to effect and maintain human-divine relation—was wrong, but that it was wrongly conducted. What kind of sacrifice was fitting? And what was its suitable manner? Philosophical schools developed a counter-concept of the *logike thusia*, spiritual sacrifice. It was a perspective to be found across the spectrum of religious intellectuals. The Epicurean Lucretius decried physical sacrifice, exhorting that true piety lay "rather in possessing the ability to contemplate all things with a tranquil mind" (*On the Nature of Things* 5.1199–204; Smith 2001: 169–70). The third-century Christian philosopher Origen of Alexandria declared, "What better gift can a rational being send up to God than the fragrant word of prayer, when it is offered from a conscience untainted with the foul smell of sin?" (*On Prayer* 2.2; Greer 1979: 83).

Greek and Roman philosophers advocated a notion of sacrifice that did not so much replace it as clarify and rank its forms. To the Neoplatonist Porphyry, physical offerings were quite literally comprised of inferior (physical) matter, appropriate for lesser gods and divine powers. The finer, subtler material of spiritual nature accorded more fittingly with the one high God whose supreme divinity governed all other existence. To this supreme God, "we should offer . . . as a sacred sacrifice, the elevation of our intellect, which offering will be both a hymn and our salvation" (*On Abst.* 2.34; Wynne-Tyson and Taylor 1965: 87). Indeed, elaborate ritual could conceal base character, a corrupt heart. Porphyry urged modesty in religious performance, "The sacrifice which is attended by a small expense is pleasing to the Gods, and divinity looks more to the disposition and manners of those that sacrifice, than to the multitude of the things which are sacrificed" (*On Abst.* 2.15; Wynne-Tyson and Taylor 1965: 72).

For Porphyry's student and critic Iamblichus, all things could be set in right relation if the appropriate sacrifices were rendered to the gods accordingly, each to its proper kind: including blood sacrifice for "material gods" (*De Myst.* 5.9, 14; Clarke et al. 2004). The Neo-Pythagorean philosopher Philostratus praised the ancient sage Pythagoras as one who "never defiled altars with blood; instead honey-cakes, frankincense, and hymns were this Master's offerings to the gods." Pythagoras did so, Philostratus claimed, because "Being conversant with the gods, he had learned what makes them angry or pleased with mankind" (*Life of Apollonius*, sec. 1–2; Jones 2006: 33).

Proper worship was also a matter of appropriate reverence, rather than excessive concern that dissolved into paralyzing fear. Again, attention to the senses could mark the distinction. The first-century philosopher Plutarch disdained the anxiety of the superstitious individual: "The ridiculous actions and passions of superstition, the phrases and gestures, the charms and spells, the running around and drumming, the impure purifications and filthy sanctifications, the barbarous and shaking penances and mortifications before shrines" (*On Superstition* 12.171a–b; cited in Rives 2007: 185).

Philosophers, pagan, Jewish and Christian, shared the view that God (or the supreme high God of the pantheon) by nature did not, and indeed could not, need physical offerings, whether incense or animal sacrifice. Rather, sacrifice was the performance of relation; the rendering of honor and thereby devotion. Yet critique of sacrifice often included the scornful charge that worshippers presumed the offering (of whatever kind) was somehow necessary. Such critique was a rhetorical strategy, useful for debating conceptions of divinity, the contrasts between human and divine natures, and especially the power dynamics between competing intellectuals (Ullucci 2012: 31–118). It relied on examination of ritual practices from the perspective of their sensory qualities and effects. Performance of religious practices—including sacrifice—continued unabated. The first-century Stoic Epictetus admonished tellingly, "But it is always appropriate to make libations, and sacrifices, and to give of the firstfruits after the manner of our fathers, and to do all this with purity, and not in a slovenly or careless fashion, nor, indeed, in a niggardly way, nor yet beyond our means" (*Encheiridion* 31; Oldfather 1966, 2: 513–15).

Ancient Mediterranean religions shared a notion of worship in which offerings—physical or spiritual, material or moral—should be characterized by beauty. In rightly practiced religion, that beauty expressed the practitioner's right devotion, the deity's worthy nature and beneficent response. The sensory adornments of rituals were hence not superfluous. Shabby, lackluster rituals were sharply criticized. Libanius wrote with warm approval of a nobleman who had generously provided the sacrifices, games, and celebratory meals at the reinstitution of a festival for Artemis during the emperor Julian's pagan restoration (*Ep.* 181; Bradbury 2004: 218–19). Julian himself was horrified by the wanton neglect of religious ceremonial he found when visiting Antioch in 360 (*Misopogon* 361D–63C). Such a sensibility also fueled the objections of late antique Christian congregations to bishops who attempted to curtail civic liturgical splendor. John Chrysostom suffered harsh criticism on this score as patriarch of Constantinople (Sozomen *HE* 6.3–21; Socrates *HE* 8.3–28). Poignantly, it was the reverence signaled by such cherished adornments that pagans lamented when their sacrifices were outlawed under emperor Theodosius I in the late fourth century (Libanius, Or. 30 *pro templis*; Symmachus *Relatio* 3.3–10 [= Ambrose, Ep. 72A], Liebeschuetz 2005: 69–78).

Ideally, physical beauty was accompanied by its moral counterpart: the virtues. Sensory imagery marked the moral categories of virtue and vice, just as they marked true or false worship. In religious rhetoric, the two domains were interchangeable. When Domitian shockingly permitted a *flamen* to divorce his wife, breaking time-honored law, Plutarch claimed that the priests at the divorce ceremony had "performed many horrible, strange, and gloomy rites" (*Moralia* 276; Babbit 1984, 4: 83).

Sensory rhetoric carried powerful connotations across physical and moral contexts, marking the point at which improper religiosity shifted to religious danger. The problem was that sensory richness could yield sensuous indulgence; to the ancient mind, debauchery and moral turpitude invariably followed. A dramatic example may be seen in the Roman historian Livy's contrasting portraits of the incorporation of foreign deities into the Roman pantheon. Both events occurred some two centuries before Livy wrote. In one account, he describes the arrival in Rome, and subsequent suppression, of the rites of the Bacchanalia, a festival in honor of the god Dionysus. His is a disdainfully squalid account, involving secret nighttime rites, copious wine, promiscuous and deviant sex, kidnappings, poisonings, murder, and human sacrifice, all under cloak of darkness with loud drums and cymbals concealing the screams. In addition to moral debauchery, dire legal consequences followed: forged seals, wills, and documents; false witnesses. Afraid to banish the mighty god altogether, the Roman senate allowed the bacchanal rites to continue in Rome under severely constrained conditions (*History of Rome* 39.8–18).

Livy's account of the Bacchanalia contrasts sharply with his rendering of how the sacred rock of the Magna Mater, the great goddess Cybele, arrived in Rome in 205 BCE, carried from Asia Minor and enshrined on the Palatine Hill to aid Roman defeat of the Carthaginians. Here Livy described the scrupulous and generous ritual care by which the sacred rock was transported, continually attended by high-ranking diplomats, religious officials, noble men and women. A great festival marked its arrival. People brought lavish gifts and offerings to the temple, while great feasting and magnificent games accompanied the celebrations. If Livy's account of the Bacchanalia was a catalogue of sensory—and religious—disorder, his presentation of the arrival of the Magna Mater was the exact opposite: an account of wholly fitting order, reverence, and pious ceremonial (*History of Rome* 29.14.10–14).

Yet Rome did not easily take to "foreign" rites. Livy himself subsequently expressed grave distress regarding Cybele's priests the Galli, notorious for self-castration and ecstatic rites. The view was shared, for example, by Lucretius, who sharply criticized the tumult, frenzy, violence, and exploitation of their processions (*On the Nature of Things* 2.600–40; Smith 2001: 50–1). Apuleius provided similarly contrasting sensory portraits in his novel, *The Golden Ass (Metamorphoses)*. He portrayed the priests of the Syrian goddess as morally corrupt and physically depraved, while his rhapsodic depiction of the rites of the Egyptian goddess Isis is radiant with lush sensory splendor.

Livy's account of the Bacchanalia provided a pattern that would recur for some centuries, whenever a religious group came under serious censure (Beard *et al.* 1998, 2: 288–348). During the second and third centuries CE, various Christian groups were likewise accused of unholy rites involving rampant drunkenness, sexual orgies, child sacrifice, and cannibalism. Apologists such as Justin Martyr, Tertullian, and Minucius Felix responded to these slanders with vehement denunciations, insisting on the chaste and innocent nature of Christian ritual and its symbolic aspects. The Christian historian Socrates accused pagans of the same practices during the pagan revival under Julian (*HE* 3.13). In each case, approval or disapproval, reverence or impiety, were expressed through the sensory rhetoric used to describe the rituals at issue.

Just as sensory rhetoric provided vivid grist for religious critique, sensory attention characterized religious reform. The emperors Augustus, Constantine,

Julian, and Theodosius I were all valorized during their imperial reigns for their extensive religious reforms. These emperors refurbished sacred buildings and sacred precincts, and constructed new ones; they restored, increased and strengthened sacred offices. They established new festivals and revived others that had languished forgotten. They enhanced religious ceremonial with imperial adornments that heightened the majesty and splendor of the occasions. They strengthened priesthoods, and insisted on improved levels of religious literacy regarding sacred traditions. Such reforms involved the sensory aspects of religion by means of material practice. They also provided rhetorical tools for critique.

The contrasting literary portraits of the emperor Constantine by the fourth-century Christian Eusebius of Caesarea and the late fifth-century pagan historian Zosimas provide a good example. Each presented an overtly religious agenda. Both portraits are notable for their attention to monumental building projects, the adornment of civic communities, the tone of religious observance, the quality of law, and the tradition of imperial beneficence to the poor and needy. These socially (and sensorily) concrete activities were then characterized in morally positive or negative terms, by the use of morally coded sensory imagery: light, radiance, and beauty according to Eusebius (*Life of Constantine*), as opposed to debauchery, depravity, and decay in Zosimas (*New History* 2.29–39). All of these activities were religiously meaningful to Constantine's subjects and certainly also to his biographers. Their measure provoked praise or criticism, rendered in sensory terms, both for the materiality of Constantine's achievements and for their "spiritual" worth.

SENSORY COMPETITION

Imperial effort to reinvigorate religious practice could take a negative, and equally sensory, form: the destruction or dismantling of competing religious buildings, serious curtailment or complete prohibitions of rival religious activities, or even outright persecution. Yet persecution was an inconsistent and extreme condition in the Roman Empire. More often, the different religions of the empire co-existed as in a religious marketplace, often in an uneasy balance of agonistic interests (Beard *et al.* 1998, 2: 288–348; Rives 2007; Ullucci 2012).

Here, too, in the domain of religious competition, the senses played a functional role. In part, this was because the different religions of the empire followed many similar practices. In the second century, for example, the Christian apologist Justin Martyr complained that "wicked demons" had taught practitioners of Mithraism to imitate Christians by placing bread and water "with certain words said over them" during their own rites of initiation (*First Apology*, sec. 66). How could one distinguish between truth and falsity, if the practices seemed the same?

Lavish sensory adornments to ceremonial characterized religious activities of all kinds between the fourth and sixth centuries. In this respect, late antique religious leaders engaged the work of the senses quite literally for religious rivalry. As part of his campaign to delegitimize Christianity, Julian drew attention to the similarity between pagan and Jewish cultic activities, over and against the unholy and irreverent worship of Christians, who had "abandoned" the venerable practice of animal sacrifice (*Against the Galileans* 306A–B; on Christians and sacrifice, see Ullucci 2012: 65–136). More insidiously, Julian exploited the ambiguities of the shifting sensibilities. As Christians began during the fourth century to adorn their liturgies with abundant incense—a common Mediterranean practice they had wholly eschewed during their first centuries—Julian was able to trick Christian soldiers into offering incense unwittingly at pagan shrines, much to their grievous horror (Sozomen *HE* 5.17).

At the same time, religious leaders attended to the sensory education of their flocks: employing morally freighted rhetoric to highlight sensory

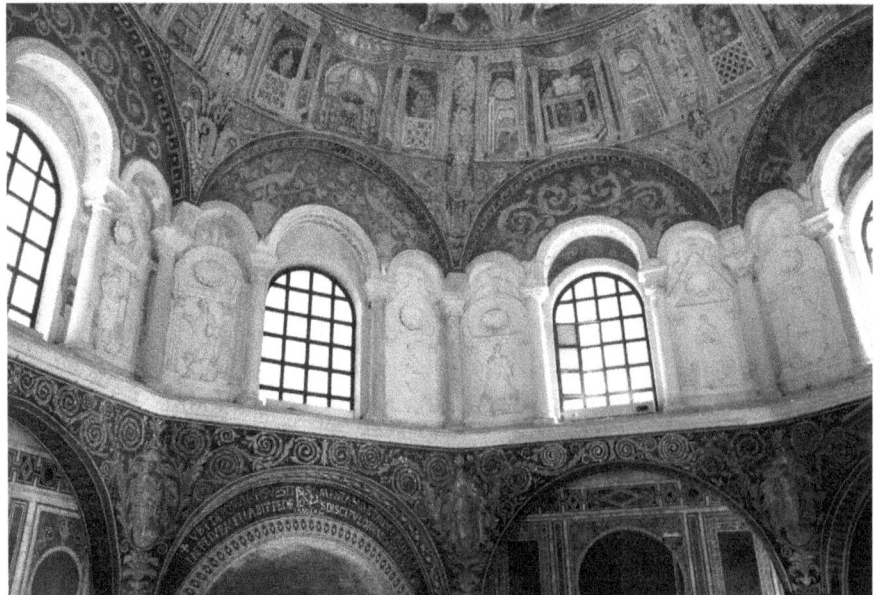

FIGURE 4.3: Baptistry of Neon, Ravenna, showing sculpted columns and arches adorned with mosaics. Copyright: Holly Hayes.

awareness, whether positively or negatively, in relation to competing religious practices and claims. Such strategies were common also between competing orthodoxies within the same religion. Cast in high relief by the political and social tensions of the times, the senses thus came to play a crucial role in the discourse of religious difference, identity, and boundaries.

The issues may be clearest from the perspective of Christians, who evidenced dramatic changes in sensory orientation between the first and sixth centuries CE. Prior to their legalization in the fourth century, Christians were a small minority in the Roman Empire, generally scorned and occasionally persecuted. Heavily focused on an awaited Second Coming of their Savior Jesus Christ, early Christian writers encouraged their audiences to remain as removed as possible from the surrounding Roman culture. While early Christian literature praised the physical beauty of the natural world as the workmanship of their creator God, such sentiments were muted during the first three Christian centuries. Similarly, descriptions of Christian rituals during these earliest centuries generally highlighted ritual actions and sequences, without comments on sensory qualities (e.g., Justin Martyr *First Apology*; Tertullian *Apology*).

The exception to this pervasive viewpoint occurred in Christian literature that looked to other worlds: to imagined tours of heaven or hell, to apocalypses with luridly detailed accounts of the dissolution and re-creation of the universe, or to accounts of dreams or visions, filled as they were with glimpses of the divine. In such literature, authors employed a sensorily dense and awe-filled rhetoric, whether of beauty, disgust, or frightening ambiguity.

Closely related are the early martyr accounts, in which the sharpest sensory evocations elicited not the horrors of death by torture—the situation in which the event took place—but rather, moments of divine–human intersection. Christian witnesses at the execution of the bishop Polycarp described a sweet scent of frankincense enfolding the martyr like a billowing shrine, dramatically unlike the stench of burning flesh (*Polycarp*, sec. 15; Musurillo 1972: 2–21). Again, Christians wrote that the martyrs of Lyons and Vienne marched to their deaths exuding the perfumed fragrance of a wedding procession, their wounds glistening as though with sweet ointments, their imprisoning chains gleaming like jewels, and their faces alight with joyful rapture (*Lyons and Vienne*; Musurillo 1972: 62–85). The visions attributed to the martyr Perpetua and her companion Saturus during their imprisonment were redolent with a Paradise of sweet honey and milk, refreshing fountains, perfumed scents, healed wounds. Perceiving their situation as combat with Satan himself, Perpetua's visions conveyed further the thrilling sensations of the gladiatorial stadium, with rippling muscles, explosive attack, mighty wrestling, and the exuberant triumph of the victorious combatant (*Perpetua and Felicitas*; Musurillo 1972: 106–31).

Christian martyr accounts were deliberate in their inversion of cultural sensory codes. In the martyrdom of Perpetua and Felicitas, the naked female bodies repulse the crowd, leaking the blood of childbirth and the milk of motherhood in a context that violated the (pagan) crowd's moral sensibilities. Yet in her dream vision, Perpetua had fought the devil himself in nakedness that was glorious with divine triumph. In imaginative literature, the inversion took on spectacular proportions. When the governor of Antioch tried to humiliate the young Thecla by parading her naked before her execution, her nakedness was suddenly shielded by a divine radiance that blinded the crowd. No weak and feeble femininity constrained the mighty Thecla, whose very toes were kissed by lions as she was cloaked in potent flower petals thrown by her admirers (*Acts of Paul and Thecla*; Elliott 1993).

The legalization and increasing political and social triumph of Christianity over the course of the fourth century brought a marked shift in Christian attitudes towards the physical world. As noted above, deliberate attention to the senses accompanied this process. At the same time, attention to the sensory aspects of worship was a fraught endeavor for Christians. How could one distinguish between beauty offered to God, and sensory indulgence (Harvey 2006: 156–221)?

For example, in his *Confessions*, Augustine of Hippo described the impact he felt when hearing hymns during the liturgy, following his conversion to Christianity. He addressed the experience to God:

> How I wept during your hymns and songs! I was deeply moved by the music of the sweet chants of your Church. The sounds flowed into my ears and the truth was distilled into my heart. This caused the feelings of devotion to overflow. Tears ran, and it was good for me to have that experience.
>
> *Conf.* IX.vi.14; Chadwick 1991: 164

Yet Augustine remained suspicious of the experience and its intensity, which he marked as both sensory and emotional in impact. Later in the *Confessions*, he reflected on the conundrum. In his view, there was danger and even sin when the beauty of the music—whether melody or singer's voice—moved him apart from the sacred words of a hymn or Psalm. The sensory pleasure seemed to him "enervating" and "deceptive" (*Conf.* X.xxxiii.49; Chadwick 1991: 208). Other Christian leaders warned against the same danger (McKinnon 1987: 106, 120,

144–5 [#228, #266, #333]). Nonetheless, Augustine recognized that omission of the music altogether was a response of "too much severity," itself sinful in nature. The conflict led him to an uneasy recognition that sometimes the weak could be helped to truth through the beauty of liturgical music (*Conf.* X.xxxiii.50, Cp. Aug. *Ep.* LV.34–5, McKinnon 1987: 163–4 [#377]).

Indeed, music was an area of common competition during late antiquity. Choirs of Christian nuns pursued the emperor Julian through the city of Antioch, loudly singing Psalms that mocked "heathen" idols and the enemies of the Lord (Theo. Cyr. *HE* III.19.1–4; in McKinnon 1987: 104–5 [#225]). With flagrant confidence, competing factions of Christians would attempt to out-sing one another, as if to demonstrate truth by volume and zeal, as happened in Constantinople between Nicene and Arian Christians during the patriarchate of John Chrysostom (Socrates *HE* 6.8; Sozomen *HE* 8.8). Or, they criticized one another's manner of worship as overly sensual. Thus Theodoret of Cyrrhus scorned the schismatic Melitians of Alexandria: "as if not bound by [canon] law, they contrived the following absurd practices: to cleanse the body with water on alternate days, to sing hymns accompanied by hand-clapping and a sort of dance, to shake a group of bells attached to a rope, and other things similar to these" (*Haer. fab. comp.* iv.7; in McKinnon 1987: 105–6 [#227]).

Theodoret implies that for the Melitians, sensory pleasure took precedence over religious propriety. Yet Augustine was mindful that the criticism worked both ways. The Donatists criticized his Catholic churches for their "rather sluggish" manner of hymnody: "so that the Donatists reproach us because in church we sing the divine songs of the prophets in a sober manner, while they inflame their revelry as if by trumpet calls for the singing of [P]salms composed by human ingenuity" (*Ep.* LV. 34–5; in McKinnon 1987: 163–4 [#377]). Here there was also tension over the validity of newly composed hymns, as opposed to the use of the biblical Psalms and canticles. This had been a perennial concern (e.g. the cases of Paul of Samosata, Eusebius, *HE* 7.30.12; or the deacon Arius, Philostorgius, *HE* 2.2), but by the later fourth century hymnography had gained its own place in a rapidly flourishing Christian aesthetic.

Christian preachers admonished sharply against the dangers of pagan music, and especially of musical instruments—the major justification for what became a general ban on musical instruments for eastern Christianity (see McKinnon 1987). Two areas of concern received particular vilification: the songs of non-Christian festivals, and the music of the theater (Quasten 1983). Both were fundamental components of late antique civic life, and both were inextricable from pagan religion in the minds of Christian leaders (e.g. Leyerle

2001; Maxwell 2006; Webb 2008). Canon law might forbid the Christian from singing pagan songs, but such a ban was not realistic (*Apos. Const.* V, X, 2; in McKinnon 1987: 111 [#241, with further citations]).

Amidst a chorus of such ecclesiastical admonitions, the fifth-century preacher and bishop Jacob of Serug reflected on the significance of hearing for the disposition of one's soul. The sounds of the city could pull one in every direction, tugging one's attention with conflicting emotions: the sounds of excitement in the marketplace, or of wailing women lamenting the dead, or of the theater with its impious debauchery, or of gossip with good news or bad. By contrast, the liturgy filled one's ears with holy hymns, the sweet voices of choirs, the cadence of sacred readings, the intoned beauty of homiletic instruction, the bodily sensation of singing responses and recitative prayers ("On Partaking"; Harrak 2009). Listening in liturgy was not, for Jacob, a passive activity but an active religious practice of molding oneself towards the (Christian) divine and away from worldly distractions or competing religious media.

Competing religions vied with one another for legitimacy—and indeed, for political supremacy—even at the same ritual events. At the famed Oak of Mamre in Palestine where angels had once appeared to the biblical patriarch Abraham, Jews, Christians, and pagans all celebrated its summer festival with their respective cultic traditions. So tumultuous did the festival season become—a sensory cacophony of prayers, hymns, incense, animal offerings,

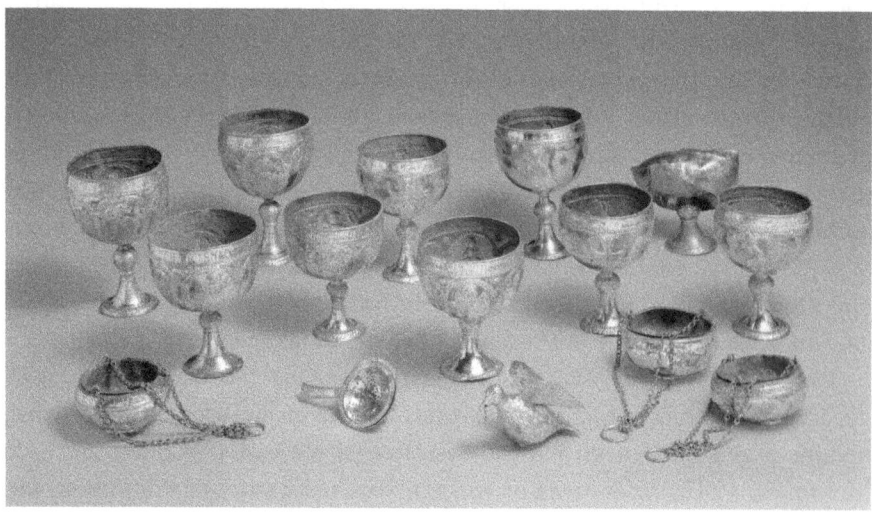

FIGURE 4.4: Christian liturgical instruments, Northern Syria, c. 500 CE: chalices, censers, wine strainer, a dove; silver, silver gilt. Photo: Metropolitan Museum of Art, New York.

libations—that the emperor Constantine intervened, abolishing all non-Christian celebrations, tearing down the existing shrine, and building a church for exclusive Christian use (Sozomen *HE* 2.4).

The rhetoric of late antique religious leaders became stereotypically shrill with the effort to distinguish the practices of one from another. Christian homilies and hymns castigate against the "stench" and "gloomy fumes" of pagan sacrifices, while extolling the "sweet fragrances" of their own incense and holy offerings. Pagans decried the "foul stink" of Christian ascetics (Harvey 2006: 204), while valorizing the (pagan) philosopher's home so fragrant with incense that it resembled "a holy temple" (Eunapius *Lives*; Wright 1968: 467).

Similar rhetoric, steeped in sensory attunement, characterized late antique literature of moral approbation or censure. In hagiography, saints wafted with the fragrance of virtue, redolent with the Holy Spirit's grace. By contrast, in "orthodox" historiography the heretic Arius died a revolting death, drowning in a latrine in his own dysentery (Theodoret *History of the Monks* 1.10), just as the emperor Julian's henchmen who had persecuted Christians died of heinous disease (Philostorgius *HE* 7.10, 7.13). Demons, heretics, and religious "others" (Jews or pagans) could be discerned by their stench, a physical trait to match their moral dissolution (in Christian eyes)—albeit sometimes so subtle that only a saint could perceive it.

Processions became a defining feature of late antique Christian worship, filling the streets and roads of the empire, and necessitating the development of ecclesiastical architecture that enabled complexly choreographed movement (Baldovin 1987; Mathews 1999). But processions were also an effective method of sensory competition. Christian liturgical processions paraded through civic communities singing their hymns, swinging their censers, clothed in vestments and festive garments, perfumed with holy oil and flowers. The same streets also rang with the songs and wafted the fragrances of pagan festival processions. It could be difficult to distinguish between them, as Christian leaders worried (e.g. Paulinus of Nola *Poems* 14, 18, 21, 25, 33; Ps.-Joshua the Stylite *Chron.* 30–1).

The great scholar and ascetic Jerome found himself defending the Christian use of scented candles, jeweled liturgical instruments, and the veneration of relics, over and against the criticism of other Christians who scorned these practices as "idolatrous." Jerome urged that similarity should not invalidate a piety that served Christian truth: "In the one case (pagan), respect was paid to the idols and therefore the ceremony is to be abhorred; in the other (Christian), the martyrs are venerated, and the same ceremony is therefore to be allowed" (*Against Vigilantius* 4–7; NPNF² 6: 418–20).

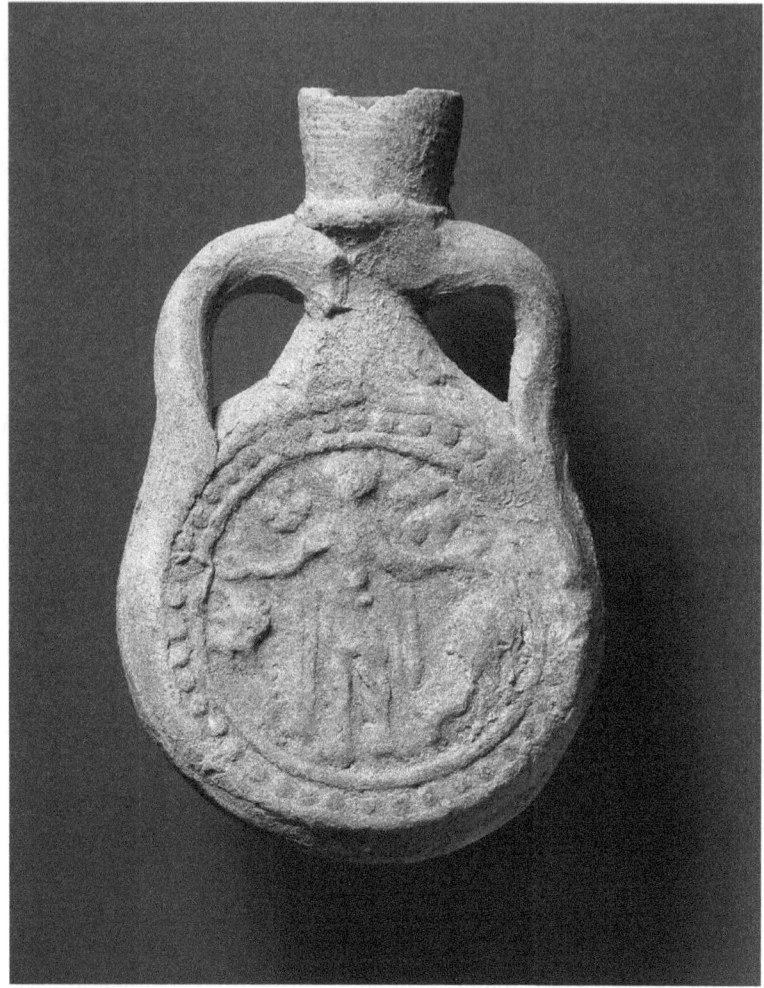

FIGURE 4.5: Terracotta pilgrim flask, Egypt, sixth century CE, to be filled with perfumed holy oil at St. Menas' shrine. Copyright: The Cleveland Museum of Art.

The competition between Jews and Christians played out famously in the city of Antioch, where John Chrysostom employed fierce sensory rhetoric to demonize the Jews, while also castigating those Christians who willfully joined their celebrations. These Christians were "diseased," struck with a "serious illness": they saw no problem in attending Jewish festivals, following prescribed Jewish fasts, joining their holiday feasts, or indeed, approaching their synagogues or even their healing shrines with awe. In turn, Chrysostom inveighed, the Jews were like animals in their gluttony and drunkenness:

"corpulent," "skittish," "fit for slaughter," "dancing with bare feet in the marketplace," a drunken rabble of "effeminate men and prostitutes" (Hom. 1; Mayer and Allen 2000: 148–67).

Thinly disguised by Chrysostom's florid rhetoric was the dilemma of the late antique person, who recognized—and apparently, responded to—common religious behaviors. In John's day, Antioch seems to have had competing shrines, Jewish and Christian, both dedicated to the Maccabean Martyrs and both, perhaps, claiming to have their relics. The shrine to Apollo, in Antioch's sacred district of Daphne, competed for similar needs. The population seemed open to a general religious participation, whereas religious leaders, like Chrysostom, sought exclusivity and absolute boundaries. Sensory rhetoric could give the impression of sharp, clear difference in a context that disallowed such certainty.

The senses were a fundamental aspect of ancient religion. Bodily practices, sensory engagement, and the cultivation of sensory awareness were common features across the different religions of the Roman Empire. Such elements not only adorned the rituals, but also provided a sensory discourse effective for religious critique (of one's own tradition, and of others), and for competition amidst the turbulent religious pluralism of the late antique empire. Attention to these aspects makes indisputably clear that ancient religion was very much a bodily matter, profoundly shaped and informed by the senses. Indeed, through the senses religion was transformed from the "merely" physical to other, far greater domains of meaning.

CHAPTER FIVE

The Senses in Philosophy and Science: Five Conceptions from Heraclitus to Plato

ASHLEY CLEMENTS

> Mind: Colour by convention, sweet by convention, bitter by convention, but in reality there are but atoms and void.
> Senses: Wretched mind, after taking from us your assurances, do you overthrow us? Our fall will be your defeat!
>
> Democr. B125 DK

This is—perhaps only a glimpse of—a remarkable dialogue written during the late fifth or early fourth century BCE by the Atomist Democritus of Abdera (born *c.* 460 BCE) in which the senses are personified as maligned disputants in a contest with the mind. The history of early Greek epistemology—traceable in its origins to as early as the sixth century BCE—is often told as the story of the challenge to which Democritus, for his part, offered this exchange by way of "compromise": the attack of "pure reason" on the epistemic authority of the senses.[1] But it is only during the fifth and fourth centuries, the period on which this chapter focuses, that the two combatants imagined here—the faculties of the mind and the senses—emerge explicitly as antagonists and co-dependents in Greek philosophical debate.

To be sure, from the earliest Greek philosophers of the fifth century the claim to philosophical wisdom involves strong assertions of the limitations of ordinary perception;[2] not to the effect that senses must be abandoned per se, but rather, that it is necessary to ply them actively, in accordance with certain principles, in order to discern what truly is. For Heraclitus (c. 540–480 BCE) and Parmenides (born c. 515 BCE), for instance, the problem with mortal thought lies both with mortals' unthinking reliance on perception and their failure to learn how to use the senses correctly in conjunction with understanding. In Anaxagoras (c. 500–428 BCE), too, we find both serious doubts about the veracity of perceptions, and a central role allocated to them in inquiry: despite the inherent weakness of the senses, he claims, it is still possible for mind (*nous*) to infer reality from the evidence provided—appearances are "a sight of the unseen" (B21, 21a). Likewise for Empedocles (c. 492–432 BCE): however limited each of our sensory capacities may be alone, by marshaling all channels of understanding together we are able to attain the insight of truly balanced thought (B3). But it is Democritus who most explicitly defends the epistemic value of sensory perception in these terms: for him, our senses provide "dark knowledge," yet knowledge without which the mind would be helpless (B11, B125). Indeed, even in the work of Plato (c. 424/3–348/7 BCE), who, against Protagoras' (c. 490–420 BCE) claim that the senses alone can be the "measure" of truth, stresses the necessity of moving beyond perceptibles in order to acquire knowledge, Greek philosophy begins with the senses.

But "the senses"—at least as we in the modern West understand them—also begin with Greek philosophy; for the beginnings in the fifth century of a debate about the epistemic authority of perception coincide with the emergence of "the senses" as a new object of inquiry in philosophy, science, and medicine. With the possible exception of Alcmaeon of Croton (*fl.* 500–450 BCE), those fifth- and fourth-century philosophers who offer detailed accounts of cognition—Anaxagoras, Empedocles, Diogenes of Apollonia (born c. 460 BCE), Democritus, and, in the form of the *Timaeus*, Plato—all accordingly participate in a tradition of inquiry into nature (*phusis*) in which the physiology of the senses forms a significant part of the wider project of explaining the origins and development of the cosmos. Their diverse physical speculations, preserved for us in a work entitled *On the Senses* (*De sensibus*) written by Aristotle's pupil and successor Theophrastus (c. 371/70–288/7 BCE), in turn, influence the theorization of the senses by the early medical writers, whose rival enumerations and physiologies similarly reflect the processes and structure of the world at large. Just as there is no clear solution to the problem of how to differentiate the powers of the mind from the capacities of the senses during this period, so, too, there is no authoritative account of the senses (Laks 1999: 257–9; Lee 2005: 5).

The purpose of this chapter is not to offer a comprehensive treatment of the competing ideas about sensory perception generated by the rise of these two debates (Beare 1906 and Laks 1999 offer surveys). Instead, I sketch a brief overview of just five different conceptions of the senses that appear in Greek philosophical and scientific thinking of the fifth and fourth centuries against the broad canvas of these theoretical concerns. My aim is, in each case, to explore the close relationship that connects early Greek ideas about senses and the larger practical, philosophical, and scientific agendas of which they are a part. From Heraclitus to Plato (and beyond), rival portrayals of the senses "embody" different cultivations of the senses, and posit, scrutinize, and advocate different sensory relations with the world. In examining these relations, this chapter therefore sets out to explore how a brief history of the senses in five conceptions might also provide the foundation for an "embodied" cultural history of philosophy itself.

SENSES AS "BAD WITNESSES"

Around the beginning of the fifth century BCE, Heraclitus of Ephesus wrote a book that sought to demonstrate how the cosmos made up of opposite qualities and processes is bound together by latent unities. Influenced by the empiricism of Xenophanes (born *c.* 570 BCE), and Hecataeus of Miletus (*c.* 550–476 BCE), Heraclitus' treatment of the senses reflects his commitment to the notion that the unified structure of the nature of things—above all the unity of opposites— is hidden, yet discernible in sense experience (B123, B54; cf. B7). For Heraclitus, the eyes and ears are "witnesses" (*martures*, B101a; B107) whose function is to furnish, from limited personal experience, apprehension that is "common" or "shared" (*xunos*, B80, 89, 103, 113, 114; Pritzl 1985: 306; cf. 308; what follows is indebted to Pritzl's fine account). But the value of their testimony is subject to the correct appropriation (*mathēsis*, B55), understanding (*noos*, B40) and judgment of a man's soul (*psuchē*), which is, at B107, for the first time in Greek philosophy, identified as the rational cognitive faculty in man:

Bad witnesses are the eyes and ears for men, if they have barbarian souls.

On one view of this fragment, the soul that is "barbarian" (*barbaros*)—literally a non-Greek speaker—is a soul that cannot understand the metaphorical "language" of the senses and so renders them poor witnesses. Another interpretation suggests that it is the latent principles of its own language that the soul must understand in order correctly to interpret the testimony of the eyes and ears (Nussbaum 1972). For just as language is a unitary system of subordinate parts, so, too, as Heraclitus reveals through all manner of linguistic games, the cosmos is unitary, although comprised of many parts.

Yet the word for "barbarian," *barbaros* in Greek, most importantly connotes (indeed, phonetically mimics) the inability to articulate according to the rules of the right language, or, to make the distinctions and connections that render speech intelligible (Kahn 1979: 107). Plato's *Protagoras* (dramatic date, *c*. late 430s BCE) offers us a playful later extrapolation of this sense of the term even to Greek dialect, when, in the midst of a debate about the meaning of Simonides' poetry, the Sophist Prodicus argues that Simonides' (Cean) text is criticizing Pittacus of Mytilene (whose father was a Thracian) because he "did not know how correctly to distinguish (*diairein*) the meaning of each word as he was from Lesbos, and nurtured in a foreign tongue (*en phonēi barbarōi*)," a phrase which pointedly also refers to the Aeolic dialect (341c). The linguistic skill—lacking in Lesbian *barbaroi*—required in order correctly to understand the meaning of Simonides' language, Prodicus implies, is the skill of division (*diairesis*). And it is this skill which, in the *Phaedrus*, as the basis for Platonic dialectical method, is further defined as the ability to carve up things "according to their natural joints (*arthra*)" (265e–6a; cf. *Statesman* 287b–c on *diairesis* "according to limbs (*kata melē*)"). Fifth- and fourth-century discussions of language exploit the same imagery of physiological articulation: the creation (or perception) of intelligible words from confused and indistinct sounds involves the action of articulating by means of "joints" (*arthra*), that is, rendering into distinct yet connected parts that which is undifferentiated or conflated.[3]

Heraclitus' image of a soul that is *barbaros*, then, perhaps evokes an inability to re-articulate that which should be distinguished and connected in the right way by "joints" (cf. B10; B19). The implication is that it is the lack of these joints and the balanced relations they constitute that makes the eyes and the ears worthless witnesses (cf. B10; Epich. B13). Indeed, at the outset of his work, Heraclitus mocks those unable to articulate—that is, understand—the testimony of their senses in this way as the *axunetoi* (not simply "ignorant" ones, but ones who are "unable to bring together," B1; B34). These are men who, like the barbarian souls they possess, "do not know how to hear or to speak" (B19), and so "do not comprehend" (or, again, "do not bring together," *ou xuniasin*, B51), and who, since they are not able to make "graspings" or "apprehensions that bring things together" (*sullapsies*, or, on a variant reading, "connections" or "joints", *sunapsies*, B10), "having heard, are like the deaf" (B34).

The soul with comprehension (*noos*), by contrast, is able to distinguish and rejoin the testimony of the ears and that of the eyes using the principles of hidden order (*logos*, B1), which, although revealed by Heraclitus' own "account" (*logos*, B1) and "common" to all (*xunos*, B2), go unrecognized by the many. Significantly, the correlates of what is heard and what is seen in Heraclitus are words (*epea*) and deeds (*erga*) (B1; Pritzl 1985: 309). As Pritzl has shown, in his first lines, Heraclitus implies that in order to understand the harmonious nature of any given thing ("how it holds together") manifest in the tension between opposing elements, one must perform an act of *diairesis* between these two dimensions of experience (*diaireō*, B1). Such a division, Heraclitus suggests, discloses how words and deeds each partially reveal the nature of a thing, but also how its complete nature can only be arrived at through their recombination. When, through a pun on the Greek words for life (*bíos*) and for bow (*biós*) Heraclitus prompts us to recognize that despite its name, which evokes life, the bow's work is death, for instance, he highlights how what is heard and what is seen can, when distinguished and recombined according to the right *logos*, reveal a unity between opposites that is otherwise hidden (B48). Indeed, throughout Heraclitus' fragments, it is only by first distinguishing and then putting together, names or words and processes, activities or deeds in this way, that philosophical wisdom can be acquired (Pritzl 1985). Heraclitus' model of philosophical inquiry thus enacts the role of the epic witness (*martus*), who must likewise coordinate his ears with his eyes to attest that oaths that are heard and subsequent actions that are seen correlate.[4]

It is in the context of this project of re-articulating the testimony of the senses in concert with Heraclitus' *logos* that his variant of the proverbial saying "the eyes are more accurate witnesses than the ears" (B101a) clearly belongs. For it further draws to the surface the sense in which the Heraclitean soul's interpretative task also implies a prefatory, conceptual *diairesis*, the separation and recombination of two kinds of experience. For the eyes, metonyms of autopsy, must be recognized as preferable to relying solely on the ears (sc. the learning received aurally from the poets, or others, cf. B40, 57), if the senses are to be plied together in concert with *logos* to serve as "good witnesses" in the rational divisions and combinations that form the basis of Heraclitean inquiry (Laks 1999: 262). As Heraclitus says at B55: "Of whatever sort of thing there is sight, hearing, learning by experience (*mathēsis*), this is what I prefer."

SENSES AS "MUCH-WANDERING LIMBS"

The hugely influential poem written by Heraclitus' contemporary from Velia in southern Italy, Parmenides, similarly implicates its audience in adjudicating against understandings of the world that derive from naïve perceptions. Parmenides' text begins by situating its audience alongside an initiate (*kouros*) on a journey characterized by the shrill sound of silence and blinding light, that culminates with a divine revelation at the site of primal adjudication and the origin of all things, the Underworld (Kingsley 1999). Here, "far away from the beaten track of men" (B1.27), past the gates of the paths of Night and Day, an unnamed goddess reveals the nature of reality (in the first part of the poem known as the *Alētheia*), and also imparts the mistaken beliefs of mortals (in the second part of the poem known as the *Doxa*), so that this initiate might never again be overtaken by mortal opinions (B8.61). Throughout, the initiate, and by extension Parmenides' audience, is enjoined to direct "mind" (*noos*) to "proofs" (*sēmata*), bear witness to and imitate the goddess' "interrogation" (*elenchos*) into what genuinely is, and to make a "judgment" (*krisis*) in favor of it, because "conviction" (*pistis*) attends only upon what-is, and the goddess Dike herself oversees our activities.

The goddess' object is to liberate her initiate from the predicament of naïve mortals whose ordinary ways of conceptualizing the world according to the misleading impressions of their senses spuriously equate their own discursive constructions of experience with reality. Her lesson will be an exposition of the only paths of inquiry open for those seeking after genuine knowledge of what really is, and it will first distinguish two: one, the pathway of what-is, leading to being and reality, the other, the "pathway" of what-is-not, leading to non-existence and so nowhere (B2).

But before the goddess reveals the natures of these routes, she first (at B6 and B7) warns of the error committed by those mortals who fail to make a clear distinction between the two paths, always imagining themselves to be on the positive route to what-is, when in fact they repeatedly stray onto the fallacious negative route, and so remain caught wandering aimlessly on a backward-turning path (*palintropos ... keleuthos*, B6.9) of their own at the point of intersection between the two. Here, with their "wandering mind" (*planktos noos*, B6.6) steered only by "helplessness" (*amēchaniē*, B6.5), mortals "two-headedly" (*dikranoi*, B6.5) vacillate on their specious third way, "knowing nothing" (*eidotes ouden*, B6.4) and "deaf and blind" (*kōphoi homōs tuphloi*, B6.7). Against this fate, the goddess exhorts, the initiate must guard by trial and judicious direction of his faculty of understanding (*noos*), judging the arguments he is given about what-is by marshaling a "much-contesting disputation" (*poludēris elenchos*) of the sort exemplified by her own account. B7:

> For never shall this prevail, that things that are not are;
> but you, restrain your thought from this route of inquiry,
> nor let much-experienced habit force you along this route,
> to direct a sightless eye and an echoing ear
> and tongue; but judge by argument (*krinai de logōi*) the much-contesting disputation
> spoken by me.

The goddess' picture of the "sightless" (*askopos*) eye and "echoing" (*ēchēeis*) ear and tongue of those who lack her divine insight draws upon wider poetic idioms of mortal helplessness (*amēchaniē*) and so recalls the predicament of the confused mortals of B6 (cf. *Hym. Hom. Herm.* 91–3; Aesch. *PV* 447–8). But Parmenides' fullest account of unthinking reliance on the senses occurs not in these opening physical evocations of mortal confusion, but more allusively in the cognitive illustration of human helplessness found in the mortal cosmology recounted in the *Doxa* section of the poem. Here the goddess warns she will speak as a mortal, setting out a "likely-seeming" (*eoikōs*, B8.60) but "deceptive world-order" (*kosmos . . . apatēlos*, B8.52) that we must negotiate using the criteria for what-genuinely-is given to us in the *Alētheia* section of the poem if we are to ensure that *noos* remains in our control and does not stray onto a path of wandering. At its outset, at B8.50–61, the goddess describes the fundamental mistake all mortals make when setting out to account for the nature of reality. Mortals err because they found their understanding of the world on the interaction of two primal forms (*morphai*), Light and Night, which they have distinguished in body (*demas*) as opposites of a particular kind. Mortals take these forms to be ontologically distinct, but the properties by which they constitute them indicate instead that their natures are co-dependent. As each form is defined as the mirror-image of its counter, and therefore the embodiment of that which the other is not, ontologically, each remains intertwined with its opposite, so that to set out to describe the nature of one inevitably implies invoking the negation of the other (Light is not-Night and Night is not-Light), and thus setting *noos* to wander on a path that only turns back on itself (*palintropos . . . keleuthos*, B6.9; Curd 2004: 104–10).

Indeed, as the goddess relates how mortals build their account of the phenomenal world in the cosmology of the *Doxa* through the practice of naming discrete things it becomes clear that there is no part of the cosmos they have conceived that is free of the forms' fallacious intermixture (for "since all has been named light and night [. . .] / all is full (*pleon*) of light and unknown night together . . .," B9). This is the crucial context for understanding Parmenides' obscure account of human cognition at B16. Here, the goddess of the *Alētheia* (who, if we are correct in assigning B16 to the *Doxa*, still speaks as a mortal), turns her attention to the nature of mortal thought and perception, alluding to a model of physical mixture (*krasis*) of "the much-wandering limbs" in order to explain the way *noos* is present to men.

> For as each man has a mixture (*krasin*) of the much-wandering limbs (sc. sense-organs) (*meleōn poluplanktōn*),
> So mind (*noos*) is present to men; for it (sc. mind) is the same thing as that which the nature (*phusis*) of the limbs (*meleōn*) (sc. sense-organs) thinks (*phroneei*) in men,
> both for each and every man; for the full (*pleon*) is thought
>
> Trans. Meijer 1997, modified

Instead of being directed to what-is (its only genuine object, B8.33–6), *noos* passively "stands by" men as each man has a mixture of the "sense-organs" or "much-wandering limbs," whose (mixed) nature (*phusis*) in turn is taken by mortals to be thought (*it* thinks, *phroneei*). Mortals thus take thinking (*phronein*) to be perception (Meijer 1997: 62–73). In their allusion to the senses as "much-wandering limbs" (*melea poluplankta*, B16.1) these lines pointedly exploit the connotations of epic physiology. The word *melos*, "limb," is only used in the plural (*melea*) in the earliest writers, where it is often simply translated as "body." This is the sense some critics read here, translating Parmenides' "mixture of the much-wandering limbs" as "a mixture of bodily states." Others read the *melea* as the constituent elements of the cosmos, Light and Night, from which the body itself is comprised (Curd 2011; Laks 1990; Vlastos 1946). But in Homer, the term *melea* connotes the bodily limbs not in their jointed and articulated plurality, which is the preserve of the term *guia*, but rather, in their plurality as separate bearers of the muscular sinuosity or tension that enables, and is made manifest in, flexibility and bending. Hence bound up in the Homeric *melea* is the notion of limbs that bend back on themselves (as, indeed, is drawn out explicitly by Aristotle's variant reading of B16.1, *meleōn polukamptōn*, "much-bent limbs").[5]

The word *krasis* "mixture," which, like the word *mixis*, also "mixture" (B12.4), is also only found in the *Doxa*, similarly implies the compresence of separate elements. It very likely recapitulates the process of "mixture" (*mixis*) orchestrated by the goddess of the *Doxa*, who, at B12, at the outset of this mortal cosmology, is said to steer the opposites mortals name in the world back together, and so provide the agent of coming-into-being and change in the phenomenal world. Indeed, in Parmenides, *krasis* connotes not only a "mixture," but also a "muddle," a joining together of things, which through the very necessity of their synthesis, demonstrate themselves to be only spuriously distinguished (cf. B12).[6] The goddess' use of *krasis* and *melea* at B16.1 therefore perhaps subtly hints at the equivalence as artifacts of mortal thought of both the *Doxastical* sense-organs to which B16 alludes and the material elements, Light and Night, of which the world they perceive is comprised, and which, in turn, engender sensation. For if, on one level, B16.3–4 suggests that mortals take thinking (*phronein*) to be solely comprised of (or the same as) their *Doxastical* sense-impressions, the fragment as a whole also implies that what mortals take to be thought (*noēma*) is merely the passively-received sum (cf. *pleon* at B9 and B16) of a twofold confusion: a "muddle of (much-wandering) limbs (sc. both the *Doxastical* senses and the primal forms), which in their plurality or separation bend back on themselves" (cf. Meijer 1997: 66).

B16 therefore completes the imagery of *Doxa*-bound mortal perception found in the *Alētheia* section of the poem at B6 and B7. Insofar as mortals mistake the "nature of the limbs" in their ever-changing mixture (*krasis*) for what-is (the only proper object of *noos*), the world they experience is thus merely the sum of a sightless eye, and an echoing ear, and reduplicating tongue (B7); for the *noos* that comes to men through the mixing of "much-wandering limbs that bend back on themselves" is itself, in turn, necessarily set "wandering" on a "backward turning course" taken only by those who are "undiscriminating," "deaf and blind" (B6). This is the lot of all mortals who fail to make the logical distinction (*krisis*) essential for all those who would direct *noos* to reality: is it or is it not? As the goddess of the *Alētheia* reveals, unlike the sum of the senses as mortals conceive of them, what-is is "whole and of a single kind" (*oulon mounogenes*, B8.4), or, perhaps even, "whole of limb" (*oulomeles*), a textual variant that may represent a later attempt to associate Parmenides' conception of the being to which *noos* is naturally drawn with the aniconic divinity of Xenophanes, who sees and thinks and hears as a whole (*oulos*, B25; this is Bryan's suggestion: Bryan 2012: 99 n.141).

Empedocles, one of the pluralist respondents to Parmenides, almost certainly responds polemically to Parmenides' portrayal of the *krasis* of the senses (*melea*), calling them instead *guia*, "articulated limbs" (or *palamai*, "palms"), and issuing his own enjoinders to perceive what-is holistically. Yet even if Parmenides issues negative portrayals of unthinking dependence on ordinary perception and those who fail to direct their senses, like Heraclitus, he still expresses an implicit optimism about the ability of mortals to transcend the limits of untutored perception. By practicing discernment by *logos* (*krinai de logōi* at Parm. B7.5; cf. Heracl. B1), both thinkers imply, it is possible to direct *noos* to reveal how things really are.

SENSES AS "NARROW PALMS" AND SENSORY PERCEPTIONS AS THE "PLEDGES OF LIMBS"

Parmenides' portrayal of ordinary sensory habits and mortal conceptions of thought and perception at the beginning of the fifth century had exposed the fallaciousness of mortal cosmologies grounded in the mixture (*krasis, mixis*) of ill-conceived opposites. But in the work of the philosopher-healer Empedocles of Acragas, a generation later, it also elicited a defense of the utility of *krasis* theory to explain the world registered by the senses and the mechanisms of cognition. Indeed, for Theophrastus, Greek philosophizing about the senses begins in earnest with the physical speculations of the *krasis*-theorizing pluralists like Empedocles (Theophr. *Sens.* 2). At the heart of Empedocles' theory is the generation and destruction of all mortal things through the mixture and separation of four divine elements (the "roots"), each positively defined and organized by the conflicting forces of Love and Strife according to the model of Parmenides' *Doxa*. Yet whilst Empedocles mobilizes a new language of the senses distancing himself from Parmenides' wandering mortals, he also warns against the poor guides the senses can be for those who fail to "articulate" them correctly.

Unlike the opening chariot ride of Parmenides' poem, which sets its audience speeding directly to an encounter with a goddess "on a route far away from the beaten track of men" (B1.27), senses filled with shrill sound of silence and blinding light, the opening of Empedocles' poem situates its audience in the ordinary mortal world, developing Parmenides' imagery of mortals "carried along" (*phorountai*), "deaf and blind," their *noos* "driven" (*ithunei*) only by *amēchaniē* (B6), by evoking the chariot ride "enjoyed" by all others, from which his fortunate addressee has just turned aside. B1–2[7]:

Pausanias, son of prudent Anchites, listen.
For narrow (*steinōpoi*) palms (*palamai*) have been poured over the limbs (*guia*)
and many wretched things crashing in dull the wits
and having observed (*athrēsantes*) a paltry share of life during their lifetimes

short-lived ones, like smoke they are lifted up and fly off,
believing only that which each happened to bump into,
whilst driven in all directions, but each boasts of having discovered the whole.
Thus these things are neither observed (*epiderkta*) by men nor heard (*epakousta*),
nor embraced by mind (*noōi*). But you, since you have turned aside here, shall understand as far as mortal resourcefulness (*mētis*) can reach.

Ordinary mortal understanding is blighted by the exercise of senses that are narrow and limited. The fragmented and partial view (*steinōpos*) they each engender as mortals are driven in all directions, assailed by worthless things, and believing whatever they "happen to bump into," is haphazard, incomplete. But even as B2 portrays this ludicrous picture of mortal experience, Empedocles' refashioning of the senses as "palms (*palamai*) that have been poured over mortal limbs (*guia*)" implies that the senses are benefactions that might yet serve as a means of ingenuity and articulation, for those who understand how to use them. Empedocles himself claims such divine wisdom, and he promises to liberate his listeners by teaching them how to use their sensory perceptions as "pledges" (*pisteis*) to the insights he will plant in them, B3.9–13 (Kingsley 2003: 508):

But come, watch (*athrei*) with every palm (*palamēi*), in what way each thing is clear,
not holding any sight (*opsin*) more reliable (*pistei pleon*) than hearing (*akouēn*),
nor resounding hearing (*akoēn*) beyond the clarifications of the tongue (*glōssēs*);
nor from any of the other limbs (*ti allōn* ... *guiōn*), by which there is a passageway to understanding (*poros esti noēsai*),
withhold assurance (*pistin*), but understand (*noei*) by what way each thing is clear.

Against the lot of those floundering mortals who have seen (*athrēsantes*) only a paltry part (*meros*) of life but mistake it for the whole (*to holon*, B2.3–6), Empedocles here urges his listener to behold (*athrei*) with *every* palm, articulating sight, hearing, and taste together as equal sources of assurance (*pistis*), along with any of the "other articulated limbs (*guia*)" through which there is a route (*poros*) to understanding. He will reveal that everything in his audience's familiar world is the sum of a deception, a grand artifice formed by harmonious mixture of the four elements by Love against the separative influence of Strife (B6, 8, 17). Empedocles repeatedly directs his listener to perceive the signs of this ongoing conflict and the cyclical pattern of which it is a part in the ordinary processes of the world around him, urging him to articulate his eyes with the understanding of his ears, so that it will no longer remain "unseen and unheard" (B2.7).[8]

He enjoins his audience to infer correctly from its own embodied experience, "to see her (sc. Love) with your mind *(noōi derkeu)*, and don't sit with bedazzled eyes" (B17.21–6). Even though mortals are aware that "she who is recognized even by mortals as innate in genitals *(arthrois)*," effects the joining-together of bodies *via* their "joints" *(arthra)*, he says, their dazed senses prevent them from appreciating the harmonizing power she likewise exerts in the cosmos at large (Palmer 2009: 274–5). Yet, at B20, Empedocles reveals that what can be felt of Love in one kind of bodily "joint" can also be apprehended in the harmony of discrete parts implicit in the very existence of the body *(sōma)* as a whole[9]:

> This is manifest in the mass *(onkon)* of mortal limbs *(broteōn meleōn)*.
> At one time our limbs *(guia)* all come together to be one in love,
> and obtain a body *(sōma)*, at the peak of blooming life;
> at another time again divided by evil strifes
> they wander each apart along the shoreline of life . . .

Empedocles' portrayal of the body as a composite of articulate limbs *(guia)* brought together ("harmonized") under the reign of Love but before and after wandering separate from one another during the ascendancy of Strife, suggestively rewrites the imagery of the much-wandering limbs *(melea)* brought together by mortals into a "muddle" *(krasis)* at Parmenides B16. With his opening enjoinder to perceive what is manifest in the "mass *(onkon)* of mortal limbs *(broteōn meleōn)*," Empedocles allies his evocation of the body *(sōma)* as an articulated composite of joined-up limbs *(guia)* with Parmenides' description of being itself (also called "whole of limb," *oulomeles*, B8.4) as like the "mass *(onkōi)* of a well-rounded Sphere" (B8.43). He thereby subtly implies that in the divinely joined-together mass of the mortal limbs *(melea)*, which is directly perceptible through the senses *(guia)*, there is to be grasped that which is beyond our perception: the perfect, changeless unity into which all things comprised of the separate four elements eventually meld when Love's work finds its highest form of completion.

Reciprocally, having taught his audience to see Love's harmony at the level of the microcosm, Empedocles goes on to evoke her equivalent effects at the macrocosmic level too (Palmer 2009: 275). As Love reaches ascendancy and her mixing of the elements transforms the world into a homogenous deified Sphere, for instance, its homogeneity is signaled by its lack of separate body parts (B28, 29): when its "limbs" (*melea*), that is, its constituent elements, are alluded to, as at B20, their mention stresses only the absence of differentiating discord (*stasis, dēris*, B27a). Nor, in this phase of the cosmic cycle, are the "swift limbs" (*ōkea guia*) of the sun yet to be distinguished either; the Sphere's harmony (*harmonia*) "fixes them in deep hiding" (B27.1). Yet as soon as Strife's influence grows in the cosmos ("was nourished in the limbs (*enimmeleessin*)," B30) and the Sphere begins to be shaken, the articulated limbs (*guia*) of the god become visible once more, as the world begins again to separate back out into its four constituent elements (B31).[10] It is from this state of total Strife, which constitutes the beginning and end of Empedocles' cycle (B20.3), just as Love forces Strife's limbs (*melea*) gradually to withdraw (B35.11), that she is able to refashion what were once the constituent limbs of the Sphere into the constituent limbs of living organisms.

Empedocles' exemplary case is her crafting of the eye in a famous simile that evokes the design of a lantern, B84:

> Just as when someone, before taking to the road, constructs a lamp for himself
> A flame of gleaming fire in a stormy night,
> Fitting, as protection against all winds, lantern casings
> That scatter the breadth of the buffeting winds,
> While the light, finer as it is, leaping through to the outside,
> Shines on the threshold with its unimpaired beams,
> Thus, after Aphrodite had fitted the ogygian fire enclosed in membranes with pegs
> Of love, she poured round-eyed (*kuklopa*) Kore (water) in filmy veils; these kept off the depth of water
> Flowing round about them but allowed the fire to pass through to the outside, in that
> It is finer, where they had been bored through with marvelous funnels.
>   Text and trans. Rashed 2007

Here, recapitulating the processes Empedocles prompts his listener to see in the allusively "spherical" "mass" of the body at B20, and the divine Sphere itself, Aphrodite's crafting of the spherical (*kuklōps*) limb of the eye is achieved through the harmonious combination of disparate parts. At its center, Aphrodite fastens fire in membranes. But this she carefully surrounds with water held back from the fire by filmy veils of aither, whose function is to allow the fire within the eye to pass through without being smothered by the surrounding moisture. The eye is thus the product of Aphrodite's ingenious joining together of the four primal constituents of Empedocles' cosmos: most explicitly, the divine elements of fire and water, but, allusively, also aither ("filmy veils"), and earth ("membranes," "pegs"; Rashed 2007: 30; cf. Theophr. *Sens.* 7).

Yet Theophrastus' account suggests that the eye is not only a sense-organ in which one thus sees Love's harmony, but also a device (*palamē*) designed to see the proportions of her harmony, indeed, to see *in* those balanced compositions (cf. B109). He describes how the surface of the eye is comprised of alternating passageways (*poroi*) commensurate with the two elements necessary for sight, fire and water, and designed to receive the stream of fiery and watery particles that emanates from visible objects (*Sens.* 7). The eye's perception of color (the object of vision) depends upon its ability to register the proportionate mixture of such particles of fire and water, which, in their differing ratio, as brightness and darkness, engender color sensation (see Ierodiakonou 2005). Yet even as the eye is naturally attuned to the harmonious compositions of Love in this way (B23), it can perceive the fiery and watery elements that stream from objects only because they are drawn by the influence of Strife to separate out from visible things as part of the cosmic quest of all the elements to reunite with their like (B109; cf. B90). The eye is thus a device (*palamē*) perfectly designed for grasping a cosmos comprised of visible things created by the antagonism of Love and Strife.

The principles visible in the structure and mechanics of the eye also inform Empedocles' physiological explanation of perception as a whole. Each sense-organ is similarly comprised of "passageways" (*poroi*) that register sensation only as appropriately sized "effluences" (*aporroai*, B89, 90; Pl. *Meno* 76c) that stream from all objects in the world and "fit into" (*enarmottein*, Theophr. *Sens.* 7) their narrow channels. On this model, even as each sense perception tacitly registers the work of Love *via* the influence of Strife, the physiology of the sense-organs themselves entails that they can register only that "object" (e.g. color) engendered by the elemental effluences commensurate to their pores (e.g. in the case of the eye, visual particles of fire and water). Even if each sense referred to at B3 has the power to constitute a form of *pistis*, then, the senses are not only intrinsically separate, and their perceptions mutually exclusive, but also individually limited in their registration of the elements. And herein lies the importance of Empedocles' enjoinder at B3 to perceive holistically, to overcome the "narrow means of grasping" (*steinōpoi palamai*) of the sense-organs, and use every *poros* there is for understanding (*poros esti noēsai*, B3.12); it is only by marshaling all the pathways of perception together that the particular selection of elements received through each of the senses (the elemental causes of perceptions of color, taste, etc.) can be united as whole in reconstitution of the complete nature of the object from which they have come. The evidence is sparse, but it is possible at least that Empedocles situates this final process of blending in the tides of blood that wash around the heart and flow up to each of the sense-organs in channels (Rhees 2004: 52; Wright 1981: 252, cf. 162–3; for a different view, see Long 1966). As the most harmonious composition of the four elements in man, this blood constitutes the stuff of thought (*noēma*, B105.3). Thus just as at every level of Empedocles' account, the harmonious blending of fragmented parts into mortal mixtures is the cunning achievement of Aphrodite's "palms" (B75.2, 95; cf. B23), so the key to transcending the "narrow vision" of each our separate senses and attaining the harmony of balanced thought lies in the harmonious deployment of the palms she has given us as our own.[11] Parmenides had denigrated the "way of inquiry" (B6.3–4) on which mortals make *noos* dependent only upon the "*krasis* of (one sort of) much-wandering limbs," the sense-organs that in Parmenides are called *melea* (B16). Empedocles' poem, by contrast, reinstates the value of thought (*noēma*) engendered by the *krasis* that arises from the harmonious use of another sort, the grasping and articulated "limbs" he called *palamai* and *guia* (Lesher 1999: 242; Palmer 2009: 70–1, 275).

THE "SEVEN FORMS FOR SENSORY PERCEPTIONS"

Our best example of a fifth-century Hippocratic work that reflects the tradition of cosmological explanation of thought and the senses exemplified by Empedocles is the treatise *Fleshes* (*De Carne*) (Jouanna 1999: 277–84; Schiefsky 2005: 19–22). Here, in a cosmological anthropology that eclectically combines earlier philosophical ideas, the origin, morphology, and functioning of the body is explained as due to the effect of the hot on the cold (two of the three elements) which first engenders gluey and fatty organic putrefactions, and then, through a process of further heating, physiological structures and organs of all kinds (cf. Pl. *Phd.* 96a–c). Heat itself is associated with cognition and, in a characterization that perhaps draws upon the epic portrayal of the sun "who hears all and sees all" (*Il.* 3.277), is depicted as a divine entity that "understands (*noein*) all things, and sees (*horēn*), hears (*akouein*), and knows (*eidenai*) all existent things and all the things that are going to be" (*Fleshes* 2).

The operation of the senses (15–18) reflects this formative struggle between the hot and the cold, but also incorporates anatomical ideas concerning the involvement of the brain in sensory perception likely drawn from Alcmaeon. After discussing hearing, smell, and sight, the author finally turns to the physiology of speech (*dialexis*), highlighting the role of the tongue as an organ that articulates intelligible speech from sounds produced by the expulsion of breath (*pneuma*) from the body.[12] Thought itself is not explicitly discussed, but when the author identifies the heart and its vessels as the hottest parts in the body and those which draw into the body the breath (*pneuma*) used for speech, Empedoclean influence seems likely. Instead, *Fleshes* concludes by offering a Pythagorean discursus on the significance of septenary biological cycles.

In all these respects, *Fleshes* provides an instructive comparandum for the remarkable account of sensory perception found in the treatise the *Regimen*, (*De Victu*) usually dated *c*. 400 BCE. There, after establishing that the nature of man is composed of two elements (fire and water) whose mingling and separation accounts for change in the cosmos, the author turns to the way in which arts and crafts also unconsciously replicate the workings of nature. At the end of a series of illustrations, he argues that just as knowledge (*gnōsis*) comes to man through seven "forms," "figures," or "structures" (*schēmata*) in the case of writing (*grammatikē*), so, too, the body has seven "structures" for sensory perceptions.

> Through seven structures (*schēmata*) also come perceptions (*aisthēseis*) for men: hearing (sc. the ear) for sounds, sight (sc. the eye) for the visible, nostril for smell, tongue for pleasant or unpleasant tastes, mouth for speech, body for touch, passages outwards and inwards for hot or cold breath: through these there is knowledge (*gnōsis*) for men or lack of it (*agnōsiē*). (*Regimen* 1.23; for *akoē* and *opsis* as the ear and the eye in the Hippocratics, see Jouanna 2003: 12–14)

The author's invocation of seven figures of writing (presumed to be the Greek vowels) alongside seven physiological "structures" for perceptions (*aisthēseis*) recalls the analogous pairing of the voice's "sevenfold articulation" and the seven functions of the head, which comprise inhalation and exhalation, hearing, sight, smell, but also ingestion and taste, found in the Pythagorean cosmology of a treatise entitled *Sevens* (*De Hebdomadibus*, *c*. 500–450 BCE; West 1971: 379–80). But *Regimen*'s inclusion among its perceptual *schēmata* of the mouth for speech (*dialektos*) and passages for hot and cold breath, alongside the five senses later to become canonical in Greek thought, points not simply to Pythagorean borrowing, but, rather, to wider assumptions about the relationship of physiology and cognition which also inform the treatment of speech alongside senses in *Fleshes*.

In the Hippocratics, the word *schēma* denotes the various physiological structures of the body through which the perceptions penetrate the body and affect the soul and which determine the function of the body's parts—here, the physiological forms of the eye, ear, nose, tongue, mouth, body, and airways (see Hippoc. *VM* 22). Here, the perceptions (*aisthēseis*) that together give rise to knowledge (*gnōsis*), and indeed, knowledge itself, are therefore "product[s] of the body's morphology" (Presti 2007: 140). Indeed, it is the author's emphasis on the permeability of the body to reciprocal traffic from the outside and inside through such *schēmata* that explains the classification of speech as a concrete perceptible (*aisthēsis*) produced by its own *schēma* (for *aisthēsis* as a concrete perception see Presti 2007: 140). Just as the drawing in of cold air and the expulsion of hot air by means of bodily passages effects a physical product, sensation, speech itself is formed at the intersection of body and world, shaped, as the author of *Fleshes* describes, by the mouth from air drawn into and expelled from the body.[13] Indeed, the relationship between respiration, heat, and cognition implicit in *Fleshes*' cognate treatment of speech (here also, the product of air drawn into the body, heated by the heart, expelled through the head and shaped by the tongue), is in the *Regimen* given explicit elaboration. The fiery blended soul that circulates within the body is identified specifically as a faculty of all things that breathe (1.25), and as such it operates hearing, and sight, and touch, when the body is awake (1.35; Presti 2007: 142). Respiration, heat, perceptual faculties, and knowledge, are all biological concomitants.

The Hippocratic texts owe much to the eclectic exploitation of concepts and approaches belonging also to early philosophical explications of perception. But they also hint at the plurality of competing ideas about the number and epistemic value of the senses that emerge in philosophy and science during the fifth and fourth centuries. *Fleshes*' treatment of the mechanics of speaking (*dialegomai*) alongside hearing, seeing, and smelling, and the *Regimen*'s striking enumeration of "seven forms for sensory perceptions" as conduits of human knowledge (*gnōsis*), are kindred products of a period of physical theorizing to which also belongs Democritus' famously obscure claim that "there are more senses (sc. than five) for irrational creatures and wise men and gods" (A116), and his assertion, in stark contrast to the medical writers, that five senses (sight, hearing, smell, taste, and touch) should be opposed to "genuine knowledge" (*gnēsiē gnōmē*) as sources of "dark knowledge" (*skotiē gnōmē*) for men (B11).[14]

SENSES AS "INSTRUMENTS" OF THE SOUL

The breadth of the term *aisthēsis*, "sensation," "perception," "sense," "awareness," "feeling," which facilitated enumerations of the perceptions such as the one we find in the *Regimen* is perhaps no better illustrated by the list of "perceptions" given in Plato's *Theaetetus* (written c. 369–367 BCE). Here, in the midst of interrogating the claim that knowledge is perception, Plato has Socrates observe that (156b): "the perceptions (*aisthēseis*) are variously named: there are hearings, seeings, smellings, and perceptions of heat and cold, pleasure, pain, desire, fear, and many more which have names, as well as innumerable others which have no name."

On Socrates' "Secret Doctrine" theory of perception from which this passage is taken, perceptions ("hearings," "seeings," "smellings"), along with their "twins," the sensible qualities of an external object, are born from the fleeting encounter of two "parents," the sense-organ and the external object (156c–e). Yet, as the ensuing dialogue reveals, because in a Heraclitean world of flux, external objects and the sense-organs are both perpetually changing, their parentage can only yield twin offspring that are themselves unstable. Hence, as purely relational and changeable phenomena, perceptions and sensible qualities cannot meet the criteria necessary for the apprehension of "being" (*ousia*) that is necessary for grasping truth and acquiring knowledge. Rather, this requires an active process of reasoning and judging which is the exclusive preserve of the soul (186b6–d5).

Socrates lays the foundation for this relation between the soul and the senses at 184d1–5 with a striking image (Arist. *Metaph*. Γ^5. 1009^{b}12–110^a; *DA* III. 427^{a}18–27^{b}6; Theophr. *Sens*. 4; Lee 2005: 154 ff). Having established that the senses cannot perceive each other's objects, he points to the logical need for an active unifying mind able to coordinate and assess the perceptions, for, he says,

> it would be a very strange thing if there were a number of senses (*aisthēseis*) sitting inside us as if we were Wooden Horses, and there were not some single form, soul or whatever one ought to call it, to which all these converge—something with which, through the senses (*dia tōn aisthēseōn*), as if they were instruments (*organa*), we perceive all that is perceptible.

Plato's portrayal of the soul (*psuchē*) perceiving "through the senses" (*dia tōn aisthēseōn*) recalls the popular model of perception also exploited in the

Regimen, where similarly, the soul is affected by perceptions "through" the eyes and the ears (1.35.59). But unlike the *schēmata* of the senses in that text, Plato's use of the word *organa* here describes the senses not as identified with the physical "sense-organs" of the body, but rather, in their role as "utilities" of the soul (Burnyeat 1976: 41–2). The implication is that even if perceptions arise from passive affections of the body and necessarily fall short of the status of knowledge, and the senses do not perceive on their own, they can yet be used by the soul actively to ascertain the sensible qualities of things.[15]

Plato's fullest treatment of sensible qualities and the mechanics of perception is given in the *Timaeus*, a text that stands at the end of the grand tradition of Presocratic cosmologizing (it was probably written *c*. 350s BCE). In response to the challenges of Parmenides' *Doxa*, it presents a "likely" or "probable" (*eikōs*) creation account that, within the constraints of Platonic metaphysics, redeems the value of cosmology, and the world of perceptibles that it describes, as a likeness of intelligible reality (Bryan 2012: 174–5). Its account of perception is physicalist: perceptions are engendered when "affections" (*pathēmata*) caused by objects impinging upon the body from outside are transmitted through a receptive sense-organ to the mortal part of the *Timaeus*' tripartite soul (on Plato's *pathēmata*, see O'Brien 1984: 124–43). Sound, for instance, is defined as "a stroke transmitted through the ears, by the action of the air upon the brain and the blood, and reaching to the (sc. rational) soul"; and "hearing" is therefore "the motion caused thereby, which begins in the head, and ends about the seat of the liver" where the non-rational mortal part of the soul in charge of perception resides (67b). Of the three other senses Timaeus theorizes (sight, smell, taste), sight is unique because its organ is said to contribute to this physical process by emitting a visual ray (sight, the most active of Plato's senses, provides the model for intellection, see Nightingale 2004). It is when this ray meets a stream of light whose structure is complementary to it and both coalesce that external "movements" (*kinēseis*) are transmitted to the soul and the sensation (*aisthēsis*) called "seeing" (*horan*) occurs (45b–d). In parallel to the *Theaetetus*, Timaeus' account of sensible qualities, in turn, stresses that what is actually seen, the perceptible, is itself merely a product of the physical interaction of the sense-organ and the elemental properties of the object. Colors are thus generated only when there are differences between the flame projecting from the eye and the proportions of the flame emanating from external bodies (and similar physical explanations are given for tastes, odors, and sounds).

Yet the *Timaeus*' physiological account of perception also emphasizes the initially disturbing impact upon the immortal reasoning soul of the "affections" or "movements" implicated in sensation. This part of the soul is housed in the spherical head—the location also of four senses—and whilst naturally inclined to mimic the divine revolutions of the world soul, it is constantly shaken off course by the "affections" or "movements" received by the senses. Here, as in the *Phaedo* (65a–66a; 99e), the (here, singularly) rational soul is frequently distracted by the body's perceptions. But whilst the *Phaedo* consequently accords value to the senses only insofar as the rational mind might use them to identify the instability and deficiencies of the sensible world (74d–e; cf. *Rep.* 523a–b) or to furnish perceptual stimuli that, although deficient, prompt the "recollection" of knowledge (75a), the *Timaeus* presents sight and hearing as "instruments" through which to contemplate likenesses that can help remedy the disruptions suffered by the rational soul in the course of its embodiment.

The purpose of vision is to enable humans to reattune the distorted movements of the rational soul to the celestial revolutions of the divine world soul (47a–c), which are picked out from the night sky for human viewers by the fiery stars that illuminate the motion of divine intelligence (40a). Consequently, astronomy, practiced first imperfectly through the senses (47a), then pursued in its purest form by means of mathematics, is the route to reacquiring the revolutions of divine thought (cf. *Rep.* 528d5–30c1). Similarly, the purpose of hearing is to facilitate the acquisition of philosophical skills through speech (*logos*), and the study of musical harmonies, which likewise restore the inner order of the soul (47c–e; Nightingale 2004: 173–80; Sedley 2007: 124–5). A plausible—if necessarily speculative—sketch of the process by which the rational soul contemplates the imitations of divine harmony discernible in the movements of music can be reconstructed from Timaeus' later accounts of the physiology of hearing and the function of the liver (67b–c, 71a–72b, 80a–b; see Barker 2000). The remarkable purpose of this organ, which is located in the region of the non-rational soul, and which receives the movements of hearing after the impacts that effect sounds have shaken the reasoning soul in the head, is to discern the concordant and discordant relations of the movements that strike it (*tupoi*), and deliver them up as (visual) "likenesses" or "images" (*eidōla* or *phantasmata*) on its surface for the non-rational soul to enjoy (cf. 67b–c, 71b–d, 80a–b; Barker 2000). As the non-rational soul, intoxicated by these emotionally-charged mimetic images, issues its own "mantic" responses to them, the reasoning soul encounters the patterns of musical harmonies preserved therein and can subject music to rational analysis (Barker 2000: 96–7). The Platonic philosopher's ideal passage from the perceptibles of the phenomenal world to the intelligibles of the world of the forms *via* captivating likenesses or images, which is enacted in several Platonic texts, is, thus, in the *Timaeus*, "embodied" in the "likely" or "probable" account of Timaeus' physiology of perception.[16]

The teleologies of the *Timaeus* thereby also elucidate what is not outlined in the *Theaetetus*' treatment of the senses as *organa*: the best use to which the soul can put the senses in a world of likenesses such as ours. The key to the salvation of the embodied rational soul, Plato's cosmology makes clear, is not the abandonment of the senses per se, but rather the intelligent recruitment of them as its philosophical *organa*.

POSTSCRIPT: THE CYRENAICS, ARISTOTLE, AND BEYOND

The central role of "affections" (*pathēmata*) and "movements" (*kinēseis*) in Plato's treatment of perception finds a fascinating correlative in the epistemology of the Cyrenaic school, a school founded by Plato's fellow Socratic Aristippus (*c*. 435–356 BCE). In a doctrine thought to have been developed by Aristippus' grandson, Aristippus the Younger (born *c*. 380 BC), the Cyrenaics posit that knowledge of external objects is entirely unattainable, but subjective truth founded upon the "affections" (*pathē*) that are created in the interaction of our senses with "movements" (*kinēseis*) from objects is possible. Hence, they state, we should not say that we are "seeing something red," but rather, that we are "reddened," that is, our sight is being "affected redly" (Plut. *Col.* 1120e). Cyrenaic physiology bolsters this epistemological stance. As a concomitant of their disavowal of the outside world, the Cyrenaics posit that our *pathē* are known only because they are perceived as bodily states within us by means of a sense of "inner touch" (*tactus interior*, or *tactus intumus*, Cic. *Luc.* 20; 76). Cyrenaic thought thus marks perhaps the most remarkable application to the physiology of the senses of Socratic claims of ignorance, and the Delphic maxim adopted by Socrates to "know thyself" (Tsouna 1998: 139–41).

The notion of a sense of "inner touch" as an extra sensory faculty used to monitor the condition of the separate senses associated with the Cyrenaics is found also during the Hellenistic period in Epicurean and Stoic treatments of the senses, where doxographers liken it to Aristotle's (*c*. 384–322 BCE) idea of the "common sense" (*koinē aisthēsis*; Aetius *Plac*. 4.8.7 (= SVF 2.852)). By that surprisingly flexible term, in fact, Aristotle seems to have designated several different perceptual capacities (Gregoric 2006: 202–4, cf. 206). But his most famous treatment occurs in the context of his discussion of the soul (*De anima*) and in the solution of the problem resolved quite differently at *Theaetetus* 184d (where the thinking soul is posited as the unifying perceiving consciousness): the problem of the unity of the senses. At *De anima* III.2, having authorized—against those who posit a greater number—only five senses, and, with various success, sought to individuate them by medium, proper object, and sense-organ, Aristotle turns to the problem of complex perceptions. If the individual senses perceive only within the spectra of their proper objects, Aristotle asks, how is it possible to discriminate between, unify, and coordinate perceptions? Indeed, how is it that one senses that one is sensing at all?[17] Aristotle's influential answer was to posit the existence of a higher-order perceptual (that is, non-rational) power of the soul, a kind of "common sense" (*koinē aisthēsis*) which accompanies the five senses, and is responsible for the unification and control of their perceptions from the central sense-organ, the heart.

Aristotle's theories, whilst developed by the Peripatetic school, were challenged in the Hellenistic and Roman periods by the rise of Epicurean, Stoic and, subsequently, Neoplatonic, models of perception. But during Late Antiquity and the Medieval period, his *De anima* and *De sensu* claimed ascendancy, alongside the medical writings of Galen (c. 129–?, 199–216 CE), as the most influential discussions of the senses bestowed by Antiquity. From the work entitled *On the Nature of Man* written by Nemesius of Emesa (fl. c. 400 CE) at the end of the fourth century CE, to the treatises on the soul written by the classical Islamic and Jewish philosophers of the ninth and tenth centuries CE, to the commentaries on Aristotle's works written by Averroës (c. 1126–98 CE), and by the Latin medieval commentators, it is using Aristotle and Galen as their starting points that later thinkers formulate their questions into the nature, objects, number, and internal orchestration of the senses.[18] Their treatises, in turn, testify not to the simple adoption of Aristotelian and Galenic doctrine, but to its selective appropriation, further development, and creative fusion with Platonic, Stoic, and Neoplatonic elements, as well as post-Galenic medical ideas, to form new models of the senses. When Nemesius posits three post-sensationary faculties (to become known as the "inner senses" in the medieval period) localized in different ventricles of the brain to complement the five external senses, for instance, he likely draws upon the ideas of the medical writer Posidonius of Byzantium (fl. c. 370 CE) in order to develop Galen's physiological claims about the suitability of the brain to house the triad of "imagination," "memory," and "cogitation" familiar from Aristotelian psychology.[19] His innovative elaboration of earlier Greek ideas further to assert the status of the body and its parts as "instruments" (*organa*) of the soul (an idea shared by Aristotle and Galen), finds parallels in the work of the earliest Arabic and Hebrew students of Aristotle in the ninth and tenth centuries CE, who also draw upon Aristotelian psychology and Galenic thought about the cognitive primacy of the brain in order to theorize their own three "internal senses" located in separate ventricles of the brain.[20] Their enumerations are, again, successively revised and expanded in the early eleventh century by the Persian philosopher Avicenna (c. 980–1037 CE) to four or five inner senses. That 500 years later, Avicenna's doctrine appears in London in the popular English vernacular form of the "five wits" dramatized in Shakespeare's 141st sonnet, in turn, nicely illustrates the passage back to Europe of his ideas, which could not be ignored by Aristotle's twelfth- and thirteenth-century Latin commentators (Heller-Roazen 2007: 164). By that time at least, Antiquity's competing theories of perception had become part of not one but several conjoined cultural histories of the senses.

CHAPTER SIX

Medicine and the Senses: Humors, Potions, and Spells

HELEN KING AND JERRY TONER

"I find that a bad head cold clears up if the sufferer kisses a mule on the nose," advises Pliny the Elder (*Natural Histories* 30.31). This kind of homespun remedy is not perhaps the kind of treatment we imagine when we think of ancient medicine. We expect cool and rational observations from the first men to have come close to what we call physicians, men such as Hippocrates, the "Father of Medicine." However, the figure of Hippocrates himself, idealized over much of the subsequent history of Western medicine as the clinical observer *par excellence*, envisaged sitting at the patient's bedside watching and working out what to do (with the resulting case histories providing a model of the inductive method), is more of a fabrication than a reality. Only a few hundred years after his death, stories already circulated in which Hippocrates cured the plague of Athens, found out why the philosopher Democritus behaved so oddly, and was approached by the king of Persia to heal a disease ravaging his empire (Pinault 1992). In fact, not one treatise of the seventy or so in the "Hippocratic corpus" can be attributed to the historical Hippocrates with any certainty, while his persona has been created by our expectations of what a doctor should be like. Central to these expectations is the assumption that physicians will use their senses as the interface between the confusion of symptoms and the secure diagnosis of a disease.

Pliny, of course, was not a Greek doctor, but a Roman putting together the information that every elite man should be able to possess. Despite our image of what ancient medicine should be, the stories about the "Father of Medicine," and the recommendations of Pliny show that, in reality, ancient medicine encompassed a huge array of different types of knowledge and practice. Many of these involved potions derived from traditional folklore, or practices that formed part of what we today see as a separate area, "religion." As well as asking doctors—if one was available, an issue for those living outside major urban centers—people sought treatments from the healing god, Asclepius, and they visited magicians to buy various spells or amulets to heal or ward off disease. All of these medical practices relied heavily on the senses for access to the body, and often used substances in treatment because of their sensory dimensions. Being ill and undergoing diagnosis and therapy was a fully embodied experience, and the aim of this chapter is to look at how integral the senses were to the whole range of ancient healing. This approach is informed by a wider shift in studying the ancient world; the emerging focus on the way that all the senses would have been used in the past even, for example, to navigate one's way through an ancient city (Betts 2011).

ANCIENT HUMORAL MEDICINE

People in antiquity seem to have worried about their health just as much as we do today, but they had very different ways of understanding health and illness. Physical sensations were generally conceptualized as being one of the main causes of illness in the first place. It was believed that the senses, which were often likened to the five gates of a city, could act as entrances to the individual's inner being. In this way, sensations were believed to have a direct impact on the individual receiver, which meant that exposing oneself to the right kinds of sensory stimuli became a critical issue for personal well-being. Smells, for example, were not seen as just a byproduct of an object or person, they were "agents in and of themselves" (Harvey 2006: 30). The boundaries of the body were thought to be permeable, enabling sensations to penetrate and affect the individual in a variety of ways. Bad air, for example, could cause internal corruption if drawn into the body. An ancient Greek or Roman was what he or she *sensed*.

While Pliny emerges from a strong Roman tradition that argued that medicine should be carried out within the household, by the male household head, the huge number of medical texts we know about in the ancient world shows that many believed that treatment should be sought elsewhere. The great doctor Galen, who served as the Roman emperor Marcus Aurelius' personal physician, is known to have written over 350 treatises. But Galen was not alone. Medical writings ranged from the early Hippocratic treatises to those of later writers under the Roman Empire, such as Aretaeus, Caelius Aurelianus (who produced a Latin version of the Greek work of Soranus), Celsus, Alexander of Tralles, and Paul of Aegina. These named individuals are the exception, in that their work was copied, and survives in part today; far more ancient medicine was lost. Broadly speaking, these writers all shared a theory that viewed the human body as a collection of liquids, not of organs. The body was thought to contain four humors—named in the most influential text of humoral medicine, the Hippocratic *On the Nature of Man*, as black bile, yellow bile, blood, and phlegm—as well as other fluids such as sweat, semen, urine, and spit. Illness resulted primarily from an imbalance among the body's fluids (King 2013). Before Galen, in the second century CE, decided that

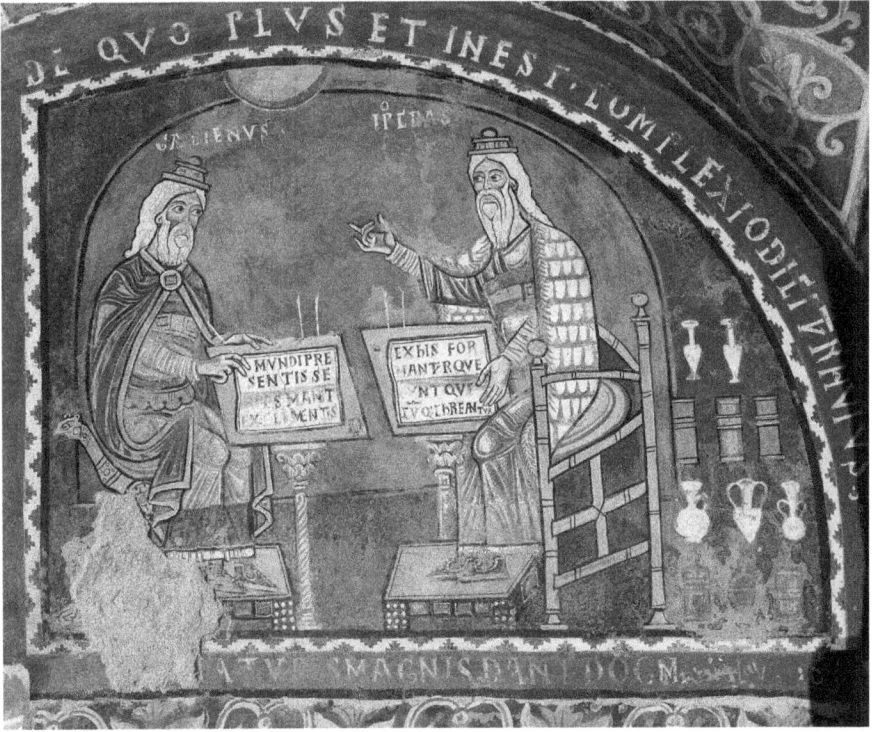

FIGURE 6.1: Hippocrates and Galen, early thirteenth-century fresco, in the Crypt of St. Mary Cathedral, Anagni, Lazio. Getty Images.

he liked the four-humor theory of *On the Nature of Man*, and so argued that it must be by the "real" Hippocrates, many other versions of the fluids of the body existed. In all cases, these theories suggested that the types of illness a patient suffered reflected different levels of heat and moisture within the body. Thus mania, for example, was characterized by heat, dryness and an excess of yellow bile; melancholia by the cold dampness of black bile.

Beyond this, there was little on which ancient medical writers agreed. They worked in a competitive marketplace and had to attract customers to their own particular theory or therapy (Nutton 1992). While they did not so label themselves, the history of medicine has divided them into three different approaches to disease and healing. The group we label as the Methodists—because they believed there was a very simple, easily learned "method" of categorizing all diseases as those caused by constriction, by relaxation, or by a mixture of the two—saw medicine as consisting of a few simple principles, which could be applied to all types of ailment. Empiricists saw things differently. Their view was that it was best to respond to and treat the particular symptoms of the patient. It was impossible to know catch-all theories which would be universally applicable; all was contingent. The Rationalists held that it was necessary to understand the underlying causes of diseases, as well as the more obvious symptoms. While he had nothing but scorn for the Methodists, the great Galen drew on both these last two sects, making use of direct observation of symptoms as well as coming to logical conclusions about how they originated and were connected.

The competitive nature of ancient medicine is reflected in the Hippocratic text, *Regimen*, which details how the author has alone discovered how to tell when a patient is about to fall ill (1.2). But it also raises the question of what medicine really is. The text discusses medicine as a specialist skill, a *technê*, arguing that like divination it knows the unseen by means of the seen (1.11). It privileges the power of observation to reveal a true understanding. Such specialist skills were characterized as activities requiring intellectual competence, scientific knowledge, and manual dexterity; they were governed by rules, could be taught, and produced verifiable results (King 1998: 40–1). However, the comparison with divination underlines that we should not understand this statement of medicine as a *technê* as being equivalent to a modern concept like "science."

But observation was not the same as seeing. The text goes on to list the means by which the doctor can carry out such detailed observation of the patient's symptoms. It takes place through seven senses. There are the familiar five—hearing, sight, smell, taste, and touch—to which are added speech and breath.

These are the sensory means that together bring knowledge to the trained healer (1.23). The role of the senses in ancient medicine was therefore fundamental. The body, like a book, could be "read" by those with knowledge of its basic sensory language. The senses provided the main way for accessing the otherwise hidden interior of the body in order to come to diagnostic judgments, which in turn determined treatment (King 1998: 45–6; Nutton 1993).

Sensory engagement with the body by its interpreter, the doctor, could be all-encompassing. Taste could be important in diagnosis: "wax in people's ears, if it is sweet, it foretells death, but if bitter, not" (*Epidemics* 6.5.12). So could hearing: for example, in cases of lung inflammation, the doctor shakes the patient and listens to the sound of his chest before cutting to let out the accumulated pus (*Diseases* 2.47), while the words of the patient or his or her carers, heard by the doctor, could provide the clues to diagnosis. The power of speech could move in the opposite direction when the doctor persuaded the patient to accept a certain course of treatment. But it is fair to say that for the followers of Hippocrates sight was the dominant sense when it came to diagnosis. The third book of *Epidemics* shows the detailed level of continuous, largely sight-based observation that Hippocratic doctors were writing up in their case notes (excerpts adapted from the Loeb translation):

Case 4
Philistes in Thasos had for a long time pain in the head, and at last fell into a state of stupor and took to his bed. Heavy drinking having caused continuous fevers the pain grew worse. At night he grew hot.
Day 1: Vomited bilious matters, scanty, at first yellow, afterwards increasing and of the colour verdigris; solid motions from the bowels; an uncomfortable night.
Day 2: Urine thin, transparent, with a small quantity of substance, like semen, floating in it. About midday became raving.
Day 4: Convulsions, exacerbation.
Day 5: Died early in the morning.

The doctor considers temperature, excretions, movements, and sleep, using hearing (the patient's story of this pain having affected him for "a long time"); touch (he was hot); and sight. While here taste and smell are not as prominent as the other senses, he is expected to use all material available to his senses, to complete a 360-degree evaluation. His analysis will also include the patient's physical surroundings, his or her manner, thoughts, dreams, stools, urine, breathing, and belching to name but a few (see *Epidemics* 1 for other factors).

Moreover, physicians also had to be able to apply judgment to this mound of accumulated data. Reason was seen by some doctors as the sixth sense; on the only occasion when Galen mentions the five senses explicitly, it is alongside the need for intellect to make sense of their evidence (K18B.632–57; Nutton 1993: 10). In his treatise on identifying the best doctor, Galen says that the "complete physician who is skilled in prognosis" needs "a general mental image of all the events in advance, thus visualizing them before making a diagnosis through the senses" (Iskandar 1988: 87.2–3, 6–8). For this reason medicine remained close to philosophy since it formed its judgments on the use of logic rather than experiment. Galen saw himself as both a physician and a philosopher, as he explained in his treatise *The Best Physician is also a Philosopher*.

The earliest Hippocratic texts date from the late fifth century BCE. By the time Galen was writing in the second and early third centuries CE, the non-visual senses had acquired a more prominent role (Mattern 2008b: 149–55). Galen sometimes boasts he can diagnose a patient simply by looking at him (e.g. K10.673–4) and certainly seems to view sight as the initial means of approaching diagnosis. But he also uses the odors of such things as urine, faeces, ulcers, and breath as indicators of ill-health. Taste can be important and he advises that the doctor "should lick the sweat of a patient that has collected on his finger during examination to see if it is sweet or salty or variously acrid" (K11.445; Nutton 1993: 11). Listening to the sounds the patient's body makes and to the patient's responses, even to the tone of his voice, can all reveal the inner causes of the illness. The words of the patient and the patient's family were held to be of particular importance in giving diagnostic clues.

But it is to touch that Galen gives perhaps the highest importance as a diagnostic tool. The skin, he wrote, was created by Nature as "the instrument of assessment" (*Mixtures* 1.9). Touch was used to take the temperature and the pulse, as well as to feel the patient's body to ascertain what troubles lay within. Of these, it was the pulse which was most revealing and helped "see" inside the abdomen. Galen's fourteen books on the subject are reduced to a brief sketch in one surviving text (K8.504–6) but all emphasize what minute distinctions he felt he could isolate when taking the pulse. While these distinctions were not unique to Galen, he seems to have developed pulse lore to a particularly high level. Awareness of pulsation goes back to the Hippocratic treatises and to Aristotle; Praxagoras noted that only the arteries, not the veins, move in this way. Herophilus, the third-century BCE doctor whose work only survives when it is quoted by others (Galen among them), distinguished between different speeds, rhythms, strengths, and "sizes" of pulse. He took a water-clock with him when he visited patients, adjusting it according to the age of the patient and then determining whether the pulse was out of alignment with age (von Staden 1989: 262–88).

The fine gradations of pulse which Galen believed he could detect by listening to the diseased body can be hard for us to understand, when modern medicine has reduced the pulse to a matter of numbers. With one patient we read that "the fever was rather high, but that his pulse was regular, very large, swift, frequent and vigorous; that the heat was not of the type that is biting to the touch" (K10.610; Mattern 2008b: 144). One of Galen's most famous cases from his treatise *On Prognosis* involved the wife of Justus, who lay awake at night constantly tossing and turning. He surmised that she was either suffering from a depression caused by black bile or from some worry she was unwilling to confess. Female patients were often thought to be withholding information out of modesty and she is portrayed as barely speaking, avoiding eye contact by covering her head. Taking her pulse, Galen noticed that it raced when the name of the famous (and probably inappropriately low-status) dancer Pylades was mentioned. He concluded, rightly, that she was infatuated with him. Like some ancient medical Sherlock Holmes, Galen is able to feel what her body is telling him, despite her silence. Her body speaks to the trained reader, even when her mouth remains firmly shut (K14.631; King 1998: 47). Galen's comments on the pulse show that a very sophisticated use of non-visual senses existed and played a vital role in diagnosis in antiquity; however, the clue that led him to mention dancers was a chance remark by another member of the household.

Here again, then, intellect is needed to accompany the evidence of the senses and to understand what they are telling him. This recalls the Hippocratic *On the Art* (11) where we are told that the eye of the mind (*opsei gnômês*) can see what the eyes alone do not. Touch, for example, does not inherently lead to accurate diagnosis. Galen described how temperature could be detected by touch alone but, to discern the degree of wetness or dryness of the body, this must be combined with sight and reason (*Mixtures* 2.2). It is what we could call "informed touch"—touching the vein by taking the pulse, also feeling the abdomen, and knowing what the sensations mean—that reduces the likelihood of being deceived. This was a danger of which the earlier Hippocratic texts were also aware. One warns, for example, that postures of patients with spinal problems can deceive the unwary doctor (*Joints* 46). The body was deceptive; the senses could lie; and the skilled practitioner had to weigh up the evidence.

Even sight could deceive. The Hippocratic texts warn the doctor of this. A tumor in the ear may "deceive a healer into expecting it to contain excess humoral fluids, so that he cuts into it in order to release them" (*Joints* 40).

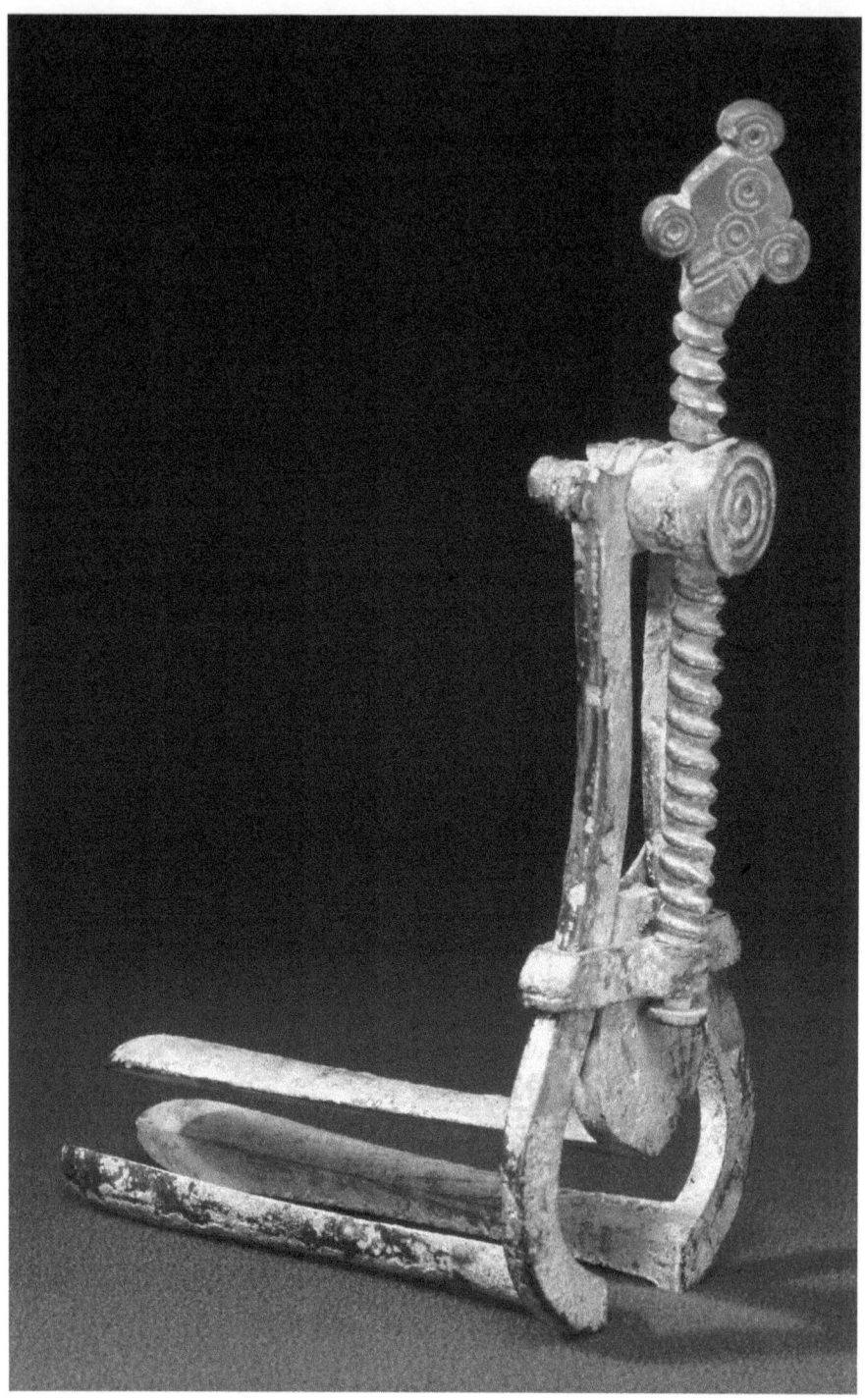

FIGURE 6.2: Roman vaginal speculum, 100 BCE–400 CE. Getty Images.

Specialist instruments, such as the vaginal speculum and anal probes, were developed to enhance the sense of sight and allow the physician to see into orifices. But even these could mislead. With the anal speculum, the very instrument intended to allow access to the inside of the body could, when it was opened up, act to obscure the lump that it was supposed to reveal; hence, this attempt to enhance the sense of sight could be counterproductive. There was criticism, therefore, of the evidence provided by the senses as providing a less-than-perfect guide to the body.

A further aspect to the senses was the ancient doctor's attempt to create a good sensory impression to increase confidence in his clients. The Hippocratic treatise *The Doctor* states that he should have a good color and be plump to show he can look after himself, be clean, well-dressed, and anointed with sweet-smelling unguents; but these should be "beyond suspicion." Simplicity appears to be the aim; all these factors "are pleasing to people who are ill." He should be silent and thoughtful, to show that he is intelligent and considering his diagnosis.

The simplicity of the ancient bedside manner could contrast with a tendency in the patients themselves to be deceptive. An appendix to the *Seven Books of Paul of Aegina (Appendix to Book 5)* entitled "On feigned diseases and their detection," warns that such malingering is often discovered by experience or the doctor's natural sagacity. It was hard to detect the inner pains, safe from the prying senses of the doctor, that people usually claimed to be suffering. But the senses too could play a role and the faker is only discovered by his aversion to swallowing medicines he would be anxious to take if actually ill.

And doctors too could play tricks to deceive people into thinking they had witnessed impressive medical procedures. The same text describes how some practitioners pretended to be able to cure epilepsy, and having made a small incision in the back of the head, they "extract something from the wound which they hold in their hands which impresses people." We might think that such quackery was rare but the text also warns that such professional imposters were "more numerous than could be contained in this whole work." Perhaps seeing an object apparently taken from the body could have a healing effect on the patient.

Being a patient in antiquity was in any case a strongly sensory experience. Pain relief was minimal and the suffering of illness was probably for the most part seen as an inescapable feature of human existence; one of the ancient Greek words for pain, *ponos*, is also used for hard agricultural labor. From toothache to tumors, most people suffered extremes of physical sensation through the sicknesses they suffered, the treatment of which then often caused even greater pain. Sometimes the patient was acutely aware of the sensory signs, as when Aretaeus described how a dying person could not endure his own smell (*SA* 1.9.5–6). In other situations, the sensory experience of illness was a disordered version of normality. We find various examples of patients suffering from delusions and hallucinations. Galen describes patients who pluck at loose pieces of thread on their clothes or try to pick up non-existent hairs. He is unsure whether such behavior resulted from the wrong association of sense data or the mind had temporarily gone beyond the limits of reason. Some of these sufferers were able to recall why they had been acting so neurotically when they came to their senses. One said that the nap of the woolen cloth seemed to stick out, another that chaff seemed to be hanging on the walls of the sick room, and another that little animals seemed to fly near his eyes which he tried to chase away (K18B.75). This kind of delusion also affected other senses. Galen relates the illness of the physician Theophilus who was able to discuss and judge things correctly but was under the illusion that some flute players had taken up residence in the corner of his house, where they played continually, even during the night. Even when Theophilus shouted at them to go, they stayed put (K7.60–2).

The treatment of mental health disorders of this type in antiquity is illuminating because it shows how closely interconnected were medical concepts of mind, body, and the senses (on mental health in ancient Rome, see Toner 2009: 54–91). Medical writers have numerous accounts of patients suffering from various kinds of mental disorder which affected their sensory perceptions. Galen describes a patient who thought he was a pot and was scared he would break (K8.190). Alexander of Tralles mentions a patient who bound up her little finger because she was worried that the world would collapse if she bent it (*Twelve Books on Medicine* 1.605, 607). Medical treatments of all kinds were concerned with maintaining humoral balance by carefully controlling the physical sensations that were working on the body. This also applied to the brain. So music might be played to an individual suffering from madness to bring harmony back to the humoral misalignment because the sounds acted on the body as a whole (Horden 2000).

In cases of mental disturbance, doctors examined the shape and features of the head to see if an imbalance in temperature or fluid within the skull was affecting the brain's function. Excessive heat or moisture would lead to madness and would be reflected in "thick, strong, black hair." Bald people, by contrast, were thought to have cool, dry brains which made the hair thin, but helped keep them sane (Galen K1.325–6). Treatments would seek to restore balance by physically altering the environment in which the brain was operating. The head might be shaved to allow heat to escape or strong-smelling compounds of pepper, frankincense, or oil of roses might be employed to cool the brain (Caelius Aurelianus 1.5.167). Caelius argued that the causes of mental illness could also lie in other physical factors, such as indigestion, drunkenness, sleeplessness, love-sickness, anger, grief, anxiety, superstitious fear, shock or blow, intense straining in study, business or other ambitious pursuits, love potions, the removal of long-standing hemorrhoids, or the suppression of menses in women (1.5). Aretaeus argues that visual imagery can cause mental illness; excessive visual stimulation encouraged people to suffer delusions and hallucinations that would lead them "away from what is real." He advises that there should be no paintings or bright colors in the rooms of sufferers from brain-fever (*On the Causes and Symptoms of Chronic Diseases* 2.3). This was a strongly somatic culture. All illness and anxiety was seen in purely physical terms, so it seemed perfectly natural to apply physical remedies to try and solve mental problems.

FIGURE 6.3: Bas-relief depicting surgical instruments, from the Catacomb of Praetextatus, Rome. Getty Images.

The senses were a key way for the competing factions within ancient medicine to differentiate themselves from each other. In what amounted to a medical supermarket, each doctor or group of doctors set out alternative cures based on a variety of physical factors. These included treatments based on diet, drink, drugs, sleeping, sweating, hydrotherapy, blood-letting, and purges. White hellebore was widely used as a vomitive, while black hellebore was prescribed as a powerful laxative. Caelius Aurelianus attacks other medical sects for recommending treatments for epilepsy that included tying up the patient, eating weasel and the testes of beavers, or placing a flame close to the patient's eye and tickling him (1.116). Some of these treatments went to even greater physical extremes. Celsus advises that the insane are "best treated by certain tortures." So whenever the patient said or did anything wrong, he was to be "coerced by starvation, fetters, and flogging" (3.18.21). Caelius recommends far more gentle and sympathetic treatments, including massaging the patient and keeping him free from stress. Those who were depressed should see a comedy: those who were euphoric should watch a tragedy (1.58).

The physicality of these treatments for mental disorder is striking. It was taken as read that a mental problem required a physical remedy. But since there was no easy access to the brain itself, trepanation being a highly dangerous and rare course of action, treatments were prescribed which would operate through the senses to restore balance to the head. All served to counteract imbalance in humors, temperature, or liquidity by either bringing them back into alignment or evacuating the excess.

As well as showing the extent of sensory treatments in ancient medicine, these various approaches serve to underline the importance of smell, touch, and taste in premodern medicine, senses which have been significantly downplayed in modern medicine. The move towards clinical observation and anatomical dissection in the eighteenth century and beyond has meant that sight has returned to its original Hippocratic position and become far more dominant. Advances in medical technology have exacerbated this sensory shift. Instruments such as thermometers and x-ray machines have reduced the role of the doctor in sensing the patient's pulse or feeling his way into the inner body by means of touching the outside. The "minor" senses have been largely confined to various alternative therapies; for example, the focus on smell in aromatherapy, or on the healing power of touch in massage.

Most of the patients Galen describes were men (see Mattern 2008a). But women also received medical treatment, and the senses were invoked in their therapy, perhaps most strikingly in the use of opposed pleasant and foul odors in treatment. Women were believed to suffer their own gender-specific form of mental disorder, known as hysterical suffocation, meaning "suffocation coming from the womb." Found mainly in virgins and widows, depending on where the womb moved to within the body, the symptoms included shortness of breath, chest pain, pain in the legs or groin, and seizure. The treatments prescribed involved trying to coax or coerce the wandering womb back into its proper place. Strong odors were thought to be particularly effective in this task. A foul smell placed under the woman's nose would repel a uterus that had risen high up in the body. Conversely, fragrant aromas could be applied to the sufferer's vagina to try and entice the womb into returning to its proper place.

Roman society placed an enormous pressure on women to reproduce and rear children. Perhaps the stress caused by this was one factor that led some women to exhibit symptoms of mental disorder. Male writers medicalized these expressions of disorder according to their own preconceptions of how a woman should behave. They believed that the only permanent cure was for a woman to fulfill her core role in society: being a wife, having sex, giving birth, and childrearing (Soranus *Gynaecology* 3.26). Galen also thought that dramatic seizures in women were caused by lack of intercourse leading to the retention of "female seed," which would then become poisonous (K8.420). The sensory cures could only act as stop-gaps, because female health was understood as being reliant on reproductive activity. For the woman, perhaps the emotional outbursts, pains and seizures of the "wandering womb" offered a way to gain some temporary relief from those very same social pressures, acting as a physical representation of her resistance to society's norms. While women were supposed to settle down into their socially-ordained roles, their wombs could resist and travel around the body in search of moisture (King 1998).

Ancient medicine as practiced by doctors like Hippocrates and Galen was not available to all. A doctor like Galen—who was expected to act like a modern personal trainer, advising on every aspect of diet and lifestyle—while willing to demonstrate his skills in public on any available patient, would normally treat the wealthier members of ancient society; typically, urban males, aged between 25 and 40, members of the leisured class who exercised in the gymnasium (Mattern 2008a). He generally practiced in the urban centers of Pergamum and Rome, where physicians of many different approaches competed for patients. We should not imagine that everyone in antiquity believed in their theories or turned to such practitioners for treatment in times of illness.

There is no evidence that Galen charged a fee—although he was not above receiving generous gifts from satisfied clients—but further down the medical food-chain things would have been very different, making the cost of medical treatment an issue for many people. There is evidence that some better-off members of the non-elite did seek treatment. Galen refers to one joiner who was a skillful artisan. Caelius also recommends that if mentally ill patients are unacquainted with literature, the doctor should give them problems appropriate to their particular craft, such as agricultural problems for a farmer. But that suggests that being unacquainted with literature was not the norm for his patients. We must realize, then, that ancient society contained many other forms of belief concerning illness and the correct form of medical treatment.

THE CULT OF ASCLEPIUS

The cult of Asclepius offered a popular religious alternative to the treatments of medical theorists. Temples to this god of healing flourished across the Mediterranean world. Galen's home, Pergamum, contained a widely popular Asclepieion, as did Epidauros. A common form of treatment was for patients to sleep within the temple precinct, during which the god was expected to come to them, either healing them on the spot or advising what they had to do to be cured. At Epidauros, short narratives of these divine cures were engraved and set in a wall. One, from the fourth century BCE, reads:

> A man who had his toe healed by a serpent. He was taken outside by the temple servants with a malignant sore on his toe and set upon a seat. While he slept a snake [a symbol of the god] crawled out of the shrine and licked his toe. The patient woke up and was healed. He said that in a dream he had seen a beautiful youth put a drug on his toe.
> Quoted in Phillips 1973: 199

Five hundred years later, the cult was still thriving. The orator Aelius Aristides had a lifelong devotion to the Asclepieion, keeping a detailed journal of his numerous treatments. It is a relentless account of what to modern readers feels like an almost neurotic attention to physical, sensory detail:

> On the following day I bathed again. I dreamt my food had not digested properly. I consulted the priest and I vomited in the evening. The god ordered us to do many strange things . . . when the harbour waves were

swollen by the South wind and ships were in distress, I had to sail across to the opposite side, whilst eating honey and acorns, and then vomit.

Sacred Tales 1.65

When the god commanded him to bathe in snow, he "gladly obeyed" (4.11). It is easy to imagine that receiving the detailed attention of the temple priests and attendants within a healing context delivered a placebo effect that was powerful enough to cause an improvement in many cases.

No simple dichotomy existed between these religious treatments and those of humoral medicine. Physicians worked at the temples of Asclepius. Nor was there any straightforward opposition between medicine and science, and faith-based healing. Galen himself trained as a doctor following a dream in which Asclepius appeared to his father, attributed to the god a healed abscess, and later used him to avoid going on campaign with the imperial household to Germany by claiming that he had been told by Asclepius in a dream not to travel. Aristides also tells us how certain dreams appeared to him at the time when a physician had arrived to treat him. Aristides has no doubt whose advice to follow. The doctor would only be able to help him "as much as he knows how." And even the doctor, when he heard about the dreams, being "a sensible

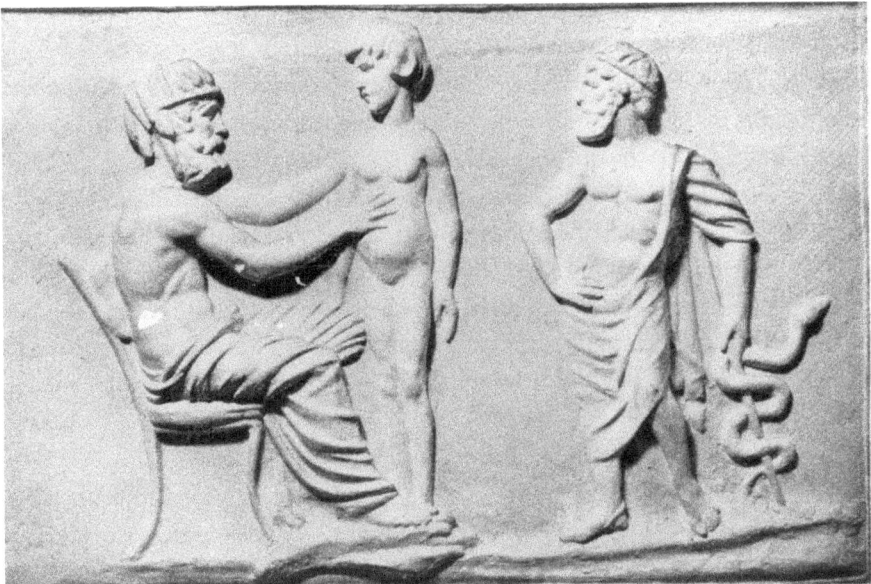

FIGURE 6.4: A cast taken from an ancient Greek intaglio gem, depicting a physician examining a patient while Asclepius, the god of healing, stands nearby holding the symbol of medicine, a snake coiled round a staff. Getty Images.

man," also yielded to the god. They both recognized the "true and proper doctor" and did what he commanded. The result was that his night was "wholly endurable and everything was without pain" (*Sacred Tales* 1.57).

FOLK MEDICINE

As noted above, most patients who visited physicians came from the top section of society. The popular culture mocked some of these physicians' high-status theories. In one joke, a patient said to a doctor, "I've got the runs, something must be wrong with my humors"; the doctor replied, "you can disappear down the toilet and you won't spoil my good humor." Many people, in fact, had to turn to their own more homespun, traditional beliefs and remedies when looking for a cure.

Traditional folk medicine contained a plethora of sometimes contradictory beliefs about what caused illness, which often involved a combination of both natural and supernatural causes. Most people would customarily spit on an insane person if one crossed their path, because spitting was believed to repel any mental contagion (Pliny *Natural Histories* 28.7; Plautus *Captives* 547–55). Some people put spit behind their ears to "calm mental anxiety" (Pliny *Natural Histories* 28.24–7). The passing of time did not bring about a decline in these kinds of belief, even as Greek humoral medicine became more widely practiced throughout the Roman empire. Many Romans seem to have maintained their ancestors' early distrust of these "fancy," foreign humoral theories from the East. Traditional Roman folk medicine saw no need for medicine itself. Nature herself was seen as having provided all the remedies people needed (Pliny *Natural Histories* 2.155). Treatments were based on a small number of ingredients which could be easily found on an average farm, such as wool and eggs. Cato the Elder eulogized the medicinal properties of the humble cabbage (*On Agriculture* 156–7). It is the cabbage, he believes, which surpasses all other vegetables: "It promotes digestion marvelously and is an excellent laxative, and the urine is wholesome for everything." The different varieties of cabbage contain all the virtues necessary for health, and "constantly changes its nature along with the heat, being moist and dry, sweet, bitter, and acid." Here, however, we should perhaps be cautious in proposing a contrast between simple, homely Roman medicine and complicated, philosophical Greek medicine; we know that the Greek doctor Chrysippus wrote a book on the healing powers of cabbage, so Cato's comments may come from literate rather than folk medicine.

In other cases, folk remedies mixed together the different sensory properties of everyday objects and living things into a powerful healing cocktail. Pliny, for example, describes the various ways to cure jaundice (*Natural Histories* 30.93–4). "Jaundice," he says,

> is combated by dirt from the ears or teats of a sheep, the dose being a coin by weight with a morsel of myrrh and two measures of wine; or by the ash of a dog's head in honey wine . . . or by earthworms in oxymel with myrrh, or by drinking wine that has rinsed a hen's feet—they must be yellow . . . or by the brain of a partridge or eagle in wine.

Finally, he explains, there is a bird called "Jaundice" from its color. "If a sufferer looks at it he is cured, we are told, and the bird dies" (Loeb translation adapted). Here, healing comes through the sense of seeing.

Such folk medicine belonged to an oral tradition that was handed down from generation to generation. Instead of the philosophical theories of Greek humoral medicine, it relied for its effect on placing ordinary matter in extraordinary situations, acting as a metaphor for the disorder of illness itself. Normal colors and smells in strange places disrupted the proper ordering of the universe in the same way that disease did, but then served to counteract the disorder as a way to return to normality. Again it is easy for us to see a sharp divide between these superstitious folk practices and the medical theories of men like Galen. The lived reality seems to have been far messier. Dung therapy performed by doctors exploited the power of smell (von Staden 1992), while Pliny even claims that spitting accompanied by a threefold curse is customary in all medicine (*Natural Histories* 28.36).

MEDICAL MAGIC

The language of curses brings us to another widely popular source of medical diagnosis and cure: magic. Magic too confounded the experiences of daily life by playing with texture, color and smell to subvert the normal sensory world. A simple spell for a cough, for example, involved writing in black ink on hyena parchment. But many spells were far more complicated. A sense of their complexity can be seen in dream interpretation, where woolen garlands signify witchcraft and spells because they are "intricate and multicolored." So we find in a magical cure for gout a whole array of sense perceptions being used to transform the world into a strange and unfamiliar place:

> You should make the man sit down and place clay under his feet . . . Afterwards you should bring an ant; you should cook it in henna oil; and

you should anoint his foot with it. When you have finished, you should bring Alexandrian figs, dried grapes, and potentilla. You should pound them with wine and anoint him. In addition to this, you should breathe at him with your mouth.

PDM 14.985–92 in Betz 1992

Even a matter as simple as breathing acquires a mystical significance, as the individual's body becomes a conduit through which magical powers can flow.

Magic loved to create new verbal sounds that meant nothing but charmed the speaker's and listener's ear. So for a headache, write "ABRASAX" on scarlet parchment, make it into a plaster and then place it on the side of head. These sounds transformed into writing were the way to communicate with the powers of the underworld. Like "abracadabra," they spoke directly to the demonic powers in their own language. The words became progressively more complicated as time went on, presumably as familiarity meant that it took more novelty to impress people buying spells. An amulet for a gouty man has far more complicated magical voices: "You should write these names on a strip of silver or tin. You should put it on a deerskin and bind it to the foot of the man named, on his two feet: 'THEMBARATHEM OUREMBRENOUTIPE AIOXTHOU SEMMARATHEMMOU NAIOOU, let [insert name], whom [insert name] bore, recover from every pain which is in his knees and two feet'" (*PDM* 14.1003–14). In some spells the sounds captured in writing last for many lines of text. Try reading them and it is impossible not to falter, even when they repeat many times.

Magic also reflected a competitive world where people had to work hard to secure their position in society, however humble. Most ordinary folk seem to have seen life as a zero-sum game. So if a neighbor was doing well, it was at someone else's expense, and that someone could be you. Many spells involve acts of sensory aggression to help persuade the demonic powers to reverse this imbalance in fortune. Or they try to persuade others to come over to the curser's point of view. One spell offers a way to afflict a rival with insomnia:

Take a living bat and on the right wing paint with myrrh the following figure, and on the left write the 7 names of the god as well as: "Let her, [insert name] whom [insert name] bore, lie awake until she consents." And so release the bat again. Perform this spell at the waning of the moon when the goddess is in her third night, and the woman will die for lack of sleep, without lasting 7 days.

PGM 12.376–96

Magic worked to disorientate the senses and overturn sensory norms. The more extreme the request, the harder the spell often seems to try to subvert sensory experience. A contraceptive spell, labeled the "only one in the world," advises:

> Take as many bittervetch seeds as you want for the number of years you wish to remain sterile. Steep them in the menses of a menstruating woman. Let her steep them in her own genitals. And take a frog that is alive and throw the bittervetch seeds into its mouth so that the frog swallows them ... And take a seed of henbane, steep it in mare's milk, and take the nasal mucus of an ox, with grains of barley, put these into a leather skin made from a fawn and on the outside bind it up with mulehide skin, and attach it as an amulet ... Mix in also with the barley grains wax from the ear of a mule.
>
> PGM 36.320–2

By combining the mundane in strange new forms, magic sought to create sensory disarray. Putting the everyday in strange places created a disordered world which paralleled the error that the spell was trying to redress. It summoned up a netherworld of demonic forces, which would be attracted by the disordered extremes and powerful sensory features of the spell. Magic changed the form of normal objects by grinding and mixing, then incorporated them into a new authoritative text. By specifying in exact, minute detail the ways in which particular items were to be used in the ritual, magic placed the individual in a new relationship with his or her senses.

It is difficult to establish any clear division between magical and folk medicine. Folk healing frequently contains magical features. Cato, for example, advises a combination of touch and chant to cure dislocation of the joints: "Take a green reed four or five feet long and split it down the middle, and let two men hold it to your hips. Begin to chant, 'motas uaeta daries dardares astataries dissunapiter' ... If the pieces are applied to the dislocation or the fracture, it will heal" (*On Agriculture* 160). Here we have a combination of chant, sympathetic magic, and mystical voices all being used in the context of folk medicine. Similarly, putting out a fire by throwing wine over it was thought to reduce fever. Pliny discusses the magical properties of metal, especially iron (*Natural Histories* 34.151). *Ex voto* offerings to the gods were also widely used, which often consisted of small clay representations of the part of the body which was afflicted by illness, often giving an exaggerated sense of the affected part, and perhaps reflecting the sensory experience of the sufferer.

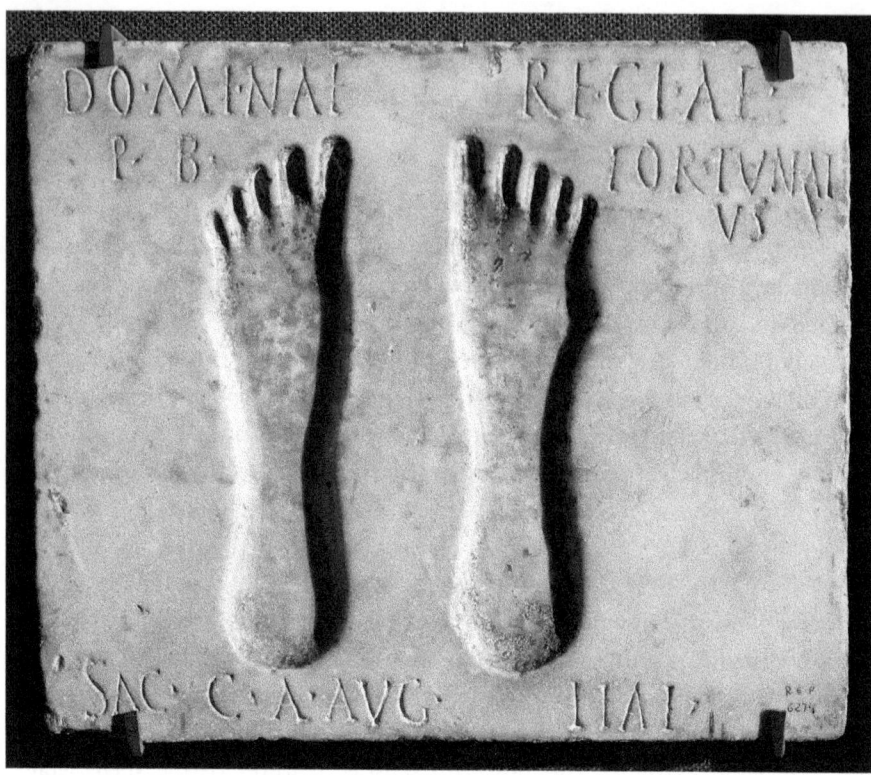

FIGURE 6.5: Imperial-age *ex-voto* depicting footprints uncovered in Italica, Spain. Getty Images.

All these examples come from Roman folk medicine. We should be careful not to draw a harsh distinction between Greek rationality and Roman superstition, since Greek folk medicine was simply less recorded than the Roman tradition. The Hippocratic corpus also contains some folk and magical practices. Amulets, for example, were used to speed up labor: "smear fruit of the wild cucumber, which is already white, on wax, then wind up in red wool, and tie it to her loin" (*Diseases of Women* 1.77).

Nonetheless, exponents of traditional Roman folk medicine were keen to make a strong distinction between their own practices and magic. Pliny advises for the treatment of brain-fever, "wrapping a warm sheep's lung round the patient's head" (*Natural Histories* 30.96). He then goes on to mock the various magical cures for this condition. Whether it is taking the brain of a mouse in water, or the ash of a weasel, or the eyes of a horned owl reduced to ash, Pliny is adamant that he is "inclined to treat this remedy as one of the frauds with which magicians mock mankind." This is particularly so because magical treatments often linked their efficacy with the phase of the moon or the sign of the zodiac, "so," he explains, "if the sun is passing through Gemini then the sick should be rubbed with the burnt comb, ears and claws of a cock, but its spurs and wattles if it is passing through the moon." But he cannot distinguish between folk and magical treatments on the grounds of their content or their extreme use of everyday materials in alternative sensory contexts.

All forms of ancient medicine structured the healing event, especially its spoken component, to help the healer acquire the authority to intervene (Gordon 1992). Treatment then sought to restore order through shared assumptions, whether they related to the humors or the ordering of the universe. There was significant overlap between different kinds of medicine, even when practitioners sought to differentiate their own particular area of expertise. We find this also in the treatment of animals. Several texts survive dealing with veterinary medicine, especially relating to horses (see Adams 1995). The horse served a vital role in the army, the chariot-racing of the circus, transport, and the official communication network, the *cursus publicus*. Horse doctors were therefore important. A fourth century CE text by Pelagonius, *On the Veterinary Art*, details the kinds of injuries horses could sustain in the circus. It includes blows to the eyes from an opponent's whip, cuts to the tongue from pulling too hard on the bit, and injuries from being hit by a chariot wheel. In line with Greek medicine, Pelagonius sees equine disease as being caused by factors such as heat, cold, or damp (e.g. 33.2, 30.4). Treatment includes surgical procedures, poultices, evacuations, but also incantations and amulets. One papyrus, surviving from the second century, is a letter to a Roman cavalryman in Egypt. It ends with the wish that his horse may not be suffering from the evil eye (*O. Florida* 15). Magic had a deep-rooted place in all forms of traditional treatment and medical writers did not reject it entirely.

FROM DEMONS AND MIRACLES TO THE UNTREATABLE

Demons played an important role in magical treatments. They also dominated popular ideas about mental disorder. One explanation for mental disorder was that demons entered their victims and possessed them. These demons represented creatures who lived halfway between heaven and earth, but who could be found anywhere. No one knew exactly what a demon was, but it was commonly thought that they were either unclean spirits of the underworld or the souls of those who had met a violent, untimely death. The popular understanding of mental disorder, therefore, saw it as a disruption of the proper ordering between the individual and the divine. Mental disturbance happened when the fabric of the universe was torn, allowing chaotic, demonic powers to break free from their correct place and pour into the human sphere. The result was a comparable sensory chaos.

The invasion of evil spirits into the body was an intensely physical experience. Demons could enter the body through orifices such as a yawning mouth. When stirred up by St. Hypatius in the fourth century, these spirits appeared like "bright phantoms" and a "great howling arose" (*Life of Hypatius* 18). The victims of this possession ceased to inhabit the world of ordinary sensations, like the Gerasene demoniac in the Bible, who escaped from the chains he had been kept in, fled to the desert and lived among the tombs, naked, crying and bruising himself with stones (Luke 8:26, 29). Treatment consisted of physically and sensorially attempting to entice the demons back out. Remedies ranged from beatings, drilling holes in the head and bloodletting, to incantations and exorcisms.

The power to perform exorcism acquired a peculiarly dramatic role in the later Christian Roman Empire. Through the healing touch of the holy man, the possessed were able to have their sanity restored. These holy men acted in imitation of Jesus himself who cast out demons from the afflicted. The power of touch was central to Jesus' healing miracles. In one, a woman who had suffered blood-loss for twelve years was cured simply by touching the hem of His clothes (Luke 8:46). This was a power that was passed on to His most devout followers. Touch allowed the divine to pass through its human conduits into the bodies of the ill. Thus sufferers were able to be cured when they merely touched face cloths that had themselves touched St. Paul: "their diseases left them and the evil spirits came out of them" (Acts 19:11–12).

Illness acquired a metaphorical role in the Christian world. Just as Jesus' touch could deliver an individual from sickness, so could His spiritual embrace deliver the sinner from eternal damnation in the fires of hell. The arrival of the bubonic plague in 541 CE offered an example of an illness which was beyond any form of medical treatment, whether humoral, folk, magical, or religious. It was hard for the Christians not to see this as a divine message (see Toner 2013). Images of plague created a world where all the normal rules of society had been turned on their head (see, for example, John of Ephesus 543–4 for an account of the Great Plague). Accounts linger on the massive sensorial assault the disease launched on its victims: its vivid colors, dreadful stench, and the bitter cries of the sick (see Jones 1996). The plague was "a fearsome and terrible scene for onlookers," who had to gaze on piles of rotting, stinking corpses. The normally solid body liquefied. Streams of putrid matter flowed from the skin, the bowels, and nostrils. Many of these plague deaths took place in the home, normally a place of safety. As a result, extremes of sensory experience occurred where there should have been normality and routine.

In this dystopia, where the human body was beyond medical help, the extremes of plague contrasted with the moderation of the Christian life. All the normal sensory rules were inverted. The dead, through their liquefaction and vivid coloring, lost their human identity. What should have been respected remains became repugnant to the senses. They became emblematic of the profound moral decay which had in Christian writers' eyes caused so great a disaster in the first place. It was a terrifying call from God for repentance. Here, in all its stinking, gruesome detail, was a terrifying foretaste of the eternal punishments of hell that awaited the unrepentant sinner. All the sick could do was pray for forgiveness.

CHAPTER SEVEN

The Senses in Literature: Falling in Love in an Ancient Greek Novel

SILVIA MONTIGLIO

INTRODUCTION

Greek literature is sensuous. As the product of a largely aural culture, it is meant for the ears, for their pleasure. Poetry is sung and accompanied by music. Since Homer, raconteurs and public speakers enchant their audiences not only by what they say but also by the sound of their words and voices. Nestor, one of the best speakers, boasts of a clear and resonant voice (*ligys*), a voice "that flows sweeter than honey,"[1] perhaps slightly high pitched. Menelaus speaks "very sonorously," but the sound of Odysseus' voice is even more impressive: "when he let out his powerful voice from his chest, and words like snowflakes in the winter, then no other mortal could compete with [him]" (see *Iliad* 3.214 and 221–3; I have discussed the aesthetics of the voice in Homer in more detail in Montiglio 2000, especially pp. 68–77). Euphony is in the spotlight of Greek literary criticism. Questions include: what effects do the beautiful sounds of poetry have on the hearers? How to create those beautiful sounds? Which vowels and consonants go together and which ones do not (see Stanford 1967)? Prose writers such as historians, philosophers, or orators ask how much auditory beauty should their non-fictional projects afford their audiences: is the pleasure of hearing conducive to learning or does it lull the mind?

Greek literature caresses not only the ears. Verbal persuasion could be felt to work through other senses as well, to have an impact on sight and even touch as well as hearing (see the discussion of Gorgias' theory of poetry in Worman 2002: 161–5). A common rhetorical figure in Greek poetry is the cross-sensory metaphor, synaesthesia. We have just encountered Nestor's voice, "flowing sweeter than honey": a voice with a taste and a smooth, fluid texture. Another, striking, example, still from Homer: the voice of the Trojan elders who give good counsel is "lily-like" as is the voice of the cicadas (*Iliad* 3.151–2). In this image the shrill and high-pitched sound of the insect's singing blends with the whiteness of the flower, as in the Italian expression *voce bianca*, white voice, for the voice, not yet broken, of a pre-pubescent singer. A lily-like voice is seen as much as heard, or it is heard through the eyes.

Which takes me to a major sensory function of words in Greek literature: to create or reproduce images. A fundamental quality of good style was "vividness," *enargeia*, the ability to make audiences see through words. Again, Homeric epic provides the prototypical expression of the visualizing power of words: when Achilles decides to go back to fighting, the god Hephaistos fabricates a full armor for him, including a shield with engraved images, of the cosmos, life in peace, and life in war. As if vying with the artwork, the poet carefully describes every image, to put it before the eyes of audiences turned spectators. Such descriptions of artworks, called *ekphraseis*, multiply in later literature (the bibliography on *ekphrasis* is vast: see, recently, Webb 2009). Greek drama is yet another verbal spectacle: because of the relatively rudimentary stage décor, Greek audiences were asked to see many things that they physically did not see. And they saw the invisible through the "vividness" of the dramatist's words.

LOVE AND THE SENSES IN GREEK LITERATURE: A BRIEF OVERVIEW

The ambition of much Greek literature to fashion images through words is just one aspect of the premium Greek culture at large put on sight as the highest of the senses (but see now Butler and Purves 2013).

"To live" in Greek is to "see the light" (Hades, the Greek underworld, is the realm of darkness). To know is to have seen (the main verb for "to know," *oida*, is a perfect build on a root (*-id*) meaning "to see"). We "see" a dream. And we fall in love through our eyes. Popular etymologizing connected *erân* (to love, to desire) to *horân* (to see) or explained the former as the flowing (*rein*) of beauty into (*eis*) the eyes.² Countless literary texts depict love as a painful condition caused by the sight of beauty, as in this lapidary statement: "no one has escaped or will escape love as long as there is beauty and eyes can see" (Longus *Daphnis and Chloe* preface).

As we have just noted, however, the Greeks were also strongly susceptible to the seduction of words, voices, and sounds. The one temptation Odysseus knows from the start that he cannot resist is a song, the beauty of a voice without a body. The seduction of aural impressions extends to the erotic domain. Love itself is accompanied by persuasion (*Peithô*) since Homer, as in the phrase, "but she did not persuade my heart in my breast" (see *Iliad* 6.162; *Odyssey* 7.258; 9.33). Hesiod embellishes Pandora with a voice and persuasive speech, two of her dangerous gifts (see *Works and Days* 73f; on these sources see Gross 1979: 305). Likewise on Aphrodite's girdle are figured "the whispered endearments that steal the heart away even from the thoughtful" (*Iliad* 14. 216–17 in Lattimore's translation). Odysseus, with his vocal and verbal charms, his "honeyed words," attracts Nausicaa when they first meet, in spite of his weathered appearance. After hearing those words she compliments the filthy shipwrecked, telling him that he is not a bad man. An ancient commentator thought that Nausicaa fell in love with Odysseus right then, before he bathed and Athena beautified him.³ Another heroine, Medea, not only keeps seeing the man she loves after he leaves, but "ever in her ears rung his voice and his honey-sweet words" (Apollonius of Rhodes *Argonautica* 3.457–8). Virgil's Dido, largely inspired by the figure of Medea, drinks in Aeneas' long story of woes, and, with it, drinks love. Her love begins as a passion for hearing: "And unhappy Dido was protracting the night with varied talk, and drinking long sips of love, asking many a thing of Priam, many of Hector" (*Aeneid* 1.748–50). Aeneas' words are engraved in her heart as much as his face (*Aeneid* 4.4–5: *haerunt infixi pectore vultus/verbaque* [his face and words cling fixedly to her heart]). The love-smitten queen rehearses his words, wants to hear them again and again. When he departs, "far away she hears him and sees him far away."⁴

In the same epic, Venus lures her husband Vulcan by "words that breathe divine love" (*Aeneid* 8.373: *dictis divinum aspirat amorem*). The voice of Eros himself is like honey, sings another poet (Moschus 1.9). And so is the beloved's voice. The moralist Plutarch deems a woman's auditory appeal part and parcel of her seductiveness: "Just as poetry adds to prose the sweetness of song and meter and rhythm, making its educational powers more forceful and its capacity for doing harm more irresistible; just so nature has endowed women with a charming appearance and a persuasive voice" (Plutarch *Dialogue on Love* 769 C). Poets repeatedly sing of a beloved's vocal and verbal charms: "Oh you of the beautiful face, of the golden locks, Galatea, of the charming voice, child of the Loves." Or: "I'd rather hear Heliodora's voice in my ears than the harp of the son of Leto." A girl is praised for having "more magic in her voice than there is in the girdle of Aphrodite;" and yet another one for possessing both persuasion and a voice as charming as that of the Muse Calliope, who embodies vocal beauty in her very name (*kalê-ops*, fair-voiced): "You have the beauty of Cypris, the mouth of Peitho, the form and bloom of the spring Hours, the voice of Calliope."[5] In contrast, of a woman who has lost her charms it is specified that her voice is "senile" (*Palatine Anthology* 5.273).

Hearing can be even more enthralling than sight for the lover because it marks closer proximity to the object of desire, as in this line: "blessed is he who sees her, but three times as blessed is he who hears her" (*Palatine Anthology* 5. 94). Not surprisingly, then, the perfect life of lovers could be described as uninterrupted talking and hearing: "He had no other business than loving Anthia and being loved by her, than talking to her and hearing her talk" (Xenophon of Ephesus, *An Ephesian Story* 1.4.1).

Touch and smell also play into love's beginnings: "And look at Ariadne, or rather at her sleep; for her breast is bare to the waist, and her neck is bent back and her throat is soft . . . How fair a sight, Dionysus, and how sweet her breath! Whether the fragrance is of apples or of grapes, you can tell after you have kissed her!" (Philostratus *Imagines* 1.15.3). This *ekphrasis*, which describes the painted image of Sleeping Ariadne, rivals the image by appealing to touch, smell, and even taste. The writer seems to be feeling the impact of Ariadne's charm in that image through the perception of Dionysus, who is becoming her lover and is allured not just by visual beauty but also by olfactory and tactile sensations, a fragrant breath and delicate skin, and by the anticipation of aromatic kisses. Another writer, of erotic letters, dwells even more emphatically on love's olfactory enticements: "Her throat smells like ambrosia, and her breath is sweet. If it has the fragrance of apples or roses mixed in a drink, you will tell me when you kiss her."[6]

Touch, a modulation of which is kissing, both marks a progression in the lovers' intimacy and fuels the passion. Writers who list the senses involved in the arousal of love place touch near the climax: one falls in love first by seeing, then conversing, touching, kissing, and finally intercourse (Donatus *On Terence Eunuch* 640; thanks to Gareth Schmeling for this reference). Or, in a variation: "it's not enough to look at the loved one or listen to his voice as he sits facing you, but love has, as it were, made itself a ladder of pleasure, and has for its first step that of sight . . . and, once it beholds, it wishes to come nearer and to touch." There follows kissing, fondling, and finally intercourse.⁷

THE NOVEL: LOVE AT FIRST SIGHT

We now move to the core of this chapter: the role of the senses in the arousal of love as described in the Greek novels. How do the Greek novels fit in a culture that puts a premium on sight in the ignition of love but acknowledges the importance of the other senses as well?

We call "Greek novels," or, as some prefer, "romances," a number of fictional narratives written between the first and the third or fourth century CE. Those fully extant are Chariton's *Callirhoe*, probably the oldest, *An Ephesian Story* by Xenophon of Ephesus, *Leucippe and Clitophon* by Achilles Tatius, Longus' *Daphnis and Chloe*, and Heliodorus' *Aethiopica*, the latest.⁸ Except for *Daphnis and Chloe*, these narratives follow a similar plotline: a lad and a maiden of extraordinary beauty fall in love, are married or pledged to each other, but before they can "live happily ever after," they are violently separated and shuffled around the world, where they face all kinds of dangers: pirates, shipwrecks, enslavement, executions and, the most threatening of all, rival suitors.

The protagonists of these novels generally fall in love at first sight.⁹ Callirhoe is on her way to a temple, Chaereas is coming back from the gymnasium, when "at the corner of a narrow street the two walked straight into each other; the god [Eros] had contrived the meeting so that each should see the other. At once they were both smitten with love" (*Callirhoe* 1.1.6). From the earliest novel to the latest one:

> at the moment when they set eyes on one another, the young pair fell in love, as if the soul recognized its kin at the very first encounter and sped to meet that which was worthily its own. For a brief moment full of emotion they stood motionless; then slowly, so slowly, she handed him the torch and he took it from her, and all the while they gazed hard into one another's eyes, as if calling to mind a previous acquaintance or meeting.
>
> *Aethiopica* 3.5.4–5

Love is born at the contact of two gazes. This is a familiar motif, which we know from myriads of such scenes in literature, melodrama, or film. In rare cases the ignition of love is deflected toward the voice: the first strong stirrings of passion Count Andrei feels for Natasha in *War and Peace* are caused by her voice and words, heard in a splendid moonlit night; Gabrielle, the maiden who falls in love with Étienne in Balzac's *L'enfant maudit*, is first drawn to a voice, his, singing in the darkness, and he to another voice, hers, echoing his song. But these episodes are preparatory for the meeting of the eyes; they prefigure that meeting.[10] Though falling in love at first sight is a literary commonplace, however, a noticeable feature of the two Greek scenes cited above is that no words are exchanged between the boy and the girl.[11] There are external reasons for this: the encounter takes place in a ritual context (in Heliodorus) with its rigid protocol, or the girl's mother is present (in Chariton).[12] A spontaneous conversation would hardly be possible in such circumstances, especially considering the relative segregation of the sexes in the upper class (to which the novels' protagonists always belong). Yet, the absence of words from those scenes of love at first sight puts the burden of the passion entirely on the encounter of the eyes. The lovers become lovers without hearing each other speak, what words, with what voice. They are not overwhelmed by the power of sound together with that of sight, as in the opening lines of this Irish song: "When first I saw you, I saw beauty . . . when first I heard you, I heard sweetness . . ." (*The Wishing Well*, by Connie Dover, in *Celtic Voices* 1995). A movie director who would wish to render the spirit of those scenes should perhaps, at the moment when the protagonists' eyes meet, silence all noises occurring in the background, interrupt or muffle any musical accompaniment, and zoom in on the lovers' expression of wonder as they take in each other's beauty.[13]

Once ignited by the touch of two gazes, love is the same forever. In more modern literature or film, the scene of first encounter is often not "the end of the story" but marks the beginning of an infatuation that grows and evolves into more profound love as the two meet again and again (take, for instance, Eric Segal's *Love Story*). There is no such development in the Greek novels.[14] This is perhaps best explained by invoking ancient conceptions of selfhood, which, even in the Hellenistic and Roman periods, are not centered on the inner world of the individual but are structured by the position of the individual in society.[15] Novelistic love does not grow because the lovers do not look inside themselves. An additional explanation for this lack of growth in erotic passion is, however, possible: the perfect and perfectly mutual love of the novels' protagonists cannot grow because perfection does not. Love, to be sure, is put to the test; but the tests confirm it, they do not change its intensity. The first sight has the last word. That the protagonists' love cannot grow because of its inborn perfection and perfect mutuality seems suggested by the different treatment accorded to non-mutual love. Though our characters' sense of self is generally not centered on their interiority, of one of them (not a protagonist) we are told that his passion deepened along with his increasing intimacy with the loved one (*Callirhoe* 5.9.8–9): and that character is unhappy in his love. The same is true of lovers who do not fall in love at first sight. The idea that love can be kindled by "seeing the other again and again" is not alien to the novels; yet those who fall in love after some time are the rivals, whose love is and remains unrequited (see *An Ephesian Story* 1.14.7; 2.3.2; 2.11.1; 2.13.6). Mutual love, it seems, needs no more than a glance to bloom.[16]

The power of that glance in the ignition of love is demonstrated by negative evidence as well: those who do not love do not "see" the other at their first encounter. When Callirhoe, the protagonist of Chariton's novel, meets Dionysius, a noble man of Miletus who falls madly in love with her, only he is described as "seeing" the woman before him. The scene is one of first encounter, but not one in which four eyes meet. Callirhoe, though she turns her head towards Dionysius, and obviously must catch sight of him, is not the subject of a gaze: she only moves, lowers her head, cries, and finally speaks (*Callirhoe* 2.3.6–7). Her eyes do not see Dionysius because she has no eyes for him: because she is not falling in love.

THE CHARM OF HER VOICE AND WORDS

Is sight alone, then, the cause of love in the Greek novels? What happens to hearing, touch, and smell, which also play an important role in Greek erotics?

Only *Daphnis and Chloe* includes touch and smell in the arousal of love. While Chloe is asleep at noon, Daphnis takes in her scent alongside her beauty: "What eyes are sleeping there, what a sweet breath comes from her mouth! Apples do not give off such fragrance, nor do pears." Shortly beforehand Chloe, since then ignorant of love's sting, first feels it as she watches—and touches—Daphnis whom she is washing in a spring: "It seemed to [her], as she gazed at him, that Daphnis was beautiful . . . his flesh yielded so gently to her touch that she surreptitiously felt her own several times to see if his was more delicate than hers." And she persuades him to bathe again: "she watched him, and after watching she touched him; then again she went away approving, and that approval was the beginning of love" (see, respectively, 1.25.2; 1.13.2; 1.13.5). This exceptional emphasis on touch and smell is in keeping with the naturalness and innocence with which Daphnis and Chloe first experience love: unlike the hero and the heroine of the other novels, when they fall in love they do not know even the name of love. Their ignorance of social expectations and taboos allows them to be more spontaneously "physical" than the other novelistic heroes and heroines. As a counterpoint we can take *Callirhoe*, which titillates the readers by suggesting the feel of the heroine's skin but not through the words of her lover. As Callirhoe is being bathed by maidservants, the author comments: "Her skin gleamed white, sparkling just like some shining substance; her flesh was so soft that you were afraid even the touch of a finger would cause a bad wound" (*Callirhoe* 2.2.2). Not even Clitophon, the uninhibited hero of Achilles Tatius, dwells on the softness of his beloved's skin or on the sweetness of her breath. In his dream he touches her (*Leucippe and Clitophon* 1.6.5), but his waking words touch only on her appearance. When the girl sings a song about the fragrant rose, which she calls "a breath of love," he "saw the rose upon her lips" but does not imagine smelling it (*Leucippe and Clitophon* 2.1.3). Women's scents and boys' more natural odors feature in a debate (at the end of Book 2) on whether heterosexual or homosexual love is more exciting; but the hero is in male company, and both he, who defends the love of girls, and his challenger speak in purely abstract terms: we don't find out how sweet the skin of their beloved smells.

While the eroticism of touch and smell makes timid appearances in the novels, hearing is front-stage in their representation of love: we have already noted that Xenophon of Ephesus calls the blessed life of lovers one of uninterrupted talking and listening. Daphnis' music beautifies him in the eyes and ears of Chloe, who is falling in love and does not know it (*Daphnis and Chloe* 1.13). Of all the novels, however, Chariton's *Callirhoe* seems to pay special attention to the erotic power of auditory impressions. Though no words are exchanged between the protagonists when they fall in love, the heroine's voice has strong erotic effects, and so do the "voices," the rumors, that spread news of her ineffable beauty. In the remainder of this chapter, I shall investigate the ways in which this novel articulates the auditory and the visual in narrating love's beginnings.

Callirhoe, a wonder to behold, makes everyone who sees her fall in love. With formulaic repetitiveness, her god-like epiphanies are received by silence, amazement, adoring gestures, fainting....[17] When Dionysius first meets her, he takes her for Aphrodite as most people do (alternatives include Artemis, a Nereid, and Athena); but he also deems her voice as godlike as her appearance: "As she spoke, her voice seemed the voice of a deity to Dionysius; it had a musical sound, with the effect of a lyre's note. He did not know what to do; he was too embarrassed to continue talking to her; so he went off to his house, already aflame with love" (*Callirhoe* 2.3.9). Beauty for the ears strikes the final blow. We are sent back to Sappho's famous poem 31:

> He seems similar to the gods to me,
> That man who sits before you,
> And nearby listens to your sweet voice,
>
> And lovely laughter. Truly that
> Sets my heart a-flutter in my breast.
> For when I look at you for a brief moment,
> It is no longer possible for me to speak . . .

Hearing is even more unbearable than seeing for the woman who is watching the scene. It is the contrast between the irresistible beauty of the girl's voice and laughter and the apparently Olympian detachment with which the man listens to them that makes the speaker's heart tremble. To his serene listening she opposes her loss of control as she looks at the girl even briefly, building a contrast that endows sound with a power stronger than sight (in his rewriting of the poem (51) Catullus adds sight—*spectat et audit*). We also note Sappho's emphasis on the erotic power of pure sounds, with no sense attached. The girl's voice is "sweet" as her laughter is "lovely": what she says does not matter. If Greek culture, like its Western descendants, has shown anxiety vis-à-vis the enchantment of voices without sense, or exceeding sense, or opposing sense, and has tried in many ways to ban or regulate those voices,[18] Sappho's poem is a painful celebration of the seduction of a voice without words.

Which takes me back to Dionysius. He, too, is overwhelmed by a voice, regardless of what it says. Callirhoe speaks to counter his fantasy that she is a goddess: "Stop making fun of me! Stop calling me a goddess—I am not even a happy mortal!" Dionysius hears the words but is all taken by their sound, by a musical charm that reduces him to silence. Still during the restless night that follows the encounter, when he recalls Callirhoe's words along with her voice, that voice, which took his own away, has first place in his memory ("her voice . . . her words"; see *Callirhoe* 2.4.3–4).

To Callirhoe's vocal charm, however, is soon added "persuasiveness of speech" (*logôn peithô*) as one more blow to Dionysius' heart. At their first meeting Callirhoe is vaguely reminiscent of Odysseus: like him she is surrounded by a mysterious aura. When she and Dionysius meet again, she is reluctant to speak of herself as Odysseus (ostensibly at least) is at the court of Alcinous, and, when she finally speaks, she asks Dionysius for conveyance, invoking Alcinous as the model to follow. Dionysius gives her his word. Back in his house, though, he unburdens his heart, for he understands that he is not loved: "I was hoping she was Aphrodite's gift to me and I was painting for myself a life happier than that of Menelaus, Spartan Helen's husband—even Helen, I imagine, was not as beautiful as she is. And she is persuasive, too" (*Callirhoe* 2.6.1). Though Callirhoe is not trying to seduce Dionysius erotically but is only employing, in Odysseus' fashion, her speaking skills and education to convince him to go along with her wishes, her persuasive speech works yet another erotic charm on him.

When at first Callirhoe was reluctant to speak for fear that the story of her past fortune (she is the daughter of the famous Syracusan general Hermocrates, who defeated the Athenians when they attacked Sicily during the Peloponnesian War) might not be believed given her present state (she has become a slave), Dionysius encouraged her by reassuring her that no story would be "too much" compared to her beauty: "Impressive though your story be, nothing you can tell us will measure up to you" (*Callirhoe* 2.5.10). Her Odysseus-like plea, however, makes Dionysius revise his judgment and attribute to his beloved beauty of words in addition to beauty of body. The added compliment can be taken as one more analogy with Helen, the persuasive, almost poet-like beauty.[19]

Dionysius is sensitive to the power of Callirhoe's words once again when she, forced by circumstances (she has discovered she is carrying Chaereas' child), reluctantly agrees to marry him. At hearing the happy news, Dionysius, thunderstruck, loses consciousness. When at last he recovers his senses, he still cannot believe the news and urges his servant, who insists that Callirhoe has sent her to talk about marriage, to relate her words with journalistic precision: "Talk about it then ... and tell me her actual words; do not omit or add anything, report exactly what she said" (*Callirhoe* 3.1.5–6). Dionysius' request is not just owing to his disbelief, but also conveys his desire to hear Callirhoe speak, her live words. The servant obliges, for her report is in Callirhoe's own voice: "I want to marry him to keep my family pride and become a mother," she allegedly said, "in order to give my illustrious father a grandson!" These last words "inflamed Dionysius all the more," so much so that, oblivious of his dignity, he runs to Callirhoe's quarters and for a moment even thinks of falling at her feet. It is the news that makes him fly. But to hear it in Callirhoe's "own" words adds speed to his wings (the irony of the scene is that the servant makes up Callirhoe's speech. Though true to her motives, the wording is not hers, the servant cunningly turning Callirhoe's timid and unwilling acceptance of marriage into a passionate expression of pride and honor.)

It is worth noting that the lover enchanted by Callirhoe's voice and words is Dionysius, not Chaereas. About Chaereas we are only told that he fell in love at first sight. This difference seems to be related to a main difference in the configuration of the two lovers' passion: Chaereas is loved in return while Dionysius is not. Whereas sight can be perfectly mutual, hearing cannot: one speaks, one listens. Hearing builds a mutual exchange if both lovers speak and hear in turn, but it can also increase asymmetry in a relationship. This might be one reason why, in the Greek novels at large, the perfect and reciprocal love of the protagonists, ignited by sight, has no use of seductive words. Though the heroine of Xenophon's novel thinks of attracting the lad she loves by speaking as well as by displaying her beauty, she in fact has no need of her moves to kindle desire in her beloved, who already loves her (see below). (The one exception is *Leucippe and Clitophon*, where love apparently flares at first sight for the boy but not for the girl. I say "apparently" because the story's narrator is Clitophon himself, so we cannot know Leucippe's feelings with absolute certainty. Whatever Clitophon's thoughts or knowledge might be, however, to the readers Leucippe seems to develop an erotic interest in him only after he has displayed his oratorical talents, improvising an imaginative essay on the universal power of love, over animals, plants, rivers, stones.) In light of this pattern (see also *Aethiopica* 1.23, where the heroine's words cast a Siren-like spell on an unwanted suitor), Dionysius' keen sensitivity to Callirhoe's auditory charms underscores the one-sidedness of his love, already hinted at in the lack of a mutual gaze that marked their first encounter.

The same is true for Artaxerxes, the king of Persia, the last man to fall in love with Callirhoe. He, too, experiences love in his ears as in his eyes when he recalls, in a sleepless night, Callirhoe's features: in addition to her face and eyes, "her hair, her walk, her voice; the way she entered the courtroom, the way she stood; her manner of speaking, her manner of not speaking; her blushes, her tears" (*Callirhoe* 6.7.1). Earlier on that day, in an attempt to fight against his passion, Artaxerxes had organized a hunting expedition in grand style. Sounds and sights had filled the landscape and everyone's senses; but not his:

> Soon the mountains were full of people shouting and running, dogs barking, horses neighing, game fleeing ... But the King saw no horse, though so many horses were galloping alongside him; no animal, though so many were being pursued; he heard no dog, when so many were barking; no man, though all were shouting. All he could see was Callirhoe—who was not there; he could hear her, though she was not speaking.
>
> *Callirhoe* 6.4.4–5

The sound of Callirhoe's voice enters the king's fantasy. When soon it becomes purely visual (a picture of Callirhoe hunting, her tunic tucked up, her face flushed, and her breasts heaving), it is instigated by another kind of sound: an internal voice, the voice of Eros himself, who "entered the King's thought, saying to him: 'how wonderful it would be to see Callirhoe here' . . ." The King sees by hearing the voice of desire, which guides his imagination.

THE (INDISCREET) CHARM OF RUMORS

The king's fantasy is the product of a subliminal voice, the work of love's whisper. His response to that voice, which invites him to see what is not there, takes me to the power of words to foster love itself. In Greek literature erotic desire finds its way through yet another auditory channel: the rumors heard about a woman's beauty. Cyrus refuses to see Panthea after hearing, or rather, because he hears, a detailed account of her charms:

> And then we had vision of most of her face and vision of her neck and arms. And let me tell you, Cyrus . . . it seemed to me, as it did to all the rest who saw her, that there never was so beautiful a woman of mortal birth in Asia. But . . . you must by all means see her for yourself.
> Xenophon *Cyropaedia* 5.1.7

By clustering verbs of seeing and appearing, this description brings Panthea's beauty before Cyrus' eyes. Cyrus, however, resists the invitation to see the woman because the power of beauty, he knows, cannot be kept at bay. He stops at hearing, aware as he is of the stronger emotional impact of sight.[20] Conversely, the protagonists of several episodes from later literature follow the appeal of the rumor. So for instance do Helen and Achilles in this account: "Though the act of desire lies in the eyes, and poets celebrate desire in song as deriving from this, Achilles and Helen, since they had never seen each other but she was in Egypt, he at Troy, were the first to start desiring each other, finding in the ears the origin of their longing for the body" (Philostratus *Heroicus* 54.4–5). We read a similar story about the Athenian statesman Alcibiades, who, "seized with desire from hearsay, became a lover" (Athenaeus, *Wise Men at Dinner* 13.574e).

Chariton's novel turns the widespread belief in the seductiveness of rumors into a motif to advance its plot. Earlier I mentioned how Callirhoe's beauty has godlike powers when it manifests itself. On a couple of occasions her epiphanies occur after the terrain has been prepared by swift rumor spreading news of her incredible beauty. Each time this happens, however, the physical appearance beats the rumor: Callirhoe is even more beautiful than any report can make her out to be; or, from the perspective of sensory ranking, vision is more effective and accurate than words (see *Callirhoe* 4.1.8; 4.7.5–6). This same assumption, in the variant "sight is the appropriate sense to fall in love," is conveyed more subtly by a pattern in the use of the rumor-motif: though reports of Callirhoe's beauty spark erotic passion by enticing those who hear them into seeing the celebrated woman, Chariton suggests that this is not the right manner of falling in love. For those who actively respond to reports of Callirhoe's beauty do not become "true" lovers, which in turn seems to demonstrate that the ideal channel of love is sight unadulterated by rumors.

Let me start with listing the relevant episodes. Rumors of Callirhoe's divine beauty set the plot in motion while drawing much unwanted attention to her: "report of the astonishing beauty spread everywhere, and suitors flocked to Syracuse" (*Callirhoe* 1.1.2). Soon after Callirhoe is married the second time, to Dionysius, she receives the news that Chaereas, whom she still loves, is dead (which of course is not true). Though the "dead" man's body has disappeared, Dionysius, to try to distract Callirhoe from her grief, offers to build a magnificent cenotaph and to celebrate a magnificent funeral. Two Persian satraps, Mithridates and Pharnaces, attend the ceremony, "ostensibly to show respect to Dionysius, but in fact to see Callirhoe; her reputation was indeed great throughout all Asia, and by now her name had reached the King of Persia and was more celebrated than that of Ariadne or Leda" (*Callirhoe* 4.1.8). Both satraps fall in love with her. Finally it is the king's turn. Pharnaces writes a letter to him to urge action against Mithridates, whom Dionysius has accused of attempting to seduce his wife. The letter's last words are: "his wife's beauty is celebrated, so this outrageous behavior cannot escape notice" (*Callirhoe* 4.6.4). Those words lure the king into asking the woman to Babylon, where he will adjudicate in Dionysius' charge of adultery against Mithridates: "A different sentiment urged him to send for the beautiful woman as well; in his solitary state, wine and darkness played on the King's mind and reminded him of that part of the letter too." The king is particularly obsessed with rumors about feminine beauty. He hears another such rumor and summons the woman also to verify that one, to see if she is the famous Callirhoe or another woman even more beautiful.

> In addition, he was excited by the rumor that someone by the name of Callirhoe was the most beautiful woman in Ionia; the only reproach the King had to make against Pharnaces was that in his letter he had not

added the woman's name. Still, on the chance that another woman might turn out to be even more beautiful than the one so much talked about, he decided to summon the wife as well.

Callirhoe 4.6, 7–8

We know what happens to him when, already goaded by a conspiracy of rumors, he finally sees (and hears) Callirhoe.

Two characters from another novel, *Leucippe and Clitophon*, are even more susceptible to rumors of a woman's beauty than Chaereas' rivals: the extravagant Callisthenes, who falls in love with Leucippe just from hearing of her beauty and asks her in marriage without having caught even a glimpse of her, and the lecherous Thersander, who cannot contain desire for the same woman after his servant rhapsodizes about her beauty. When asked to "listen as if he were seeing" the girl, Thersander does indeed, for the praise fills him "with a kind of vision of beauty, a natural beauty."[21]

The narrator depicts both Callisthenes and Thersander as reckless and intemperate: Callisthenes is a profligate, and eventually plans to kidnap the girl he loves (but gets the wrong one); Thersander, the chief villain in the novel, has been a sex-addict in his youth and a slanderer ever since. Their way of falling in love, through the wrong sensory organ, is an aspect of their intemperance (for Callisthenes, see Morales 2004: 88). Socrates apparently would have reprimanded these two lovers-through-the-ears, for "when someone remarked that she [a courtesan] was very beautiful and had a breast beyond the power of any tongue to describe, he said: 'We must go to see the woman, for it is not possible to judge her beauty by hearsay'" (Athenaeus *Wise Men at Dinner* 13.588d).

Chariton's novel, I would propose, goes further than Achilles Tatius' in stigmatizing hearsay as a source of erotic love. Contrary to Callisthenes or Thersander, the characters who are enticed by rumors about Callirhoe's beauty do not fall in love with her *just* from hearsay, but only once they have *seen* her. And yet, though sight dutifully follows hearing as the proper sensory medium to fall in love, Chariton suggests that hearing should be dispensed with altogether, that true love needs no such foregrounding in rumor. This requirement can be drawn from the distribution of the episodes. For who responds to the rumors? Not Chaereas, not even Dionysius, but characters whom love forces to commit immoral deeds and who love imperfectly, when they love at all.

The royal suitors rest content with sheer rumors. Like Callisthenes, they are eager to marry the beautiful woman they hear praised without even needing to see her. But do they love? There is no mention of any such passion. More likely they aspire to marry the celebrated beauty because she is the daughter of a powerful leader and as a "trophy wife," to add veneer to their own power. And their failure to obtain her causes them to scheme against her marriage, which they ruin, if not for good, then for some years.

As to Mithridates and Pharnaces, their passion likewise leads them to vile thoughts and actions. Mithridates ostensibly offers to help Chaereas to recover his wife, but his hidden motive is the hope to antagonize the two husbands and profit from the situation to get the woman himself. When he is charged with attempted adultery, his first thought is to attack Dionysius and kidnap Callirhoe. Pharnaces is a paler figure, almost a figurant, but he also acts dishonestly to further his passion: it is for its sake that he agrees to take Dionysius' side against Mithridates and writes to the king. Artaxerxes is a more complex and sympathetic character. He does not wish to rape Callirhoe and respects the laws against adultery he has himself put in place. He initially does not take advantage of his power to act like a tyrant. Yet, as his passion grows fiercer, he puts more and more pressure on Callirhoe and she is saved only by the providential outbreak of a war. Furthermore, his passion might be better termed lust than love (*erôs* is notoriously ambiguous), because he makes it clear that he is not thinking of marrying her but only of enjoying her body. None of these "lovers" originally sensitive to rumors of Callirhoe's beauty love with the devotion of Chaereas or Dionysius (see *Callirhoe* 4.4.1; 4.7.1–2; 4.6.2; 6.7.7).

But is not Dionysius also susceptible to praise of Callirhoe? He also hears of her beauty before seeing her, though in his case the interplay of the two senses is subtler. First he has—sees (*eidon*)—a dream in which his dead wife (Dionysius has been recently widowed) appears taller and more beautiful. They are celebrating their marriage, with his servant singing the wedding song. As he reports the dream to the same servant, the latter exclaims: "you will hear what you have seen," with an intriguing reversal of the normal epistemological pattern, according to which sight is asked to confirm hearing as a more compelling and reliable sense. The servant means that Dionysius will hear from him how he bought a very beautiful woman, which narrative will prove Dionysius' dream (his vision) to correspond to the truth. Dionysius rejoices at "hearing" (*êkouse*) of the woman's beauty but is reluctant to believe what he hears, because "a person not freeborn cannot be beautiful" (*Callirhoe* 2.1.2–5). She will have appeared beautiful compared to peasant women, that's all. Rumors of Callirhoe's beauty multiply, however. The maidservants who bathe her and discover her secret parts and the gleam and delicacy of her skin whisper to each other: "Our mistress was beautiful, and celebrated for it; but she would have looked like this woman's maidservant" (*Callirhoe* 2.2.3). The comment pains Callirhoe: "it was ominous." Does Dionysius hear report of the bath scene? We cannot tell. But if he does, he shows no eagerness to take a look at the rumored beauty. Shortly after the bath episode Dionysius' servant tries to entice him into going to his country estate, where Callirhoe is staying, and mentions the woman casually and last, with the obvious goal of tickling his master's curiosity: "And if you are pleased with some herdsman or shepherd, you can give him the woman I just bought" (*Callirhoe* 2.3.2). But Dionysius, at least ostensibly, does not bite on the hint and makes no reference to the woman anymore. When he finally sees her, he seems as unprepared as Chaereas was at his first encounter with the same woman. At any rate, even supposing that Dionysius is enticed by the words he hears, he does not act on the enticement.

Chaereas is even less contaminated by words when he falls in love. Curiously, he who lives next door, in the same town as Callirhoe, does not seem to have heard at all of the girl's beauty in spite of the far-reaching rumors. When the two meet, he sees her only with his eyes as she sees him with hers. This is not true of every novelistic pair. Though the hero and heroine fall in love at first sight, in one case they do not come to their first encounter unprepared but are already eager to see each other. Anthia and Habrocomes, the protagonists of Xenophon's novel, are taking part in a grand procession in honor of Artemis when all the watchers take to admiring and loudly praising their incomparable beauty. And "Already some added, 'What a match Habrocomes and Anthia would make!'" The youngsters hear praises of each other and respond to them: "They quickly learned each other's reputation. Anthia longed to see Habrocomes; and Habrocomes, up to now impervious to love, wanted to see Anthia" (*An Ephesian Story* 1.2.9). The encounter is an intensely sensual experience, for the eyes but also, to a lesser degree, the ears:

> he kept looking at the girl ... could not take his eyes off her ... Anthia ... let his appearance sink in, with rapt attention and eyes wide open; and already she paid no attention to modesty: what she said was for Habrocomes to hear, and she revealed what she could of her body for Habrocomes to see. And he was captivated at the sight and was a prisoner of the god.
>
> *An Ephesian Story* 1.3.1–2

Habrocomes and Anthia are not as naïve as Chaereas and Callirhoe. Anthia might even have come to the procession ready for a romantic encounter, for all the girls taking part in it are dressed "as if to receive a lover." Her daring in exposing her charms and in attracting attention even by words (which, though not addressed to Habrocomes directly, are meant for him) is unusual for the novels' standard. Novelistic heroines, when they fall in love, do not seek to enhance their desirability before their loved one by either gestures or words. The relative "immodesty" of this scene is in keeping with the protagonists' eagerness to see each other, which was kindled by the rumors they heard of each other's beauty.

Chariton's novel, in contrast, wants the protagonist's passion to be immediate and uncontrived, clear of external means of enticement, among which rumors are a major one, and instead relegates such means to less deserving lovers: and, I will now add, to non-Greeks. Except for the Italian suitors who compete for Callirhoe's hand at the beginning (and who, however, are neither lovers nor even individualized characters), those who follow the voice of rumors and subsequently fall in love with her are all Persians. This might suggest that, in the thought-world of Chariton's novel, to be erotically excited by mentions or descriptions of a woman's beauty is at odds with Greek values. Dionysius' behavior further supports this line of reasoning. For, as we have seen, he does not act on the praise he hears, or rather, he doubts it. As the most civilized (*pepaideumenos*) character in the novel, the worshipper of moderation and self-control, Dionysius is the best representative of Greek aristocratic ideals, and, no matter how much a "lover of women" he is (*Callirhoe* 2.1.5), he does not let himself be carried away by rumors of a woman's beauty.

The male protagonist himself, however, risks behaving like those "bad" (or non-Greek) lovers in the climactic sequence that prepares for his reunion with Callirhoe. Though the text is lacunose, it is clear that Chaereas becomes curious to see the allegedly beautiful woman who will turn out to be his wife, but of whom he only knows that she is a prisoner of war. Let me give a little context. Cheareas has become the successful admiral of the Egyptians in a war waged against the Persians, and has captured the Persian retinue, which includes Callirhoe. An Egyptian soldier reports to him that among the prisoners is an extraordinarily beautiful woman. Chaereas sends the Egyptian for her, but in spite of his promises, including marriage with the victorious admiral, the woman refuses to follow him. At hearing of her refusal Chaereas reproaches the Egyptian for not having used persuasion but force. As the other protests, claiming that he has "done everything [Chaereas] said" and has even gone further, by proposing marriage, but that the stranger has forcefully rejected every advance, Chaereas decides to abstain from further attempts because "she seems a woman of dignity. No one is to offer her violence; let her do as she pleases; self-respect deserves my respect. Perhaps she is mourning a husband herself" (*Callirhoe* 7.6.10–12).

Chaereas seems to have developed into a worldly connoisseur of women, who masters the standard verbal techniques of seduction ("flatter the woman and make her feel she is loved," reads his recommendation to the Egyptian). He also seems to have opened his heart to the possibility of a romantic affair (if not marriage), and this *just by hearing* of the stranger's beauty. But Chariton does not want to sully the purity of his protagonist's manner of loving and blocks the way traced by the words that seduced him. The novelist needs the couple to be reunited, but does not want the reunion to happen in this way, by having Chaereas try again to entice the woman subsequent to the rumor that enticed him. Instead, the generally impulsive and overly emotional Chaereas now displays a level of moderation (*sôphrosynê*) worthy of Dionysius.

The reunion of the lovers will happen in another way—and in a way most effective to counter Chaereas' worldly attempts at seduction and the enticement kindled in him by rumors. As he is walking by the quarters where the Persian women are kept, the Egyptian tries again to push him to meet the beautiful stranger: "perhaps you can persuade her (*peiseis*) to get up—why leave behind the choicest of the spoils?" Urged also by his best friend, at last Chaereas goes in.

> When he saw her stretched out on the ground with her head covered, he felt his heart stirred at once by the way she breathed and the look of her, and felt a thrill of excitement; he would certainly have recognized her had he not been thoroughly convinced that Dionysius had taken Callirhoe for himself. He went up to her quietly. "Don't be frightened, lady," he said, "whoever you are. We are not going to use force on you. You shall have the husband you want." Before he had finished speaking, Callirhoe recognized his voice and threw the covering from her face. They both cried out at the same time: "Chaereas!", "Callirhoe!"
>
> *Callirhoe* 8.1.6–8

Instead of *peithô*, persuasive words forged to obtain a woman whom sheer reports have made desirable, Chaereas applies a lover's instinct and "feels" his wife before talking to her. To the immediacy of his intuition responds the immediacy of the recognition, triggered by his voice alone (on voice and recognition, see Montiglio 2013: 16–30). The voice of love (in a metaphorical sense) and a loved voice (in the literal one) have replaced the contrivances of rhetorical persuasion and made the reader forget that Chaereas might have never recovered Callirhoe if he had not been initially instigated by report of a woman's beauty.

CONCLUSIONS

Like the other Greek novelists, Chariton privileges sight in erotic contexts. In endorsing sight as the channel of love he goes even further than his fellow novelists, by severing true love from the influence of rumors. While the hero and the heroine of Xenophon's *Ephesian Story* hear about each other's beauty before they meet, Chariton's protagonists come to the first encounter unprepared. True love is a visual shock.

At the same time, however, Chariton is uniquely sensitized to vocal charms. If he joins the other novelists, with the exception of Longus, in downplaying the eroticism of the "lower" senses, smell and touch, he alone underscores the power of the heroine's voice to ignite love. At least Dionysius would apply to his experience of love the opening words of the Irish song I quoted earlier in this chapter: "When first I saw you, I saw beauty . . . when first I heard you, I heard sweetness . . ."

CHAPTER EIGHT

Art and the Senses: The Artistry of Bodies, Stages, and Cities in the Greco-Roman World

MARK BRADLEY

INTRODUCTION

In the early third century, the sophist Philostratus produced the *Imagines*, a set of creative descriptions of paintings of mythical figures, events and landscapes which he had encountered set into panels in a seafront portico in his lodgings at Naples. Typically, Philostratus' imaginative ekphrasis aimed to out-perform the painter himself in bringing his subjects to life, but his *Imagines* offer us a glimpse of the multi-sensory aesthetics that could be deployed in the description, appreciation, and evaluation of ancient art. *Imagines* 1.2 describes a painting of personified Revelry, in drunken slumber outside a wedding party: he is flushed (*eruthros*) with wine, leaning away from the heat of the torch in his hand, wearing a crown of roses that are at the same time tender, delicate, dewy, and fragrant (*meta tēs osmēs*), while music, singing, and cheering emanate from the revelry within. "Does the noise of the castanets, flutes and disorderly singing not strike you?", Philostratus asks his companion, who is also observing the painting. He goes on to describe the rose-crowns of the revelers which are no longer fresh, but crushed and withered under the touch, and hands about to clap and create additional din. *Imagines* 1.2 integrates sight, sound, smell, and touch in its efforts to animate the spectacle of the painting. Elsewhere, he describes the fragrance evoked by a painting of Cupids gathering apples and enjoying their color, taste, and touch (1.6), a cold, wet marsh with songbirds (1.9), the young Olympus with dry, fluffy hair playing his flute and gazing at his rippling reflection (1.22), and a tasty scene of fruits, honey, and cheese with sweet purple figs dripping with juice and disgorging their honey, and fragrant golden apples and pears, and grapes that are "good enough to eat and infused with wine" (1.31). At 2.26 a painting of gifts laid out for guests becomes a multi-sensory scene that mobilizes sight, taste (herbs and spices, sweet figs), touch ("it is not necessary to test the ducks' breasts by pinching them," prickly chestnuts, etc.), and smell ("the master of the farm . . . might smell of pressed grapes and of relaxation and might belch in the faces of the urban crowd"). By creatively deploying the senses in this way, Philostratus effectively collapses the distinction between art and reality: the expert artist (and the expert describer of art) can break beyond the boundaries of a single sense, shape and control the sensations experienced by the consumer, and bring his subject to life (recently on Philostratus, see Bowie and Elsner 2009, esp. Chapters 14–16; see also Costantini *et al.* 2006).

Philostratus was of course building on an old and competitive literary tradition of ekphrasis already established by epic poets like Homer and Vergil, as well as dramatists like Euripides and rhetoricians such as Dionysius of Halicarnassus, and the genre had also been developed with great sophistication by the sophist and polymath Lucian (for an excellent recent study of ancient ekphrasis, see Squire 2009; see also Montiglio in this volume). Of course it would be wrong to assume that ancient viewers all achieved this level of synaesthetic sophistication in their appreciation of visual arts, and poets and sophists alike set out above all to demonstrate their outstanding rhetorical skills in describing works of art. However, Philostratus' ekphrasis demonstrates three key points about aspects of ancient art appreciation: (1) the significance of *mimesis* or real-life imitation in producing art; (2) the development of a highly-educated symposiastic elite discourse committed to describing, evaluating, and animating those works of art; (3) the central role of the senses in achieving that animation. Not only sight, but also sound, smell, taste, and touch could be mobilized for the full appreciation of ancient art (even, as Philostratus shows us, art that was exclusively visual in nature).

Greco-Roman art has traditionally been characterized by distance and intangibility: cold blocks of marble admired from afar and representing the aesthetics of a bygone age, colorless figures on white backgrounds, inaudible black-and-white words on a page conjuring up ancient stagecraft, impenetrable musical traditions, or lifeless architectural landscapes. Moreover, this distance has been dominated by the art of vision: things seen, but not heard, smelled, touched, or tasted. But it is becoming increasingly clear that the arts of the Greco-Roman world engaged participants in a rich multi-sensory experience: classical statues were garishly painted, touched as well as seen; ancient clothes and cosmetics carried not only diverse colors but also striking aromatics and textures; stage plays made use of color-coded masks, musical choruses, dancers, fragrances; public spaces resounded with performances and recitals, and were animated with incense, flowing water, and cool, shaded colonnades. By scrutinizing the aesthetics of art—sculpture, handicrafts, drama, urban architecture—in the Greek and Roman world, this chapter seeks to break beyond the visual paradigm and reinstate the diverse role of the senses in the artistic experiences of classical antiquity.[1] To do this, it will examine a rich and varied corpus of material engaging with the arts in Greco-Roman antiquity: visual, archaeological, literary, and philosophical. As a starting point, it will examine the ancient artifacts themselves—what remains of statues, theaters, cosmetics and so on—to consider how we might approach an archaeology of the senses. But, as Philostratus has demonstrated, it is not enough simply to recreate and re-enact ancient sensory experiences: by examining the traditions of ancient ekphrasis, this chapter will also explore how the ancients themselves deployed their own eyes, ears, noses, tongues, and fingers in order to make sense of the art around them.

The chapter will approach this complex historical challenge by examining four key genres of ancient art. It will begin by revisiting Greco-Roman sculpture and, in the light of recent research, will reconsider the role of polychromy as part of the aesthetics of ancient statuary, as well as classical traditions and myths about animated, tactile, tangible sculpture. It will then consider the significance of the artistry applied to the real-life human body and the role of clothing, cosmetics, and perfumes in shaping, distinguishing and evaluating the identities of groups and individuals in the ancient world. It will then move on to the realm of performance and explore the multi-sensory aesthetics of ancient drama and music. Finally, the chapter will extend outwards to ask the same questions about public space and architecture more broadly within the ancient city, and explore the interplay between sight, sound, smell, and other sensory experiences in Greek and Roman life. By engaging with these four domains of ancient art, this chapter will argue not only that the arts were driven by sensory considerations, but that art itself played a formative role in shaping and packaging the ancient sensorium.

PAINTED STATUES

Perhaps a generation after Philostratus and in imitation of his *Imagines*, the sophist Callistratus compiled his *Descriptions*, a collection of fourteen short essays in Greek describing an array of contemporary statues. Like Philostratus, he aimed to blur the distinction between art and life by employing all his sophistic skills to portray masterful works of sculpture. Often his statues are about to spring to life: a satyr standing *contrapposto*, poised to leap up at the sound of the flute (1); Orpheus' hair, so luxuriant and instilled with the spirit of life that it deceived the senses into thinking it was being tossed and shaken in the wind (7); or a statue of a Bacchante so lifelike that "art carried imitation over into reality"—"so manifest upon it were the signs of sense perception (*aisthēsis*)" (2). Even the artifacts themselves sensed the world around them, as well as being the object of others' multi-sensory experiences. Appreciating sculpture was about much more than just viewing—the animation of skillfully sculpted statues was most evocatively expressed through the sense of touch: a bronze Eros which seemed to lose its hardness and become marvelously delicate, with hair that "yielded as though it was softened to the touch" (3); a marble Narcissus where the stone "became supple and malleable and delivered forth a body at variance quite different from its own essence," yielding the sensation of softness in spite of its hard nature (5); and Praxiteles' Dionysus, so delicate that the bronze was transformed into flesh and "would yield to the tips of the fingers when you touched it" (8). Some statues even appeared to speak, such as a stone Memnon (9), which conveyed the illusion of shedding tears and harbored the power of both speech and sense perception in spite of its inanimate nature. And an extraordinary bronze Orpheus with an exquisite lyre crafted just like the real thing, "obediently extending the deceit" and reproducing the sound of the notes, surrounded by bronze animals whose own sense perceptions were enchanted by their love of music (7).

Of course, Callistratus' descriptions were, like those of Philostratus before him, largely the stuff of fantasy, creative exercises that tested the limits of art appreciation, and auditory, tactile, and other non-visual encounters with sculpture were no doubt largely confined to the connoisseur's imagination. However, Callistratus' creative ekphrasis also exposes a very real phenomenon of classical sculpture that is largely lost to us through the passage of time: the subtle use of pigments and colorations to express realism that are now all but lost on figural sculpture. Callistratus alludes to the chromatic possibilities: a statue of an Indian in "marble verging on black and shifting of its own accord to the color given by nature to his race," with woolly black hair whose tips glistened with colors resembling Tyrian purple dye to reproduce its moisture (4); Dionysus' bronze thyrsus, no doubt permitted some natural erosion, glistened with the greenness of young growth (8); and the youthful Diadoumenos had his bronze cheeks imbued with a boyish blush ("a ruddiness born of the bronze"). In all these cases, Callistratus was reflecting on a genuine artistic preoccupation with chromatic subtlety that was intended to lull the senses into believing that the subject was living and breathing, and participated in the world for which it was created.

Recent research has demonstrated that the material chosen for classical sculpture was often selected for its inherent color and associations, and appropriated to suit the character and themes of the subject matter: white marble representing the pale "Venus in Bikini" in Pompeii; silver alloys used to evoke the pallid flesh of figures that were dying; bronze used to depict the tanned flesh of warriors, nude gods, and athletes; and so on. Imperial Rome made extensive use of polychrome marbles to reproduce colors appropriate to the figures: "purple" Egyptian porphyry employed for imperial statues and veined purple Phrygian marble used to represent the flowing drapery of eastern barbarians; yellow Numidian marble for a striking first-century lion in the Vatican Museum; black marbles to depict African subjects; red Docimian for statues of the flayed Marsyas. Even different types of white marble could be employed for different effects, such as translucent Parian *lychnites*, which made prestigious pieces like the Prima Porta statue of the deified Augustus (see Figure 8.3a) glow through their thinner sections (for discussion and references, see Bradley 2006).

But it is in the use of applied pigments, patinas, glazes, varnishes, gilding, and other accoutrements that the sculptor's exploitation of the senses is most evident. It is now generally accepted that most—if not all—Greek and Roman marble statuary and relief sculpture, following Egyptian and Near-Eastern precedents, received some form of supplementary coating to modify and enhance its appearance. Key facial features like eyes, hair, and lips were particularly highlighted to draw the viewer's attention to them, and drapery and accoutrements were also often picked out in different colors, sometimes with innovative metal attachments to reproduce jewelry, weapons and the like. Other sculptural materials were also often intricately colored: painted terracotta survives en masse, and sculpture in limestone, sandstone or other volcanic stones was typically covered with painted plaster or stucco, and it is likely that wooden sculpture was colored and embellished in its entirety. Chryselephantine statuary was striking in its polychromy, and even bronze statuary, as we have seen above, could have its surfaces variegated using different blends of alloys, gilding, inlays, darkened hair, painted eyes, silver-plated teeth and fingernails, and so on: a striking Hellenistic bronze statue of a bruised and battered seated boxer at the Palazzo Massimo in Rome, for example, employs complex variegated alloys to differentiate features of the body (including a dark bruise under his right eye), and utilizes copper inlays in channels and grooves across his body, as well as across the straps and stitching of his boxing gloves, to produce the effect of dripping blood and bruising after his fight (see Figure 8.1). The eyes (now lost) were probably inset with glass or stone to appear as lifelike as possible. In addition, the statue shows signs of wearing on its hands and right foot, evidence that it was frequently touched for inspiration by passers-by in the Baths of Constantine where it was probably set up (see Bradley 2009b: 441 for further details).

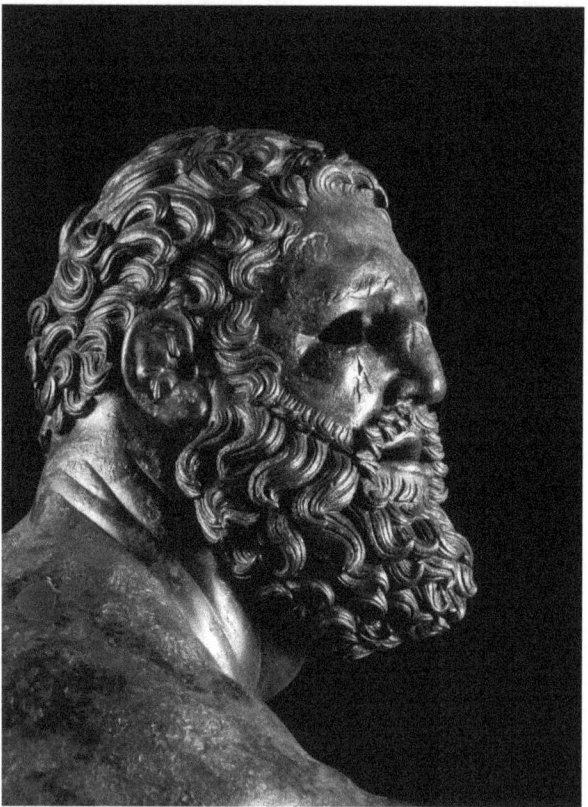

FIGURE 8.1: Bronze seated boxer, detail of face. Hellenistic period, late fourth–second century BCE. Bronze inlaid with copper, H. 128 cm. Museo Nazionale Romano—Palazzo Massimo alle Terme, inv. 1055. Image courtesy of Soprintendenza Speciale per i Beni Archeologici di Roma.

The catalog of marble sculpture with extant traces of color is now extensive, and growing, thanks to various projects, collaborations, and exhibitions across the last decade or so dedicated to identifying and reconstructing pigment traces on classical sculpture. Archaic sculpture, it has long been recognized, received particularly bold treatments of color, perhaps to underwrite the supernatural character of the figures typically represented: examples such as the Peplos Kore, vividly reconstructed in the Museum of Classical Archaeology at Cambridge, and the frieze of the Siphnian Treasury at Delphi (c. 525 BCE), retain highly visible traces of paint. A wide array of Greek sculpture from the classical period continued to be colored in varied and sophisticated ways: the Temple of Aphaia at Aegina, the buildings and sculpture of the Athenian Akropolis, the pedimental sculptures of the Temple of Zeus at Olympia, and the Mausoleum of Halicarnassus are just a few examples where research into polychromy has been carried out. The classical period was evidently marked by a more subtle and realistic use of polychromy, so that sculpted figures seemed to populate the world of the living and beguile the senses into thinking that they were real: the so-called "Alexander Sarcophagus" in the Istanbul Archaeological Museum, for example, is considered to mark a turning point in the sophistication of sculptural polychromy (see Figure 8.2).[2]

Hellenistic and Roman sculptural polychromy has been the subject of less research, but it is evident that color was applied in wide-ranging and versatile ways, especially for cult statues, garden sculpture, and portraits: a portrait of Caligula at the Copenhagen Glyptotek with a tempera technique applied to the skin and painted in its entirety; a delicately colored Amazon from Herculaneum; elaborately colored tauroctony reliefs with Mithras' face sometimes gilded as he stares back at the sun; and so on. Some artifacts, like Trajan's Column, were evidently colored to make the detail on the frieze more legible (and to pick out the emperor in his distinctive purple or red outfit). The Prima Porta statue of Augustus, on which extensive paint traces remain, has been the subject of particular scrutiny: discovered in 1863 and still retaining traces of paint across its body, it has recently been reconstructed as a painted plaster cast (see Figures 8.3a, b). This reconstruction, garish though it may seem to some, gives us a clue as to how color could transform ancient sculpture: here, the larger-than-life and brighter-than-life deified emperor was brought to life, key parts of his body picked out in bold and expensive colors such as red cinnabar and Egyptian blue; he continued to participate in the world of the living but at the same time was detached from it by his godlike appearance. What is less evident in this reconstruction is the sophistication of the finishes applied to marble

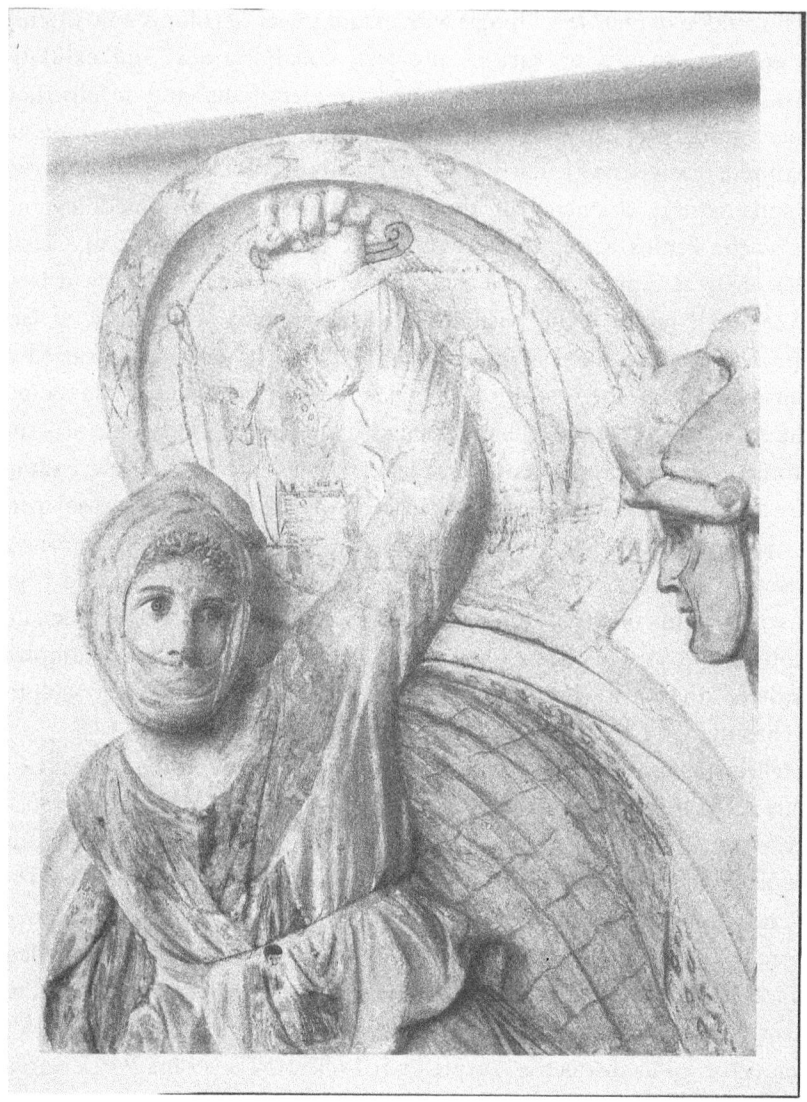

FIGURE 8.2: Detail from the color rendering of the "Alexander Sarcophagus," showing sophisticated and realistic uses of color to depict the figure of a Persian fighter. Image: F. Winter, *Der Alexandersarkophag aus Sidon*, 1912, Strassburg.

surfaces: artists made the most of the underlying marble (in this case, large-grained translucent Parian) so that particular features could be distinguished and characterized, and alongside various treatments and layers, pigments such as cinnabar penetrated the surface of the stone, allowing the artist to "suffuse" certain colors, such as the blush of cheeks (for discussion on the painted Prima

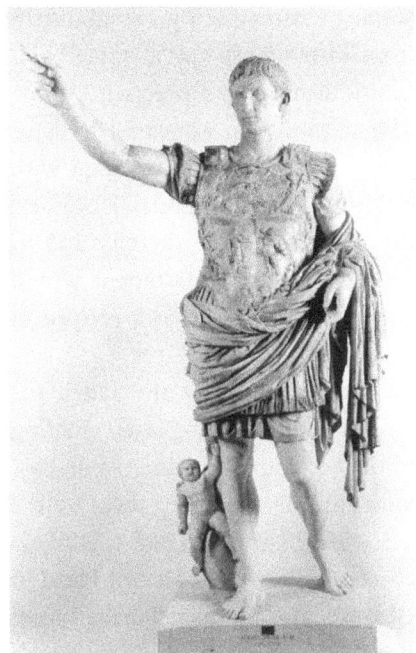 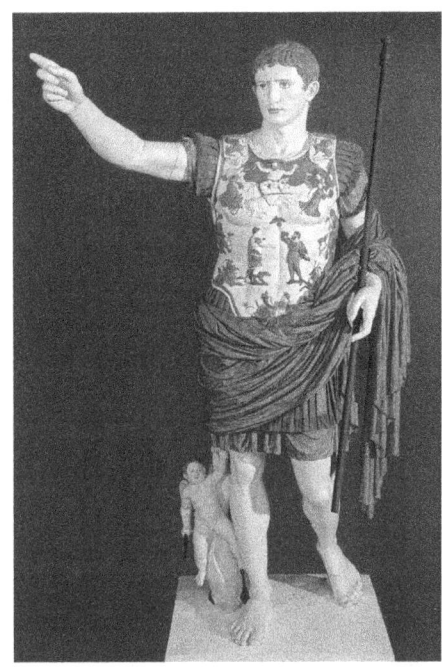

FIGURE 8.3a (left): The Prima Porta statue of Augustus, c. 15 CE. Parian marble, height 204 cm. Rome: Vatican Museums (inv. 2290). Photo: Michael Squire; 8.3b (right): The painted plaster reconstruction of the Prima Porta Augustus, 2002–3. Rome: Vatican Museums (inv. 36858). Photo: Vatican Museums.

Porta, see Bradley 2009b: 447–50; for an excellent recent study of the statue, see Squire 2013).

This idea of employing pigments to "finish" sculpture is evident throughout ancient ekphrasis: Euripides, Pliny, and Lucian, to take three examples, all comment on the significance of color for embellishing and completing statues (Euripides *Helen* 262–3; Pliny *Natural History* 35.133; Lucian *Imagines* 7–8). Finally, and perhaps most significantly, color allowed the artist to bring an otherwise monochrome figure, with white skin, hair and eyes, to life and so produce "living images" (Greek *zōa* or Latin *spirantia signa*): this, as we have seen, was the principal emphasis of Callistratus' *Descriptions*, and a section of Plato's *Republic* (4.420C) draws attention to the controlled and sober use of "correct" pigments on statues for accurate imitation. The result, it has been suggested, had more in common with the lifelike figures of a waxwork museum than the distant monochrome sculptures we experience today, and scholars sometimes speak of a *trompe l'oeil* effect that tricked the eyes of observers and passers-by, obscuring the line between art and reality. Pompeian wall paintings are littered with examples of scenes containing statuesque figures about to spring to life, or protagonists in painted scenes (often poised on a statue base) who might be either stone or flesh. This illusionism hinged precisely on the creative employment of the senses, and the statue often appeared to have sensory powers of its own, gazing back at the viewer and ready to engage with the figures around it. This idea was particularly important for cult statues, which were sometimes thought to embody the spirit of the divinity and to represent the god in shrines and temples (and which worshipers would sometimes touch for inspiration: see Introduction, p. 8), so that a reciprocal sensory relationship could be developed between object and viewer.

This artistic skill was not restricted to the visual. Pliny the Elder, for example, describes (*Natural History* 36.177) a milk-saffron plaster coating (*tectorium*) long ago applied to the surface of the temple of Minerva at Elis, which when visitors wetted their thumbs with saliva and rubbed them on the surface gave off the smell (*odor*) and taste (*sapor*) of saffron, and it is likely that some forms of sculpture, especially cult statues like the statue of Flora in Rome, were perfumed or garlanded with flowers and the like. Furthermore, touch was fundamental to statuary: the "finishing" processes applied to both relief sculpture and sculpture in-the-round involved a level of smoothing and polishing that has only recently started to be acknowledged, and it is clear that the application of complex encaustic layers of varnishes, patinas, glazes, sheens, waxes, preservatives, highlights, and metal attachments transformed both visual and tactile encounters with the artifacts (I discuss several aspects of sculptural finishing in Bradley 2006: 16–18 and Bradley 2009b: 436–40). Cult statues were regularly subjected to Greco-Roman fingertips, and in addition, the sensuality of classical sculpture has long been recognized: Pliny the Elder's story of Praxiteles' cult statue of Aphrodite of Knidos with its telltale semen stain is just the tip of the iceberg. The playful ambivalence between the statue and the living figure represented by the statue was a familiar literary topos across antiquity: Daedalus and Pygmalion are two examples of master sculptors so skilled that they could bring their subjects to life. The latter famously falls in love with an ivory statue of a woman that he has made, which Aphrodite then turns to flesh. In the nineteenth century, the French painter Jean-Léon Gérôme depicted Pygmalion in his artist's workshop, embracing the statue as it comes to life, develops a rosy hue across its skin and dark hair, and begins touching and kissing him back (see Figure 8.4), while a statuesque Cupid fires an arrow toward the besotted sculptor, and other artifacts populate the background. In fact the statue's metamorphosis from lifeless white marble to pink flesh in Gérôme's painting is something of a red herring: it is evident that

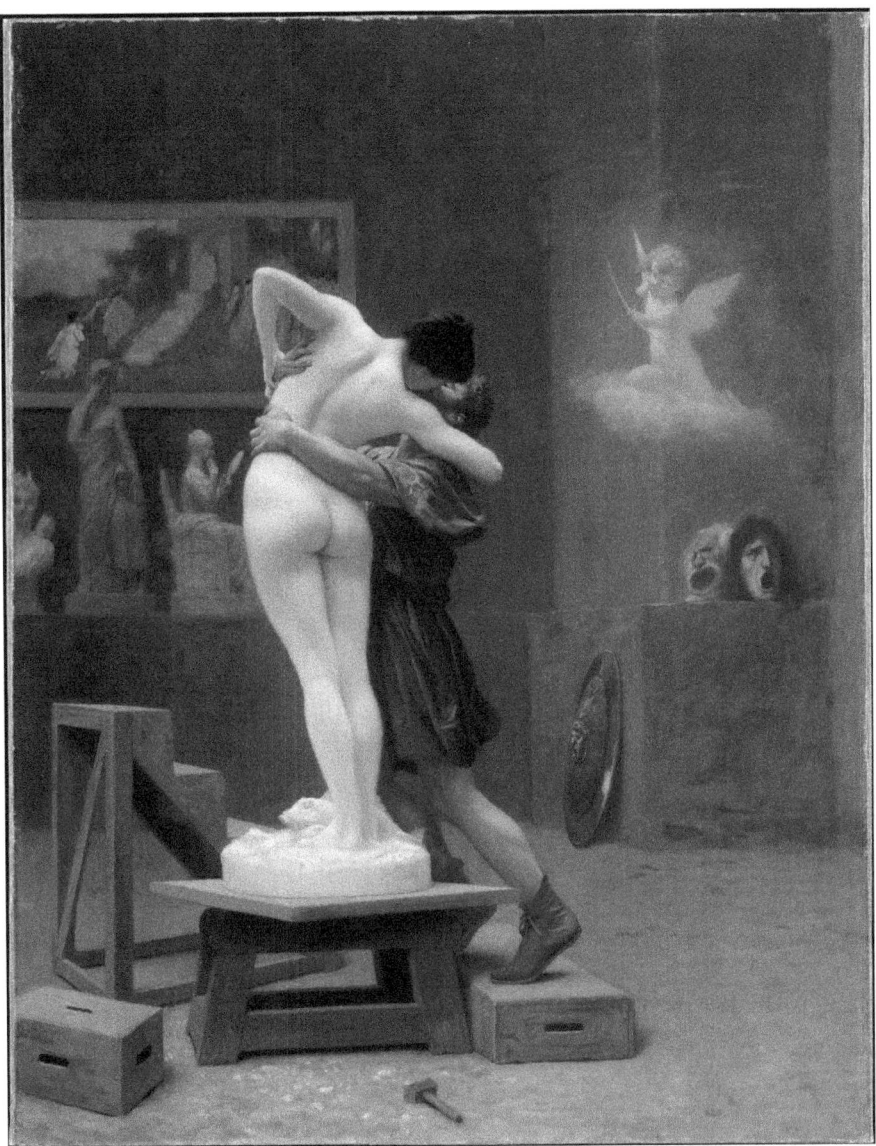

FIGURE 8.4: Jean-Léon Gérôme, *Pygmalion and Galatea* (1890). Oil on canvas, 68.6 × 88.9 cm. Metropolitan Museum of Art, New York.

the finest pieces of classical sculpture were designed from the outset to appear as lifelike as possible and captivate the senses of those who encountered them (see Ovid *Metamorphoses* 10.243–97 on Pygmalion; Pliny *Natural History* 36.21 on the stained Aphrodite; on the Pygmalion story, see Elsner 2007: 113–31).

ADORNING THE BODY

If the sculpted body mobilized complex and intense sensory experiences, the real, live classical body was no less an artifact that was subject to distortion, manipulation, and sensory modification. Bodies were naturally endowed with sensory cues: a person's skin, hair, and eye color were typical telltale signs of origin, race, behavior, character, and profession, and complex physiognomic doctrines were developed to interpret these visual signs, which became an art form in itself.

A late first-century BCE fresco from the Villa Farnesina in Rome (see Figure 8.5) shows a female figure, dressed in an elegant semi-transparent purple-tinted dress and a delicate yellow headdress around her carefully styled hair, wearing bracelets and earrings and intricately designed sandals, pouring perfume into a phial—an idealized painting setting a base standard for female adornment in a house where the womenfolk were probably expected to follow suit (see Mols and Moormann 2008: 46–50). In surrounding rooms, other frescos showed women in acts of worship or ritual, as well as goddesses and erotic scenes: a varied cameo of idealized female activity in an elite Roman *domus*. This colorful piece of domestic wall art itself toys with the viewer's senses, mirroring (or prescribing) female activities within the house itself, simultaneously clothing and revealing flesh, and promising scent but delivering none, instead relying on the actual aromas present within the house to complete the promise.

The art of the body was a subject of great interest, particularly in Hellenistic and Roman elite circles. Greek *kosmēsis* and Latin *cultus*, cultivation of the body, were well-established and much-debated activities that sometimes employed great artistry in manipulating the appearance, smell, and feel of the body in order to achieve a desired effect—exhibiting political status, appearing refined and urbane, seducing a partner, and so on. This activity, the *ars ornatrix*, was an established Hellenistic and Roman literary genre in its own right, frequently connected with female concealment, trickery, and seduction.[3] Skin color could be manipulated by activities such as tanning, which satirists like Martial derided (*Epigram* 10.12), but perhaps the most controversial form of *cultus*, and the subject of a large number of Hellenistic and Roman treatises and poems, was the use of cosmetics, particularly by women. Make-up added a fake layer of skin to the face, generated false beauty, and beguiled male viewers. Rouge could make shameless women look like they were blushing, and white lead could make others look like they were chaste indoor types (on complexions and feminine behavior, see Stewart 2007: 89–92). Ovid, suggesting cures for lovesickness (*Remedia Amoris*), advises his readers (lines 343–56):

"We are carried away by the art of adornment (*cultus*); everything is covered by gems and gold: the real girl is the least bit of herself"; the solution—"visit your mistress early in the morning and catch her in the act of smearing the concocted poisons (*composita venena*) on her face, and behold the pots of

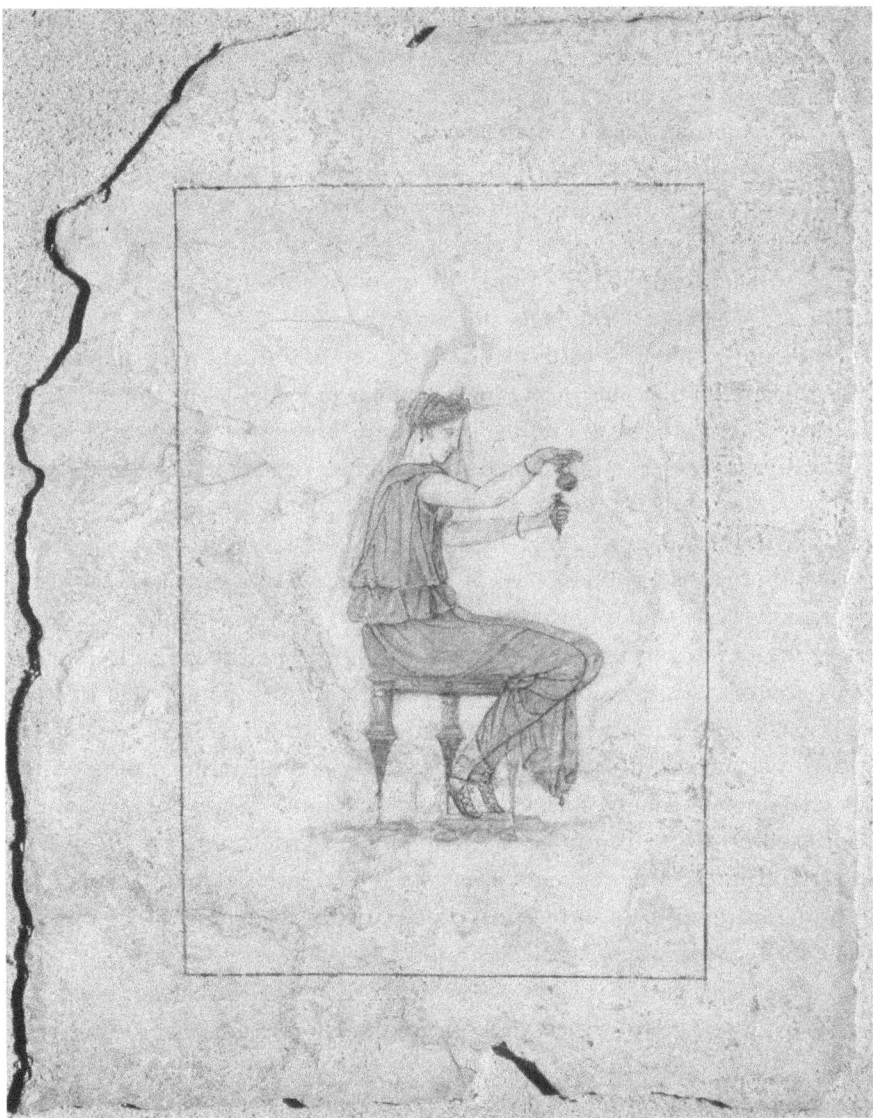

FIGURE 8.5: Fresco showing a woman pouring perfume, Villa Farnesina, Rome, late first century BCE. Museo Nazionale Romano, Terme di Diocleziano. Photo: Mark Bradley.

make-up in a thousand colors, and lanoline grease that has run down her sweaty cleavage, drugs that reek and stir your stomach to nausea."

Applying make-up was an art, but so was seeing through it, and Ovid's description is one that evokes the visible, the olfactory and the tangible. Elsewhere, Ovid extols the virtues of *cultus*: the "Art of lovemaking" (*Ars Amatoria*) and the "Cosmetics for the Female Face" (*Medicamina Faciei Femineae*) are two poems in which the *ars ornatrix* is presented as an effective and desirable art form. The latter poem provides an eloquent justification of *cultus* (in all its forms), before presenting a list of—sometimes revolting—recipes for adorning the face, designed to improve not just the *color* of the skin, but also to make it soft (*mollis*) and smooth (*levis*), and to imbue it with the various scents of myrrh, fennel, rose petals, honey, and the like. There were some extreme cases: Pliny the Elder, ever critical of extravagance, tells how Nero's wife Poppaea bathed in the milk of 500 asses on a daily basis to both soften and whiten her skin (*Natural History* 37.50).

The body could also be transformed by the use of hair dyes and wigs, a phenomenon that became increasingly popular in Rome as the empire spread its reach out to the edges of Europe and beyond, bringing back to the metropolis a range of exotic dyes and the blond and red hair of barbarian women.[4] Hair dyes were often imbued with scents such as saffron and rose oil to enhance the overall effect (see Stewart 2007: 43–5). The use of perfumes, again principally by women but also by some men of questionable character, transformed the smell of the body, and sophisticated methods were developed both to produce the scents and to discern and evaluate them. Most at stake here, at least as far as cynical conservative observers were concerned, was the question of what these perfume-wearers were setting out to conceal: vile bodies, sweat, filth, sexual obscenity, bad breath, disease—all normally discernible through the sense of smell—could be shielded from those around by perfumes, and much discussion of scents focuses on this theme (see Introduction, pp. 10–12). In Imperial Rome a wide range of scents were used, principally by women but also by men, and these were often closely tied to their provenance through name or by association (e.g. *delium* from Delos and *assyrium* from Assyria), thus advertising the far reaches of the Roman Empire, and the cosmopolitan trends of those who wore them.[5] Luxurious bath-houses offered cleansing with scented waters and perfumed oils, both to distinguish the bodies of those who could afford to use them by association with basic hygiene, and (no doubt) to conceal the unpleasant smells that would have become associated with these establishments. Lucretius (4.1174–6) captures the desperation of an old woman trying to fumigate her body with foul odors, and Martial (3.63) jibes at the elegant Cotilus, who tends assiduously to his appearance and smells continually of both balsam and cinnamon. In a similar vein, the Stoic philosopher Seneca imagines "Pleasure" as a prostitute, "slinking away in search of the dark around the baths and sweat chambers . . . soft, enervated, dripping with wine and perfume, pallid or else rouged and embalmed with drugs" (Seneca *De Vita Beata* 7.3).

Finally, it is clear that clothing—particularly on the female body—was a means of beguiling the senses with lavish and intricate colors. In the *Ars Amatoria*, Ovid describes the sheer variety of colors that the wool "drinks up": bodies "blushing with Tyrian purple," clothes "the color of sky," "the color of waves," myrtle, amethysts, chestnut, almonds, wax, and so on—and he advises that different colors are suited to different complexions (3.169–92) (a similar account, but more critical, is given in Plautus *Epidicus* 223.34; see Bradley 2009a: 179–81). And clothing was not just restricted to the visual domain: the expensive dyes that were used were closely connected to the materials from which they were derived, and so often possessed olfactory and tactile qualities which transformed the bodies that carried them. Saffron robes were popular across antiquity, and their characteristic fragrance evoked associations with flowers and femininity, and prestigious sea-purple dye (*purpura*), produced from murex snails fished from the sea across the Mediterranean basin, while it could paint the bodies of Persian monarchs, Hellenistic rulers, Roman consuls, priests, and women in a whole welter of shades in the red-blue-black range, was always recognizable through its powerful fishy stink (for references and discussion, see Bradley 2013).

Cosmetics, hair dyes, perfumes, and clothes represent just a few of the ways in which the art of adornment could be applied to the human body. Every wealthy, well-educated member of the Greek and Roman elite, for example, was expected to train in oratory, and considerable effort was applied to training the voice, posture, bearing, and gestures to suit particular circumstances, and to demonstrate their social and cultural superiority. The art of performance was critical to public self-presentation, and the following section will examine some aspects of the dramatic stage and the way in which actors, playwrights, and architects mobilized the senses to full effect within the central institution of the Greco-Roman theater.

SENSING PERFORMANCE

Just as the public presentation of the ancient body mobilized a full range of sensations, the Greco-Roman dramatic stage was a versatile and sophisticated sensory showcase. The stories, bodies, and characters on show here, as well as the theater space in which performances took place, were components of a complex audio-visual experience that was critical to public life from early classical Greece through to the end of antiquity, and which derived from traditions of singing, dancing, ritual, and celebration that were embedded in the very origins of classical civilization. The artistry of dramatic performance was wide-ranging, and developed and evolved in significant and complex ways across antiquity (see Griffith 2007 on the complex history of "theater" in Greece and Rome; see also Denard 2007); this section will outline just a few aspects of ancient drama in which sound, sight, and other senses contributed to the experience of the Greco-Roman theater.

The words that constituted tragic and comic plays expose one of the most accessible and pertinent aspects of the dramatic experience: playwrights wrote, actors spoke, and audiences listened to these words. However, it is clear that the auditory experience of drama was much more far-reaching than the transmission of words. For example, although our understanding of the role of music in drama is limited and contested, there is no doubt that the role of metrical rhythm, song, and instrumental music was commonplace in the majority of dramatic performance.[6] Nearly all ancient dramatic texts were written in verse in a wide array of meters that lent themselves to particular musical effects: iambic trimeters (which imitated the rhythms of speech), lyric (more complex rhythms normally accompanied by the pipe or kithara), or longer lines of rhythmical meter that were suited to musical chanting. By the Hellenistic period, words could even be said to be subordinate to music in drama, and a number of ancient writers berated this auditory trend (see Aristotle *Poetics* 1449b24ff. on "sweetened speech"; Aristophanes *Clouds* 966–72 on the simple virtues of "old music"; Plutarch *On Music* 1141c–2c on "old" versus "new music").

Moreover, there is evidence that playwrights and actors alike utilized highly professionalized techniques to make the most of the human voice in conveying the pertinent aspects of plays to the audience, and it is clear that (as Wiles put it) "the voice must 'convince' (or 'persuade') the audience that it is the voice of the character represented" (Wiles 1991: 218–20). Aristotle's *Rhetoric* discussed the intricacies of vocal delivery (*hypokrisis*) to match emotions, examining volume, pitch and rhythm, and in the *Problems* he linked the voice to the physiological properties of hot, cold, dry, and wet; and Vitruvius tells us about the technical precision applied to theater design to maximize the complex acoustics of dramatic performance (see also below p. 199).[7] It is likely that the use of masks (see below pp. 199–200) transformed the voices that were heard, in various different ways, and meant vocal acoustics presented a complex challenge for actor and theater architect alike (see esp. McCart 2007: 248–50). Furthermore, the well-documented hissing, booing, and clapping from spectators meant that they too made an integral contribution to the auditory experiences of ancient theater, and other sound effects such as lightning and thunder are documented in discussions of stage machinery.[8]

Ancient drama was clearly as much of a visual spectacle as it was a performance of sound, and the audience was in essence a set of spectators (the Greek word "theater" derives from a verb of "seeing"): theater worked as "a system of signs" (Wiles 1991: 14). The visual elements of ancient drama, although mostly perishable and transient, were manifold: characters moved about on stage, danced, and performed a complex set of actions and dynamic gestures, aided by a rigidly coded array of costumes and props.[9] It appears that the tragic stage became gradually more stylized and grandiose, with more elaborate masks, costumes, stage designs, and machinery, while comedy increasingly focused on a "realistic" visual performance that reproduced the appearance of everyday life.[10] Some treated this emphasis on the visual with disdain: Aristotle's *Poetics* argued that spectacle (*opsis*) was secondary and alien to the art of tragic poetry, and a matter for the costume-maker rather than the poet, while one of Horace's *Epistles* parodies contemporary tastes for tragic spectacle fueled by elaborate foreign materials that titillated the eye (sometimes forgetting altogether about the need for words).[11] Stage paintings were an art form in themselves, and Vitruvius documents the sophistication of three-dimensional stage scenery from Aeschylus onwards for illusionistic effects.[12] In Hellenistic theater, there is evidence for the use of wooden machinery which rotated painted "flats" to indicate a change of genre (Csapo and Slater 1995: 83). And in Roman theater, the increasingly imaginative use of elaborate colored and embroidered awnings (*vela*) both kept spectators cool and shaded, and created colorful effects as the sunlight passed through the red, yellow, and purple fabrics. Competitive politicians staged increasingly extravagant theater sets, and the architecture and setting of theater buildings themselves were often spectacular (see below pp. 205–6 on Pompey's Theater).[13]

Perhaps most striking of all was the system of masks (*prosōpa/personae*) that appears to have been deployed in most dramatic genres and contexts, a coded system based on a repertoire of facial expressions, colors, and features that (alongside gestures, *schemata*) was learned and understood by the majority of the population (on dramatic masks, see McCart 2007; Wiles 1991). Over 100 artifacts survive in the form of terracotta masks and painted, mosaic, and sculptural representations of masks which demonstrate a repertoire of recognizable types corresponding to character and personality (see Wiles 1991: esp. 80–3, 163–84 on the Lipari masks, and physiogmomic features characteristic of the four *genera*). Tallying closely with the surviving artifacts and in line with the traditions of physiognomy, a section of Pollux's *Onomasticon* (4.99–154) written in the late second century CE and probably derived from a range of earlier lost works on theater provides a useful taxonomic list of forty-four tragic, satyr, and New Comic mask types which demonstrates that mask shape, size, and color provided a cogent visual code, to help spectators to identify protagonists in the performance and associate them with patterns of behavior and characterization (for a good summary and discussion of Pollux's catalog, see Wiles 1991: 74–9; cf. 85–90 on physiognomics). Tragic types include pale, white-haired old men with jutting eyebrows; black men; vigorous curly-haired blond men; delicate pallid men with blond ringlets; long-haired grubby, squalid young men; lovesick men with puffy flesh and a sickly complexion; young and old women with different hair types and complexions; and rough, ruddy blond-haired slaves. Comedic characters appear to have been even more schematized and typecasted through hair color and length, beards, brows, wrinkles, fleshy folds, complexion, nose shape, and so on; slaves could be recognized by their red hair; and women were normally stereotyped according to their sexual behavior through the appearance and arrangement of their hair and the presence of jewelry, hairbands, and so on. There is also evidence that *genera* of masks from the Hellenistic period onwards employed color and form to evoke associations with the four humors and properties of hot/cold and wet/dry (further on this, see Bradley 2013; Wiles 1991: 150–2; on science and the senses, see Clements, this volume).

In addition to the masks that provided such compelling visual cues for dramatic performances, the color, shape, and fitting of costumes evoked a familiar set of associations among the audience (see Ley 2007: 270–3; Wiles 1991: Chapter 7). Corresponding closely to the character types outlined in his list of masks, Pollux provides a strikingly precise list of costume types and props (*Onomasticon* 115–20) that typically identified specific characters in different genres of play: the embroidered (*poikilon*) tragic garb, for example, with gilded, scarlet or "frog-colored" overgarments, or the dirty-white rags worn by those in distress, or the purple dress with a train worn by royal females; the animal skins, flowery *chlanis* or shaggy *chitōn* worn by satyrs; or the unfinished white *exōmis* worn by comic actors; the scarlet or purple *himation* of young men, the leather jacket of peasants, the black or grey of parasites (together with a strigil and oil bottle), yellow or blue for old women, white for priestesses, semi-transparent for young women (cf. Dio Chrysostom

32.94 on the drunken Heracles dressed inappropriately in yellow). Color-coding, then, as well as more tactile dimensions of clothing and accoutrements (rough/smooth, light/heavy, free/restricted movement), no doubt part of the learned shared experience of cultured ancient communities, appears to have been a key part of the dramatic spectacle. Pollux also discusses (at 121–32) the various props and designs of the theater stage, in such a way as to suggest that the topography of the theater layout was a familiar visual playground for spectators. Finally, it is clear that the audience itself made an increasingly important contribution to the visual experience of drama, particularly in Roman theater of the imperial period where more emphasis was placed on seating arrangements and dress (see Suetonius *Augustus* 44.1; Pollux 121ff.; Martial 5.23 on rules about knights wearing purple in the theater).

Many of the visual cues in ancient theater are evident in the frequent representations of dramatic (particularly comic) performance on pots: here, figures are generally masked (though, deliberately, this is not always clear), carry telltale costumes and accoutrements, gesture, engage physically with each other, dance, sing, or play music (see for example Csapo and Slater 1995: 64–70 on comic pots, with plates 4B–7B). One such example is the famous Attic "Pronomos" Vase from c. 410 BCE (see Figure 8.6), which shows a theatrical scene from a satyr-play, set in the sanctuary of Dionysus in which the god sits embracing his wife Ariadne surrounded by other divine figures and a total of seventeen mortal figures, including tragic actors, members of a satyr chorus, the satyr playwright, and the well-known piper Pronomos. All the actors carry their masks, except one, who is masked and dancing. Nine of the figures wear a hairy loincloth (*perizōma*) to which an erect phallus and tail are

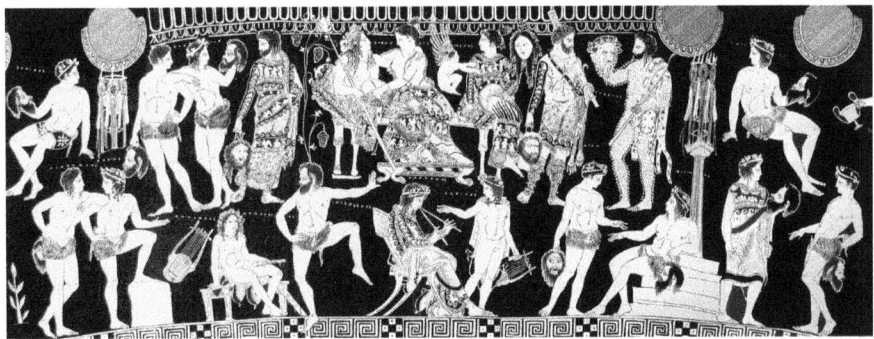

FIGURE 8.6: Drawing of a scene from the "Pronomos Vase": Dionysus and Ariadne surrounded by the actors and chorus of a satyr-play. Attic red-figure krater, c. 410 BCE. Naples: Museo Nazionale inv. 81673. Drawing reproduced by kind permission of Thomas Mannack.

attached, and the leader of the satyr chorus (second from the right) wears an elaborate embroidered outfit that is visibly thin and hugs his body. The significance of this vase painting is much discussed and debated, but it does a fine job of demonstrating that dramatic performance was elaborately visualized, coded with masks, costumes and props, and mobilized voice, music, and dance, as well as aspects of touch (embracing figures, rough/ smooth costumes etc.).[14] Some of these multi-sensory dimensions and iconography are also evident in collections of terracotta figurines of actors, or mosaics from the Roman period, such as the Dioskourides mosaics from Pompeii (see Figures 8.7a, b), which represent scenes from the plays of Menander, and which show actors in movement against an off-white stage wall, wearing colorful masks, playing a range of musical instruments, and taking breakfast together on stage (terracotta figurines: Csapo and Slater 1995: 70–3, with plates 9–10; mosaics: Green 2007: 180–2; McCart 2007: 261–2; Wiles 1991: 40, 202–3).

While various effects of sight and sound dominated the experience of ancient drama, other sensations also appear to have performed a role in certain contexts. Interaction between characters on stage could be signaled not only through words but also through touch, embrace, and physical violence: vase paintings show actors sitting in each other's laps, holding another's hair in preparation for a slaughter scene, oiling their hands in preparation for wrestling, and so on (see, for example, Csapo and Slater 1995: plates 2A and 2B, 6, and the Pronomos Vase in Figure 8.6). The religious context of a great deal of ancient drama meant that the smells of sacrifice and burning incense were never far away from the dramatic stage, and some performances appear to have integrated these olfactory experiences into their delivery: for example, Demosthenes recalls the oracles of Delphi and Dodona in c. 348 BCE which commanded the city to perform dance with song according to ancestral tradition and to fill the streets with the smoke of sacrifices and wear garlands.[15] Plays could even be set in a sanctuary, such as Euripides' *Ion* in the Delphic sanctuary and Sophocles' *Oedipus at Colonus*, which was staged in front of the local sanctuary of the Eumenides, and sacrifices sometimes took place on stage (with all the smells and noises that came with them). There is also evidence that theaters were sometimes ritually purified prior to a performance, which may have involved sacrifice, smoke, and libations (see Suda s.v. "katharison" c. 1000 CE, involving the sacrifice of small piglets; Plutarch, *Cimon* 8.7 (libations). See also Beacham 2007: 204). Dramatic performances integrated into festivals such as the Great Dionysia at Athens or the Megalesian Games in Rome were often staged in the context of religious rituals and feasting, and there is ample evidence that eating and drinking was a familiar experience during performances of comic plays, where nuts, dried fruit,

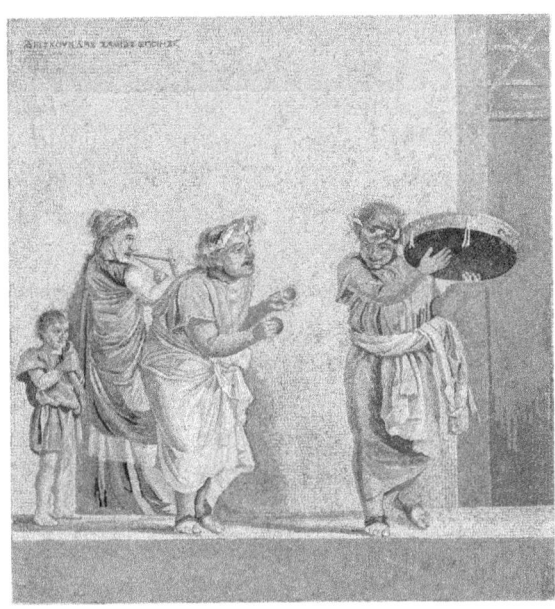

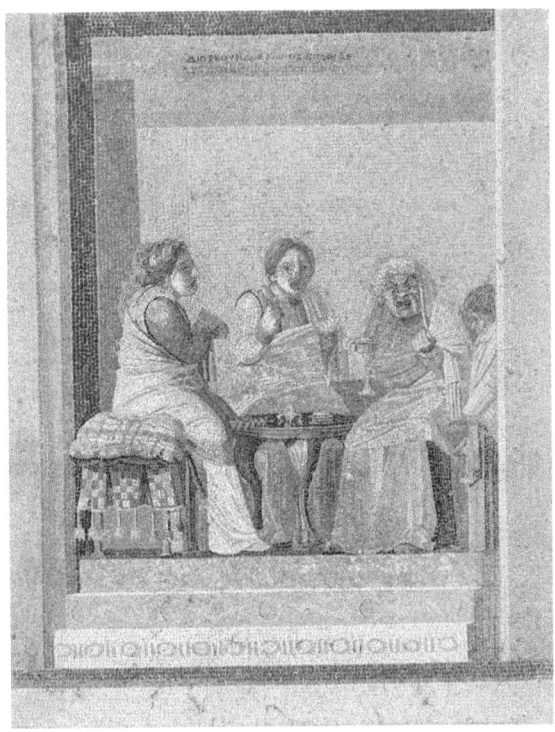

FIGURE 8.7a (top) and 8.7b (bottom): Dioskourides mosaic (c. 125–100 BCE). Museo Nazionale, Naples, inv. 9985 and 9987.

and wine were budgeted by the *chorēgos* for distribution to spectators to secure their goodwill and pander to their needs and desires.[16] Furthermore, some performances exploited food and drink in creative ways, so that taste was an essential part of the experience, and characters could eat and drink on stage (on food as a dramatic theme, see Ley 2007: 272–3; Wilkins 2000; Graf 2007: 60 on the *lectisternium* (Roman banquet of the gods) ritual integrated into dramatic performances). Pollux's *Onomasticon* (121–32) discusses the presence of "a street altar" typically set up in front of doors on the *skēnē*, as well as a table with cakes. The final act of Seneca's *Thyestes*, no doubt like earlier lost versions of the story, plays extensively on the experience of eating and drinking as the tragic king eventually realizes that he has feasted on his own sons. And Pliny the Elder describes the chewing of white myrtle berries to cure halitosis, an action that Menander built into his play the *Synaristosae* (*Women Having Lunch Together*) so that feasting and smells became an integral part of that performance (a scene represented in the Dioscourides mosaic, see Figure 8.7b) (Pliny *Natural History* 23.159, discussed in Classen *et al.* 1994: 32; Wiles 1991: 202).

Probably from the Hellenistic period onwards, scents and perfumes could be integrated into dramatic performances. Apuleius describes at length a fictional dance-drama in the Roman colony of Corinth which employed the full range of sensory stimuli, and which climaxed with an extraordinary piece of stage wizardry:

> Then from the very top of the mountain through some type of hidden pipe, a jet of saffron dissolved in wine (*vino crocus diluta*) sprayed right up, sprinkling the goats grazing around in a scented shower, until dyed to a superior appearance they exchanged their native whiteness for a yellow hue (*luteo colore*). And now, when the whole theater was filled with sweet fragrance (*tota suave fragrante cavea*), a chasm in the ground swallowed up the wooden mountain.
>
> Apuleius *Metamorphoses* 10.34

Here, the eyes, noses, and even the tastebuds of the audience were tantalized: forms and colors, movement and landscapes, interacted with the scent and taste of saffron and wine and the cool touch of the spray to transform the dramatic experience at the close of the play. Fictional though Apuleius' drama was, there is little doubt that this account mirrored the ingenuities of engineering in contemporary theater, and the warmth of flames and cool of water, along with colors, sounds, and smells, were familiar features of innovative dramatic performances (see Denard 2007: 154–6 and below).

In sum, then, ancient drama presents another pivotal form of Greco-Roman art in which the participation of bodies—actors and audience alike—exploited various sensory qualities of sight and sound, and even smell, touch, and taste, in order to heighten the dramatic experience. In all these cases, the creative artistic exploitation of the senses governed and shaped the world that ancient communities experienced, and helped them to clarify, evaluate, and understand the performances that unfolded in front of them.

SENSING THE CITY

Dramatic performances in Greek and Roman cities, then, provided a compelling context for the exploitation of sight, sound, and other senses to communicate ideas and information about society, culture, and politics to the community, and a great deal of artistic energy was channeled into the subtle and sophisticated deployment of sensory stimuli. Theater buildings themselves, as we have seen, made a major contribution to the aesthetic experience of dramatic performance, both in terms of stage design and acoustics, and they were frequently juxtaposed to temples and sanctuaries, or even integrated into them, so that the smells (and tastes) of rituals and sacrifices were part of the shared experience. The Theater of Dionysus in Athens, though its architecture changed considerably over time, was always juxtaposed to the key monuments and temples that both advertised Athenian political and imperial supremacy and commanded the visual, auditory, and olfactory attention of spectators as part of the theater's "shared experience" (see Beacham 2007: 206–7 on the significance of the monumental architecture visible from the Theater of Dionysus at Athens). Rome's first "permanent" theater, the Theater of Pompey, completed in 52 BCE, was crowned with a temple of Venus Victrix, who both oversaw and participated in the theater's activities (see Figure 8.8), and its complex was juxtaposed to four existing republican temples (the so-called "Area Sacra" of the Largo Argentina). But the complex did much more to titillate the senses of the masses for whom it was erected: its innovative enclosed design improved the theater's acoustics; the stage wall was designed with forty-six polychrome marble columns, their colored surfaces themselves a novelty for Roman eyes; water flowed down the aisles of the theater to cool the summer heat; and a fine saffron mist was sometimes sprayed over spectators to generate a truly multi-sensory experience. In between performances theater-goers could stroll around the shaded *quadriporticus* behind the stage wall, which was festooned with golden curtains from Pergamum and contained rooms exhibiting collections of painting and sculpture plundered during Pompey's campaigns, and which

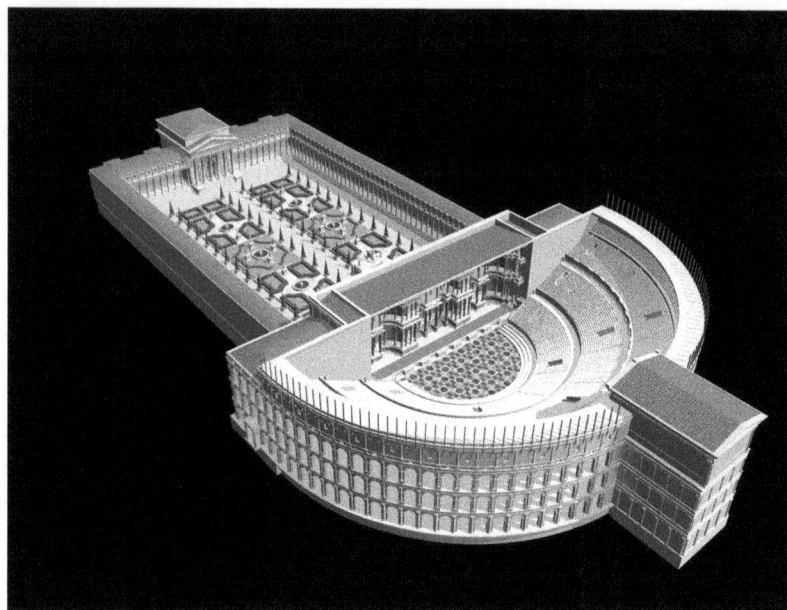

FIGURE 8.8: Digital reconstruction of the Theater of Pompey (dedicated 52 BCE). Image courtesy of Matthew Nicholls.

enclosed elaborate gardens containing lavish fountains and exhibiting exotic plants and flowers in an array of colors and fragrances. Marbles, art, and plants bore witness to the far-flung territories that Pompey had himself conquered, and along with the thriving organic genre of Latin drama performed in the theater contributed to a rich sensorium of experience that advertised Rome's cultural transformation.[17]

However, it is also clear that the architecture of Greek and Roman cities more broadly exploited the senses in order to stimulate and control the experiences of the population. Public spaces in Athens, Rome, and other cities were the product of sophisticated processes of urban design, in which monuments, sculpture, and art could dominate the line of vision with their scale, form, color, and material, the significance of which has been the subject of countless scholarly studies in recent decades. But these spaces were also the site for dramatic performances, public recitals, song, speeches, noisy processions, the clamor of crowds, animals and vehicles, as well as the spatter and trickle of water fountains, nymphaea, aqueducts, and the like. Ancient cities were, we hear, dominated by the stenches of commerce (taverns, bars, butchers) and industry (fullers and tanners), but the olfactory experience could also be manipulated by the smells of sacrifice, incense, flowers, and feasts. The cityscape was also a place for touch (the smooth feel of polished marble or the cool air of porticoes and fountains, for example)—and for taste (drinking water, public feasts, taverns, and food shops): on all this, see Potter, Aldrete, and Wallace-Hadrill, this volume.

The city was frequently described by ancient writers as a product of artistic effort and adornment. For example, a stone's throw away from Pompey's theater and just a generation later, the Campus Martius, a flood plain to the north of the city that was completely re-landscaped by Augustus with temples, theaters, baths, porticos, and gardens, was described by the Greek visitor Strabo (*Geography* 5.3.8) as the epicenter of urban *kosmēsis*, a natural spectacle conducive to social activity, sports, and general health, covered with grass and framed by the hills and river like a stage-painting (*skēnographikēn opsin*), but also striking for its gleaming marble (*leukolithos*), bronze art, and evergreen trees (see Favro 1996: Chapter 7 for an imaginary walk through the Augustan Campus Martius; cf. Vitruvius 5.9.5 on green spaces qualitatively modifying the air and clearing the vision). And in a nostalgic snapshot of the Rome from which he has been exiled, Ovid imagines a similar scene of fora, temples, marbled theaters, perfectly leveled porticos, and the grassy campus and splendid gardens, along with the pools, aqueducts, and flowing waters (*Ex Ponto* 1.8.33–8). In an earlier poem, he contrasted the Augustan present to the primitive past (*Ars Amatoria* 1.101–10), and describes awnings hung over a marble theater and stages sprayed red with saffron. Others describe the city of Augustus as "Golden Rome," in line with the new "Golden Age" heralded in Augustan propaganda, decorated with a rich array of colored marbles imported by Augustus from the territories over which he ruled. Here, theaters, amphitheaters, recital halls, and fora buzzed with the familiar sounds and voices which they produced, and the hundreds of new or restored temples, shrines, and altars set up by Augustus around the city would have filled the air with the smells of incense and sacrifice. Here, as with classical Athens, Hellenistic Alexandria or late-antique Constantinople, urban artistry evoked a full range of senses in order to stimulate the eyes, hears, noses, tongues, and fingertips of ancient perceivers.

CONCLUSION

Classical art, of course, extends far beyond the examples we have explored in this chapter, and it would be possible to tell a story about artistic engagement with the senses if one were to examine other artistic phenomena such as wall paintings, pottery, coinage, jewelry, religious processions, games, and so on.

However, the four artistic domains explored above, which are all intimately connected in various ways, demonstrate that art, artifacts and artistry in the ancient world exploited the full range of human senses. They were not just visual phenomena experienced from a distance, but products of a rich and competitive tradition of art which sought to stimulate the minds of ancient protagonists in new ways to appreciate, evaluate, and understand their social, cultural, and political history, traditions and identities. Sometimes, this manipulation of the senses met with caution and alarm: the adorned female body concealed what lay beneath, seducing and entrapping men, and the sensationalism of the stage distracted audiences from what really mattered. Other times, the production of that art, and its erudite appreciation, were symptomatic of a highly specialized, literate elite discourse which utilized the senses in very sensitive, sophisticated ways to impart cultural ideas, as well as to control the experiences of the community. But in all the instances we have examined, artist and consumer alike participated in a highly creative, competitive, and interactive process of classification, evaluation, and understanding in which the senses communicated a set of ideas about the artistic product in front of them. And these artificial sensations themselves helped to shape the world beyond art by providing a repertoire of categories, traditions, and expectations that made sense of the society in which that art was produced.

CHAPTER NINE

Sensory Media: Representation, Communication, and Performance in Ancient Literature

BENJAMIN ELDON STEVENS

Ancient sensory experience differed markedly from the experiences, practices, or media most likely encountered today. From a modern perspective, ancient sensory practices are in a way all "mixed sensory media," engaging the senses in what must seem to be at least partly unfamiliar configurations. For example, as other chapters examine in some detail, religious rites could feature animal odors alongside burning incense; market days could be indicated by ringing bells, while daily life in Greece and, to a lesser degree, Rome was marked by instrumental and vocal music; and communication across long distances could be achieved by signal fires (an example of which we shall consider below).

Attempting to recover the details of such sensory practices, in themselves and in terms of their cultural associations, is the work of a cultural history of the senses.[1] An important working principle is that sensation and perception are not the same: since physical experience is always a matter of enculturation, "the senses" are not fixed but a matter of fluid definition in culture. The effects of this work on our understanding of antiquity should be profoundly defamiliarizing: not only ancient meanings as such but also their modes of communication were very different from the modern.[2] Ancient sensory experience is thus productively understood as involving "sensory media" of material types and cultural associations quite particular to antiquity.

In this chapter I aim at giving vivid impressions of the range of sensory experiences and practices employed in antiquity, as well as of the significance they could take on in particular contexts. The examples discussed below refer to diverse practices of representation, communication, and performance. I focus on examples from the literary tradition: Homer's *Odyssey*, Plato's *Phaedrus*, Horace's *Ode* 1.9, Catullus' poem 51, and Aeschylus' *Agamemnon*. Since such literary examples are likely to be familiar, they may serve to emphasize the sorts of things that may be revealed when even well-known materials are treated in a cultural history of the senses.

Another reason for this focus is that evidence for ancient sensory experience and practice is mainly textual. This raises methodological issues. Authors operating in literary traditions will not have represented sensory experience "accurately." But we thus stand to learn how experience was entered into discourse. This is one way of emphasizing the difference between sensation as merely physical and "sensory experience" as a matter of cultural production and practice. I also note some examples perhaps less likely to be familiar. I conclude by suggesting how we might conceive of the work of a cultural history of the senses as having a sensory component of its own. This conception would, I believe, help us to develop our understanding of practices that are farther removed from the literary tradition but not therefore less characteristic of ancient sensory experience.

HELEN AND RECOGNITION AS SENSORY EXPERIENCE AND PRACTICE

Helen "of Troy" is famous—or infamous?—for her beauty: hers was "the face that launch'd a thousand ships." The speaker of that line, Marlowe's Faustus, goes on to praise Helen's beauty extravagantly: "O, thou art fairer than the evening air / Clad in the beauty of a thousand stars; / Brighter art thou than flaming Jupiter / When he appear'd to hapless Semele; / More lovely than the monarch of the sky / In wanton Arethusa's azur'd arms . . ." (12.13–18). It would seem that Helen is matchlessly beautiful by any standard of comparison.

For our purposes, however, it is significant that Marlowe's comparisons are all visual. "Fairer" than the starry night and "brighter" than lightning ("flaming Jupiter") both refer to a glow; and "more lovely than the monarch of the sky" also arguably refers to brightness. All three comparisons, then, are between Helen's appearance and other lights. For Faustus at this moment, for Marlowe in his perhaps most famous line, Helen's beauty is visual.

Helen is beautiful in Homer, too, in ways that would register on the eyes. But Homer's descriptions are not only visual. Like other characters, as well as other things, Helen is described in ways that mix the visual with other sensory qualities. The importance of such mixtures in Homer, and by extension in Greek and, *mutatis mutandis*, Latin literature, is suggested by the fact that just such a mixture marks Helen's first appearance in the *Odyssey*. That moment may serve as a first example of the sorts of things we may expect to find in ancient literature and culture with a cultural history of the senses in mind.

When Helen emerges from her chamber, the moment is not only visual but also tactile, auditory, gustatory, and olfactory.[3] Helen is "striking as Artemis with her golden shafts" (4.136), striking visually ("golden"). But there is also a tactile connotation: like Artemis' shafts, Helen's beauty somehow pierces. It is nonetheless the visual that would seem to be emphasized in what follows, as Helen's servants bring in a "carved reclining-chair," a "silver basket," a "golden spindle," and a "basket [of] solid silver polished off with rims of gold" containing "violet wool" (138–50). The visual qualities of these objects echo ("golden") and offset ("silver," "violet") Helen's own.

It makes sense that this scene would be intensely visual. Helen's guest, Telemachus, is recognized as the son of Odysseus by people who could pronounce on physical resemblance, as he himself could not. Menelaus "recognized him at once" but does not say so (131); Helen announces recognition first (she has "never seen such a likeness, / neither in man nor woman—I'm amazed at the sight"; 156–7), and then Menelaus pretends merely to agree with her ("Now that you mention it, I see the likeness too"; 164). Helen is thus doubly marked as having a special relationship to the visual: herself an object of attention, she is attentive in turn. But both Helen and Menelaus attend to the visual in a way Telemachus could not: since he has never seen Odysseus, he cannot recognize any resemblance in himself. Part of the scene's importance, then, is this visual "answer" to Telemachus' question about his paternity; in a poem deeply interested in recognition, this particular moment has a special significance indeed.[4]

But there is more to the scene in terms of sensory experience. The objects borne in by Helen's servants owe their visual effects to the richness of their material and to the high craft of their making; additional attention is thus drawn to the tactile. The "carved reclining-chair" is attractive in how its material has been treated (cf. Odysseus' and Penelope's bed (23.200 ff.) as well as the bow (21.50 ff. and 21.439 ff.)). The tactile is emphasized further in that the chair is followed directly by a "carpet of soft-piled fleece" (4.139). The metal objects, too, evoke touch through their own materials and craftsmanship. In parallel to the pairing of carved, implicitly hard chair and explicitly soft carpet, the final metal object, the hard "basket [of] solid silver polished off with rims of gold," is paired with softer yarn and wool. Helen's emergence, visually glittering, thus also emphasizes touch by contrasting objects of different materials, textures, and hardness. This tactile dimension redoubles the moment's opulence while also combining domesticity, as suggested by the materials for weaving, and sensuality, as our attention is drawn to objects of creature comfort. Again, Helen is at the focus: relaxing among the objects, she is herself a sensual object of attention.[5]

To this mixture of sight and touch is added sound. Telemachus cries quietly to himself, having covered his face with his robe (4.130).[6] Menelaus likewise keeps his own silent counsel. The next sound we are explicitly given to hear, despite the bustling servants, is Helen's voice, and that only after all the objects are placed and she has, as noted, aligned herself with them. Helen is thus indeed at the center of attention. Broadly "sensual" in that Helen is of course a *locus classicus* of desire, that attention is in Homer's language expressly and diversely sensory. Helen's emergence thus constitutes a kind of sensory practice, communicating many things including majesty, domesticity, and—insofar as she represents the past—memory.

This connection between Homer's interests as an epic poet, including memory, and mixtures of the senses is emphasized somewhat later in the scene by taste. When it comes time for drink, Helen mixes the wine not with the usual water but with a "drug" that is said to "dissolve anger" and "make us forget all our pains" (243–60). Traditionally water was used to civilize wine-drinking by reducing drunkenness; this likely also made some wine more palatable by diluting strong taste or sourness. Since the drug's purpose is to dull memory and experience, a connection is drawn between memory, in a way the goal of that highest ancient genre of epic, and, perhaps surprisingly, taste, in some traditions the basest sense.[7]

For our purposes, the adulterated wine is one more signal that, in contrast to Marlowe's visual description, Homer's description of Helen and her emergence is a mixture of different sense-perceptions, each with its own cultural associations. The nature of this mixture may—should—surprise us.

Although the visual is a focus, the tactile is ubiquitous, the auditory is used to dramatic effect, the gustatory adds an elegiac note ... and then there is the olfactory: Helen emerges from a "scented chamber." Since this would traditionally have been upstairs, Helen is represented as descending on a decreasing gradient of scent. Perhaps the scent comes with her or infuses the fabrics brought by her servants; we would love to know its odor.[8]

No matter the particular odor, the gradient reinforces the physical dynamics of the scene, charging it with sensuality quite literally before anything is said or done. Much is communicated through the senses in combinations. Focalized as the scene is through Telemachus's veiled perspective, Helen's emergence is known, and her quality perceived, before she is seen. The moment thus depends on a sensory sort of dramatic irony: Homer has us wait for Telemachus to catch up to our knowledge, and when he does we may feel our own astonishment at Helen's multi-sensuous presence confirmed. And vice versa: in this mixture of the senses, we are given very powerfully to share the scene's point, the shock of Telemachus' recognition.

PLATO ON "LITERATURE," LANGUAGE, MEMORY, AND THE SENSES

Homer's descriptions would presumably have registered more "naturally" on an ancient audience thanks to its lifelong experience of literature and the enculturated world. In this connection we may note that the literary tradition, literature itself, is a kind of sensory experience: "reading habits" comprise practices including complex configurations of the senses (see Miola 2000). The materiality of literature itself may therefore serve as a usefully defamiliarizing topic.

Despite their differences, for example, Marlowe and Homer were both intended to be heard aloud: descriptions registering on the "eye"—or other sensory organ—all do so by the proxy of the ear. Audiences were meant to hear Helen's visual beauty as well as her other sensory characteristics.[9] Strictly speaking, such transposition among sense-modalities is a kind of "synaesthesia" (see Stevens 2008: 161–3, with sources cited in n. 3). Without pushing that particular term too far, we may still expect the general notion of "mixture" to help us understand our examples more deeply.

Homer was intended for hearing, but by the time we have him he is of course written down. This situation, in which "literature" is a mixture of at least seeing and hearing, was of great interest in antiquity. Perhaps the most famous treatment is in the *Phaedrus*, where Socrates expresses concerns about writing: he suggests that, through the senses, writing has negative effects on the soul as the organ of learning and memory (e.g., 271de).[10] Socrates articulates what is of course a central Platonic notion, namely that sense-perception does not directly conduce to truth: because we may perceive only deceptive imitations, sense-perception must be ranked below intellection.[11] Writing is especially deceptive since it fixes language in place visually, while hearing is the vehicle for speech, including the properly responsive speech that is the dialectic (cf. *Phaedrus* 277e–8a).

Perhaps surprisingly, however, we also find here a rich investment in sensory language. This may be illustrated first in what is perhaps the dialogue's most famous moment, when Socrates relates how writing was offered by the Egyptian god Theuth to Thamous, king of Egyptian Thebes (274c–5b). Theuth describes writing as "a potion for memory and intelligence." Thamous thinks that "its true effect . . . will [be to] atrophy people's memories . . . writing will make the things they have learnt disappear from their minds" (275a; cf. *Protagoras* 329a, *Theaetetus* 164e, and *Statesman* 294a).

Although the fundamental problem with writing in Plato's view is not its sensory qualities as such, still we may say that his expression of its problematic effects draws attention to how it is a mixed sensory practice. Writing presents to the eye what is properly a matter for the ear. As a sort of "potion," writing, like a potent wine, results in a kind of drunkenness suitable only for "amusement" and "diversion" (276de), while serious philosophical work requires the dialectic. The dialectic is then a sort of "unmixed speech" whose simplicity—or "sobriety"?—corresponds to and conduces to that of the "simple soul," whose appetite has been properly subordinated to reason. (Writing is, however, also described as a "delicate garden" whose "diversions" are superior to precisely "*the symposia* and so on with which people amuse themselves" (276de).)

A connection may be drawn between writing as "potion" and the wine-"drug" mixture prepared by Helen: both are "Egyptian" drinks said to have an effect on the memory. Homer and Plato thus share an image of great sensory import: something as seemingly intellectual as memory is affected by something as material as a drink. We have here, then, a certain configuration of the senses, a "sensory experience" or "sensory practice," that is demonstrably shared among ancient authors.

We may now say that sensory language of this sort is characteristic of the *Phaedrus*' descriptions of speech and writing. Socrates concludes that no one who has correct knowledge would "spend time and effort writing what he knows in water—in black water—and sowing them with his pen by means of words" (276c). This image is itself a sort of mixture: of "writing in water" as proverbial for evanescence, of "black water" as a metaphor for "ink," of "sowing." Plato thus emphasizes what is, in his view, the unhelpfully evanescent nature of writing by referring to how it engages the senses: it passes us by like running water, and as black water it is, to the eye at least, unpalatable. As a sensory object, writing is indeed rather more a complex "potion" than a simple "drink."

In this connection we may turn to the dialogue's opening. The *Phaedrus* begins with Socrates wishing to hear from Phaedrus an oration by Lysias; the question arises whether it would be better heard recited from memory or read aloud. Since Phaedrus has not got the oration in memory word for word, but only in general outline, and since the excellence of Lysias' words is (part of) the point, he prefers to read it aloud.

For our purposes, it is interesting that Socrates is pleased not only by the topic of the oration ("love"; 227c) and its language but also by Phaedrus' delivery. He is pleased by reading aloud in a way that would seem to run counter to the dialogue's later argument against writing and in favor of face-to-face speech. The original speaker, Lysias himself, would of course be preferred to reading aloud and to memory. This preference for the person is complex, a variation on the Platonic theme that originals are superior to copies. But it also elevates the speaker as a perceptible body over the copy as a scroll.

At this moment, then, Socrates' pleasure centers around Phaedrus' presence, with explicit attention to sensory aspects of the experience: "I was amazed. You were the reason I felt this way, Phaedrus, because I was looking at you while you were reading, and it seemed to me that the speech made you glow with pleasure" (234d). Socrates at least does not dislike the sound, and he quite likes the look, of Phaedrus reading.[12]

These sensory aspects are an extension of, and emphasized by, the dramatic setting: a "lovely secluded spot" under a plane-tree (see Wycherley 1963). Socrates' description is worth quoting (230bc):

> This plane tree is very tall and flourishing, the agnus is tall enough to provide excellent shade too, and since it is in full bloom it will probably make the place especially fragrant. Then again, the stream under the plane tree is particularly charming, and its water is very cold, to judge by my foot ... Or again, if you like, how pleasant and utterly delightful is the freshness of the air here! The whisper of the breeze chimes in a summery, clear way with the chorus of the cicadas.

This description anticipates the pleasure Socrates takes in Phaedrus' act of reading by attending to the senses. There is sight (height and "flowering" of one tree, height and "shade" of the other), scent suggested by that sight ("full bloom, especially fragrant"), touch in terms of temperature ("cold water," perhaps also "the fresh air"), and sound that is musical and vocal ("whisper," "chimes," "chorus of cicadas").

Although sight and sound are privileged by placement, emphasis is also given to bodies both as the sites of these sense-perceptions and as they are integrated into the scene. Socrates goes on to say that "the nicest thing of all is the fact that the grass is on a gentle slope which is perfect for resting one's head on when lying down." The list of senses thus includes "proprioception," awareness of the body in space (see Ratcliffe 2008: 79–83).

In this way, a dialogue arguing that living speech and memory are superior to reading aloud is yet able to evoke and to praise the act of reading for its sensory qualities. Although from a philosophical standpoint writing is inferior to speech, the act of reading aloud is nonetheless a valuable—or, minimally, pleasurable—sensory experience. The philosophical and the sensory interact in ways that are suggestive of the complexity of sensory practices and of what we could rightly call "communication" or "representation" via the senses in combinations.

Like Homer, however, Plato also invites us to consider how the feeling that sense-perceptions "communicate naturally" is trumped by the fact that they are complex products of "culture." We are therefore invited to consider ancient associations to Plato's descriptions. Trees and their scents suggest the season, to which ancient society, attuned to an agricultural year, felt perhaps a more powerful connection. Shade and a cool stream provide refuge from the heat. There is the profound fact of "running water": made to figure "evanescence," it is also the opposite of "stagnation" linked to disease, e.g., malaria. There is the sound of cicadas in "chorus"—is the dialogue a sort of drama?—in the complete absence of machine noise.[13] Finally there is the pleasure of lying on grass. And slightly outside our passage we have an intimation of another sense: for Socrates was led outside the city walls by Phaedrus' "dangling a speech on a scroll," like a hungry animal following "greenery or a vegetable"; from this we might infer a sense, however simple, of taste.[14]

SENSE-PERCEPTION AND DEFAMILIARIZATION

If we compare the *Phaedrus*' sensory descriptions to Helen's emergence, we find a contrast between (Telemachus', our own) astonishment at the magnificence there with what seems to be (Socrates', our own) simpler enjoyment here. And the *Phaedrus* is arguably more humorous: Socrates' description of the setting leads Phaedrus to remark that Socrates is "like a complete stranger ... not a local resident" (230cd). Socrates replies that, as an "intellectual," he learns from townspeople, not from trees (275bc) (see Munson 2004: Chapter 4).

Socrates' reply emphasizes his singular behavior: he is a (self-)consciously defamiliarizing figure (famously, at *Apology* 30e he calls himself Athens' "gadfly"). For that matter, so was Helen. Just as Plato's language resonates with Homer's, so do these two extraordinary figures seem to be at the center of sensory experience. As a result, we might wonder whether the surrounding sensory experiences are somehow not representative of what was ordinary in antiquity. Certainly they are heightened, in Homer by Helen's ostentatious magnificence and in Plato by Socrates' funny irony. And of course we should expect differences between "literary" examples like these and examples from "lived experience."

But I have focused first on sense-perceptions surrounding these singular figures in literature to emphasize how all of ancient sensory experience may seem unfamiliar to us. As we pursue a cultural history of the senses, we do well not to assume that there is common ground between different sensory cultures. We are better served by adopting defamiliarization as a working principle, noting differences and peculiarities so as properly to contextualize similarities and what, if any, are "general" or "universal" features of sensory experience across human cultures.

HORACE ON SENSORY EXPERIENCE AND CULTURAL CHANGE

Horace's *Ode* 1.9 looks to a long-standing symposiastic tradition, originally Greek, and it marks a relatively recent turn in Latin literature towards the Italian landscape.[15] This combination is beloved of Horace: wine-drinking appears in many of his poems, and he is perhaps the Latin poet most responsible for a turn towards the landscape.[16] Those elements are depicted in vividly sensory terms. But both Greek and Italian traditions also figure Horace's relationship with his contemporary "Augustan" culture, including what has been called the "Augustan program of cultural renewal" and the "Roman cultural revolution" (see Zanker 1988; see also Habinek and Schiesaro 1998; Spawforth 2011; Wallace-Hadrill 2008). *Ode* 1.9 may thus exemplify how sensory experience is both a matter of culture, and, as cultural experience may be entered into discourse, a means of articulating concerns about change. Perhaps especially at a time of great change, sensory experiences are "naturally" flush with "cultural associations."

The poem begins with a direct address, and at first—until v. 8—that second person seems to be the reader. "You see," says the speaker, directing one's attention—via the proxy of the "mind's eye"—to a nature scene changed by winter. A mountain "stands gleaming with deep snow," its "forests labor under their burden and will fail," and its "streams stand fast with sharp frost." Sight is starkly emphasized first by placement and then by our realization, in the second stanza, that one is *only* "seeing" this scene from indoors, not experiencing it via other senses.

By contrast, at the end of the poem there is an implicit absence of sight, with, if not darkness as such (the scene is now "at dusk" (v. 19)), then a kind of concealment as an idealized accompaniment of love. In the final stanza, "a girl is hiding" with her lover—perhaps the addressee, perhaps the speaker in his own memory—in an "intimate corner." The girl is "betrayed" not by a sight but by a sound, her own "pleased laugh." (There have been "gentle whispers.") And there is touch in the form of physical contact: the girl and her lover play with a "bracelet to be taken from an upper arm, or a ring from an unwilling finger."

There is thus a transition in proprioception. At the beginning one only "sees" winter from indoors and may feel a sort of heat from the hearth (v. 5). Towards the end, one is exhorted to enjoy the out-of-doors (v. 18) as they conduce to shared physical activities, "dances" (v. 16) and "sweet love-affairs" (v. 15) in spring or summer. Those physical activities, alongside the play in the "intimate corner," require close proximity and imply a different kind of warmth: the dances may be male displays; the principal love affair is male-female. This ending contrasts sharply with the cold, distant sights of the poem's opening. We may imagine stark whites and blacks (the snow and wetted branches) giving way to warmer colors—although what may be torchlight to light the dark may subtly correspond to the early "fire" in the hearth, just as the "unwilling finger" may correspond to the unmoving streams.

If we are thus drawn by sensory descriptions and implications back to the beginning, we may note that from beginning to end one "fire" in fact, in the hearth, leads directly through warmth to the other in fantasy or, perhaps, memory. Just as the heat "loosens the cold" (v. 5), so is the mind—fantasy, memory—loosened, by the heat and by that "great loosener," wine: "a four-year vintage poured pure from a Sabine jar" (vv. 7–8).

Once again, then, while considering sensory experience, we find ourselves offered wine. Like Homer's wine and like Plato's "potion," this wine seems to have an effect on the memory. Here, however, the wine is "unmixed [with water]" (it is *merum*) and seems not to dull but to loosen memory by juxtaposing past and present experience. This may be emphasized by the wine being poured "freely" (*benignius*; in combination with *large*, v. 6, perhaps "copiously"). The vintage seems to emphasize the Italian setting, as it recedes into memory, and to contrast with the Roman activities that command the present time.

If the evocations that follow are less concrete than the poem's initial sensory descriptions, this is not only because they could be signaled obliquely to an ancient audience but also because they are warmer and more fluid than the winter. Their flow is not so much "sharp" (*acuto*) or painful as bittersweet or elegiac: the context is of course old age recalling youth. This, too, resonates with our passage from Homer. But Helen was glorious still, and when she looked at Telemachus she saw Odysseus and her own vivid knowledge of him. By contrast, Horace's speaker sees white snow (*candidum*, v. 1) to match his own age-whitened hair (*canities*, v. 17). Likewise when he considers his youthful drinking partner his thoughts turn to activities now unavailable to him.

The link between sensory experience and age lets us think, finally, of larger, cultural points made by the poem, and so of how sensory experience is related to the larger forces of history. For along with youth has a culture changed, as "Italy" has been made to tend towards "Rome." Thus Mt. Soracte, a natural feature virtually invisible from Rome, gives way to cultural activities placed in the city's "field [of Mars] and open spaces." And in between "Italy" and "Rome" in this poem is the sea, likewise invisible from the city but of great importance to the empire . . . even as any storms may be quelled by the gods alone. In this connection we may note that, while the poem's "Roman" activities are public, they are not political: "give the rest to the gods" (v. 9) and "take what life gives you" (vv. 13–15) are Epicurean sentiments.

We may therefore imagine a complex correspondence between the poem's sensory descriptions and the cultural and political situations of Horace's lifetime. Activities that characterize youth are, for the speaker, a matter of the past. This is consonant with the Augustan "program of cultural renewal" as it involved restrictions on what one may do, e.g., "moral legislation" against adultery. I do not wish to limit the meaning of the poem unduly, but by making this sort of connection we stand to think more precisely about the relationship between traditions and cultural changes in antiquity. Horace's beloved symposiastic tradition does not quite apply to Roman culture, especially not now, and so his complex sensory experience of it cannot but emphasize change.

As a result, the poem's sensory descriptions have an elegiac tone. The world to which they properly belonged is gone, in part "naturally" as it has become the speaker's past, in part "culturally" as the poet has lived to see some of its features legislated away. *Ode* 1.9 thus foregrounds a relationship between sensory experience and "culture." Even in the short span of an individual's lifetime, particular sensory experiences and practices can become matters of memory, while others take the fore. Horace's poem exemplifies how sensory experience may be a matter of engagement with, and critique of, culture.

CATULLUS AND SENSORY EXPERIENCE IN TRANSLATION

Ode 1.9, like many of Horace's poems, adapts a Greek original (Alcaeus fr. 338 Voight). The boundaries between cultures or traditions are thus somewhat permeable. Horace valued archaic Greek lyric, while other authors preferred other genres and periods both Greek and Latin. The resultant shared literary tradition may distort our image of ancient sensory experience by concealing what were in fact real differences between cultures, places, and times. There is nonetheless something significant in the fact that so many representations of sensory experience were shared in antiquity: *mutatis mutandis*, this confirms our impression that there is some common ground to sensory experience and practice in Greek and Roman traditions.

To develop this further we might compare works expressing similar sensory experiences, asking which practices they represent together (e.g., *Ode* 1.4, progressing virtually identically to 1.9; cf. *Ode* 1.11.3–6 and *Epode* 13.1–6). We may also compare sensory experiences as they are figured in adaptations or translations. For example we may consider Catullus 51 and Sappho 31.[17] Catullus' experience upon seeing a beloved woman is expressed in sensory terms: the sight of her "snatches away all [his] senses" (vv. 5–6), with tongue growing numb (taste but also speech), a thin flame flowing under joints (touch), ears ringing (hearing), and, in a sort of ring-structure, eyes whose sight started it all darkening over (vv. 9–12). Such is the feeling generated by the poem, its "lyric consciousness," that we take these expressions to be personal, "from the heart" if not "from life" (see, e.g., Skinner 2003; Wiseman 1985).

But of course Catullus translates Sappho's 31, whose speaker had recorded her own symptoms upon seeing a beloved woman: tongue breaks (taste and speech), fire races under skin (touch), eyes stop from seeing (sight), ears roar (hearing), sweat drenches (touch), the body trembles (proprioception) (vv. 9–14). The differences are significant (see Stevens 2013: Chapter 7). For our purposes, however, what matters is the fact, the very possibility, of the translation: Catullus evidently felt that "his" experience could be communicated in terms of another person's sensory experience.

Translation or adaptation is thus a complex sensory practice. The literary tradition allows for the expression of what may not have been "real" but is plausible in sense-perceptual terms, while images of sensory experience serve to communicate participation in that tradition. In this connection we may add Catullus 50. "I made this poem for you, my sweet" (v. 16), says Catullus to Calvus, the reason being that a day spent together laughing, drinking wine, and composing poems (vv. 4–6) has left Catullus unable to enjoy his solitude (vv. 9–10). "Inflamed" (v. 8), he is tossed about on his bed by desire to speak with and be with his absent friend (vv. 11–13).

Although "this poem" could refer reflexively to 50, certain points of contact suggest that 51 is intended. Of special interest for our purposes is how in 50 "sleep does not cover [Catullus'] little eyes with quiet" (v. 10), whereas in 51 his eyes' "twin lights are covered by darkness" (vv. 11–12). In these passages, Catullus both wishes and does not wish for a certain ecstatic darkness, sublimely beyond the bounds of ordinary sensory experience. His experience of desire, like Sappho's, verges on the anti-experience of death.

Catullus thus exemplifies a sort of ambivalence in sensory experience and/as translation: as translations, his poems stand in for an absent experience. As in the *Phaedrus*, they also signal desire for persons.[18] But if not for the distance there would be no poem and, so, no complex communication in vivid sense-perceptual terms. (Cf. how 65.15–16 introduces 66.) In this way sensory experience is valued with some ambivalence for its paradoxical capacity to represent the most personal experience in sensory terms that are public, traditional, and shared.

THE ANCIENT IDEA THAT SENSORY PRACTICES ARE ALL "MIXED MEDIA"

For all its communicative power, then, sensory experience was not regarded as a simple good. In our authors, sensory experience can have negative associations or evoke contradictory feelings. In Homer, as we have seen, experience may be considered so painful that the senses and memory are better dulled. Perhaps more neutrally, Horace puts wine to very different purposes, and as noted he returns to the "same" basic sensory experience as in *Ode* 1.9—winter outside, warmth within—in several poems, each with a different feeling. And Catullus, to take only one additional type of example, can represent alienation via exotic soundscapes (cc. 63 and 64) (see Stevens 2013: Chapter 6). In general, then, sensory practice is understood to make communication more complex: communicative intent is not perfectly matched by ordinary sensory experience, while sensory practices may complicate a message with cultural associations of their own.

For our purposes, most important is the fact of complexity in sensory experience and practice: "mixed" sensory media are the rule. Without wishing to overgeneralize, I would say that this is something of a preoccupation in ancient thought.[19] When, for example, Catullus writes that "what a woman says to her desirous lover / ought to be written in the wind and running water" (70), we need not show that he knew the *Phaedrus* as such to recognize a shared sensory experience, namely of writing as evanescent in itself and, so, as a symbol for fleeting experience in time.

Likewise, it is well-known that ancient poetry aspires towards a future beyond "a single generation" and, so, concerns itself with differences among past, passing memory, and what may be made to endure. We may say that the tradition and, to that extent, ancient culture dwells on how to "practice" beyond an individual's sensory experience and on which if any sensory media can accomplish this. The question is whether, and if so how, one sensory experience is like another.

A famous version of this is found in a story attributing the origin of painting to tracing shadows cast by an open flame (Pliny *Natural History* 35.5).[20] The story suggests that painting is a kind of "mixed media," a sensory practice that seeks to represent in one medium as fixed what in another medium is fluid and, therefore, passing in time. In this connection, Horace has helped us to see a particularly important mixture: "poetry [is] like painting" (*ut pictura poesis*; *Ars Poetica* 361). (Cf. *Phaedrus* 275d, where writing's inability to respond to questions is compared to the "aloof silence" of painting.) Both arts are thus attempts to fix into place what is fluid by representation across a boundary between media. (*Ode* 1.9 is painterly in this way.) In general, then, media that might strike us as separate are thus in fact—in ancient practice and discourse—"mixed": any sensory practice is a matter of complex construction in culture.

AESCHYLUS, LONG-DISTANCE COMMUNICATION, AND SENSORY DEPRIVATION

Although sensorial anthropological research makes clear that the "same" or similar material conditions allow for diverse sensory experiences and practices, we may nonetheless be struck by how aspects of sensory experience seem to be shared within a place, period, or culture broadly understood. The commonalities among our authors cannot be because they are all "only human." We might therefore wonder whether shared aspects of sensory experience in antiquity are due in part to material conditions shared among our authors' pre-industrial cultures. Certain aspects of what was figured in discourse as the "natural" state of sensory experience hardly changed over the centuries and spaces represented by our authors. How may we moderns work to approach these fundamentally different bases for sensory experience in antiquity?

To get at that question, for my final example I consider a sensory experience and practice explicitly in the service of something the modern world has taken as a given: long-distance communication. I draw my example from the opening scene of Aeschylus' *Agamemnon*. By drawing us back towards the traditional beginning of the literary tradition in Homer, our first example, this final example will serve to suggest how a cultural history of the senses might encourage continuous reconsideration of ancient discourse and, so, re-examination of ancient sensory experience.

The *Agamemnon* opens with a watchman stationed on the roof of the palace at Thebes to await the fire that will signal the fall of Troy and, it is hoped, the return of the king (1–39).[21] The watchman's sensory experience is strange. As we meet him, it has long been night (he is a year into his watch), and the air is cold with dew. Any signal fire will provide information but only the illusion of warmth. Nor is it clear that the fire's information will be true "signal" as opposed to "noise."[22] For information the watchman already has: visual information that is useless to him (he has learned the night sky; 4–6) as well as an excess of auditory information, the plots of Clytemnestra and Aegisthus.

Problems in communication pervade the play; here they are adumbrated in ways suggestive of sensory experience and its limits. What the watchman knows, he will not speak aloud: he says that there is "an ox on his tongue" (36–7). We do not truly know the meaning of that phrase, but we might imagine weight, thickness, a bristling odor, a taste. The phrase is also meant to evoke emotional disturbance: the watchman has had a year of "fear as his familiar" (14). The man, in a way like the ox, is superliminal, placed outside and above; he is therefore like an animal, domesticated but unhoused, as he himself says "like a dog" (3). In asserting that he will not speak he makes his own eloquent speech uncanny and, so, calls communication into question: what are the sensory aspects of communication, and what are their limits?

In a way, the watchman's restriction has made him less like an animal and more like a machine. He must only watch, he is constrained against speaking what he knows, and he is charged with reporting if and only if he sees the fire. He is effectively mechanical, the last link in a chain of long-distance communication. Part of the drama of this opening scene, then, is that a human being's rich, "natural" capacity for sensory experience is constrained by an impoverished, machine-like purpose imposed by "culture." When the watchman speaks aloud it is strictly to no one; upon receiving the signal he need only cry aloud. Language, perhaps the ancient sensory practice par excellence, is thus distilled, infused with purpose even as it is emptied of human meaning.

We may therefore say that the watchman is compelled to discriminate among sensory experiences in ways that do a kind of violence to perception, "unnaturally" separating the senses from each other and from their cultural associations. Unlike Telemachus, who also awaits a sort of "sign," the watchman goes unrecognized, and his sensory experience is one-sided. The scene is thus charged with tensions between "natural" sense-perception and "cultural" prohibitions. "What living and buried speech is always vibrating here, what howls restrain'd by decorum!" (Whitman *Song of Myself* 8).

To put it perhaps more precisely, the watchman's sensory experience is strained to the point of what we might call sensory deprivation.[23] In place of perception he has only reception of signals. And his refusal to say certain things aloud deprives us, in turn, of information: even as he speaks at length, we are kept in suspense, made to wait for information that may not come and, when it does, may not satisfy. The play's opening scene thus serves to illustrate how central was natural language to communication in antiquity as well as how contingent it was as a sensory practice.

This situation is represented symbolically by the signal-fire: when it comes, its meaning is clear but also insufficient as well as dangerous: from a literary perspective, the fire functions as a vivid symbol, suggesting for example how the destruction of one city, Troy, might rapidly spread to consume another, Thebes. But the signal-fire would have meant additional things in antiquity, implying more than a striking visual image.[24] It must also have suggested other sensory experiences including temperature, focalized as the heat desired by and denied to the only character on stage, and smell, insofar as the sun was the only "fire" that "burned" evidently without consuming an odoriferous fuel. With an eye on Troy, it may matter that the fire is not expressly "sacrificial" and, so, provides a subtle but forceful contrast to the sacrifice that began the whole Trojan affair and, with it, much of the ancient literary tradition.

SIGNAL-FIRES AND SIGNS FOR A CULTURAL HISTORY OF THE SENSES

Concrete sensory experiences in culture precede and may limit more abstract associations to a symbol-like fire. A cultural history of the senses therefore lets us approach not only an "understanding" but also something like an "experience" of ancient life. I wonder, then, whether it may be useful to take the signal-fire as a symbol of our purpose, as we seek to "experience" the ancient world more deeply and directly. How might we respond to each sign of sensory experience as it flashes to us from antiquity, constituting a sort of long-distance communication via particular sensory media?

The type of sign—signal or symbol—makes a difference (see Peirce 1991; Sebeok 1994). Ancient signs are for us perhaps mainly "symbolic," signifying arbitrarily. *Agamemnon*'s fire may thus stand in for "mixed messages" or the politics of "figured speech." Certainly it "stands in for" the end of the war, and we may feel a "natural" association of war's end with daybreak: when the sun rises, it is just as if a war has been won; sunrise suggests victory not only against Troy but also against the dark, the cold, fear, savagery, death. Thinking of a sensory experience as "symbolic" makes us ask, "What does it mean?" And of course there *were* meanings, symbolic associations, to experiences in antiquity.

But there was also the "sensory experience itself." For ancient audience-members, the same signs would have included strong "signalic" components, provoking responses that seemed "natural" insofar as they had been inculcated by culture. The signal-fire does not "stand in for" but *is* light, heat, civilization, danger, the odors of burning wood, oil, incense, fat, meat, manure. These and other cultural associations formed part of the sensory experience of fire. While fire could connote a "mixed message," among other things, it was itself a "mixed sensory medium."

We should therefore say that ancient sensory experiences of fire were different from our own. Likewise when Helen descended, or Athens let out on a plane-tree's shade; when the trees on Soracte groaned while logs crackled on the fire; or when ears rushed with blood made hot by the sight of a lover: when each of these and innumerable other events, daily or untimely, took place, they did so in systems of sensory practices and cultural associations whose complexities we must work, and do well, to recover.

CONCLUSION

What may we say is the upshot of reconsidering ancient sensory experience and practice from this perspective?

An example like Helen's emergence suggests that something as seemingly basic as entering a room is not "natural," as if determined by unmeaningful physical constraints, but "cultural." The meaning of Helen's emergence is communicated via sensory media, via material conditions which are themselves a matter of cultural production insofar as they engage the senses. The detailed attention paid to such sensory mediation by Homer serves to emphasize as well how literature is, in its turn, not a given, as if somehow prior to sensory experience, but a sensory practice with cultural associations of its own. As we have seen in the differences between Homer's and Marlowe's depictions of Helen, representations of "the same thing" in different sensory media thus result in what are in fact "different things" in terms of how their communication engages the senses.

Literature is thus one example of how, again, "the senses" are not fixed but a matter of fluid definition in culture. This should result in a working principle of profound defamiliarization. Another culture's sensory experience reaches us with something of the feeling of the watchman's experience of the signal-fire as long-distance communication. Understood as a sensory medium, the fire evokes the political organization of material conditions required to transmit information over long distances in antiquity; this gives something of a material basis to the *Agamenon*'s thematic interest in political and domestic conflict or miscommunication. As a binary signal—either it appears or it does not—the fire recalls other signals of the same order, for example the sail whose color, white or black, would indicate the success or failure of Theseus' mission to kill the Minotaur (e.g., Plutarch *Life of Theseus* 17.5). More generally the signal-fire recalls some other modes of long-distance communication, including other relays (e.g. of messengers on foot or horseback), as well as more singular acts of "communication" like that which gave the "marathon" its name.

We may therefore conclude that our experience of antiquity is itself a matter of sensory mediation: signs reach us at something like long distance, and perhaps inevitably we respond to them at least in part in terms of our own sensory culture. In this chapter I have aimed at giving vivid impressions of how literary images may be understood as reflecting or refracting, as well as embodying, a wide range of actual sensory experiences and practices; *mutatis mutandis*, the same approach can be taken to visual or plastic arts and to other material remains. Approaching antiquity in this way may seem to require speculation. There is a risk of overinterpretation, even fantasy: to get at ancient sensory experience means exercising the critical imagination. But the upshot of a careful, reconstructive cultural history is, I would say, everything: a deeper, clearer understanding of ancient experience as it was, inevitably, mediated by "the senses," which must be understood not as simply given but as matters of complex cultural definition in turn.

NOTES

Chapter One

1 *Pan.* 11.8–12 for Diocletian and Maximian, Amm. 16.10.8 on dragon standards with Syme (1968: 15–16; 16.10.9–10) on the demeanor of Constantius II; see also MacCormack (1981: 17–33) on early *adventus* ceremonies; for the evolution of court ceremonial see Potter (2012: 51–4). For issues of class and access to foods see Goody (1982: 97–153).
2 OLD s.v. *sacro; sacer; sacrosanctus*. For the problem of a lack of a simple Latin equivalent to the Greek *miasma* see Lennon (2014: 43); Fantham (2012: 60), also important on *polluo*.
3 Douglas (1996: 41–57, esp, 52–3); for discussion of the validity of her paradigm see also the useful reviews in Olyan (2008) and Bradley (2012a: 11–14).
4 Edmondson (1996). For the Augustan regulation removing women to the upper levels of the amphitheater see Suet. *Aug.* 44.2.
5 Ath. *Diep* 5.198a–c tr. Rice (1983: 9–10) and her further discussion of the overall significance on pp. 180–92; see also Schmitt Pantal (1997: 459–60).
6 Gell, *NA* 2.24.2–6 on the lex Fannia in general esp. limits on daily expenditure, Plin. *NH* 10.139 (noting techniques of evading the restriction) on the hen and Ath. *Diep.* 6.274c–e on the laws and their observation; see in general Roisevach (2006) especially pp. 6–7 on the "natural economy." The principle of limiting expenditure by day remained at the heart of later laws: see AG NA 2.24.7–15; Tac. *Ann.* 3.52–4.
7 Much of what follows owes a significant debt to Donahue (2004: 44–52).
8 Plut. *Quaest. Conv.* 2.10.642e–f with Durand (1989: 103). Though it should be noted that at some sacrifices, magistrates could get more than other people, see esp. Rhodes and Osborne (2003: n. 81 fr. B lines 10–15); see also prescriptions such as that in Rhodes and Osborne (2003: n. 62 lines 49–54) with further discussion on p. 310.

9 *SEG* 32 n. 1243 lines 16–19. See also Hadot (1982: 173–4) noting that the wedding feast may have been more elaborate since he may not have provided a full meal in conjunction with the sacrifice to Dionysius.
10 Plut. *Crass.* 12.2; *Caes.* 55.4 where Plutarch's implication that he feasted "all" the people on 22,000 *triclinia* is problematic; for the suggestion that these events influenced habits as a whole see D'Arms (1998: 32–43; 2000: 192–200, esp. 195–7); for differential seating see the relief from Amiternum, Dunbabin (2004: 82); for people per couch see the relief from Sentinum discussed in Dunbabin, pp. 76–7.
11 Dio 55.2.4. See also Dio 55.8.2 where it is senators who dine with him on the Capitolium (see Swan 2004: 48–9; 74–5). For the *ludi saeculares* see Pighi (1965: 109–36, esp. lines 32; 35; 39; 71; 81–2; 89; 101–2; 109; 117; 138 for distributions and banquets). For people on the household staff who were concerned with banquets see Donahue (2004: 24).
12 For numbers of dead at Rome see Bodel (2000: 129); for body parts see Oros. *Adv. pagan.* 7.4.1 with Bodel (2000: 129); Suet. *Vesp.* 5.4 and Mart. 10.5.11 for a beggar thinking his dead body will be eaten by dogs, with Scobie (1986: 419); on *turgaria* and *ergasteria* see Scobie (1986: 402); see also Carroll (2006: 69–78).
13 Art. *On.* 2.3 tr. Harris-McCoy (2012: 155); see also Sève (1979: 342–3) (though the woman whose funeral is described in the text Sève publishes was in purple).
14 Eus. *VC* 4.70; the issue of Constantine's burial is complex: see Grierson *et al.* (1962); Bardill (2012: 367–84). For the context of the Christian cult of relics in its sensory aspects see Harvey (2006: 227–9).

Chapter Two

1 Due to near-universal prohibitions against burying the dead within city limits, encountering such elaborate tombs forming a "city of the dead" on the outskirts of major metropolises would have been a common experience in the ancient world. Another famous example is the Kerameikos district just outside Athens.
2 On Roman tombs, burials, the treatment of corpses both rich and poor, and the dumping of various forms of refuse on the outskirts of cities, see Bodel (1986, 2000), Hope (2000), Patterson (2000), Kyle (1998), Scobie (1986), Hopkins (1983), and the collection of articles edited by Raventós and Remolà (2000).
3 The population of Rome is a much-debated topic, but some good introductions to the relevant issues can be found in Hopkins (1978), Morley (1996), and Purcell (1999).
4 Good introductions to the topic of women and their experiences in the ancient world include D'Ambra (2006), Fantham *et al.* (1994), and Vivanto (2008).
5 Perhaps to avoid such embarrassments, Nero eventually organized a private cheerleading section of 5,000 young Romans who were trained in the sophisticated applause techniques used in the city of Alexandria, which included different clapping noises produced by holding the hands flat or cupped while applauding (Suetonius *Nero* 20). On types of acclamations and applause, see Aldrete (1999).

Chapter Five

1 Cartledge (1997: 10–11) whose characterizations I borrow; Lee (2005: 5). Fragment numbers for all thinkers discussed in this chapter follow DK.
2 For sixth-century BCE exploration of this theme, cf. Xenoph. B34 DK with Hussey (1990: 37–8), Lesher (1999: 228–31); Bryan (2012: 49–51; cf. 53–5).
3 See Democr. B5.1 DK; Xen. *Mem.* 1.4.12; for vocal articulation as "the voice in joints" see Arist. *Hist. an.* 536b10–12.
4 Epic notion of the witness, see Pritzl (1985: 306); a different view, Robb (1991: 662).
5 Homeric meaning of *melea*: Wersinger (2008: 45–61, esp. 56, citing Aristotle's variant at *Metaph.* $Γ^5$. 1009^{b}22); *pace* Popper (1963: 553).
6 For the physical *krasis* of B16 DK as a "muddle," see Mourelatos 2008: 256, 348.
7 See Kingsley (2002: 362–6) for a detailed exegesis of the opening chariot ride, its epic model, and Empedocles' language of the senses.
8 Kingsley (2002: 335). Enjoinders to see and hear: B17.14 DK; B17.21 DK; but esp. B17.60–2, 68–9 DK.
9 See Sedley (2007: 37) and n.18 for the likely placement of B20 DK. after B17 DK; cf. Kingsley (2003: 509).
10 O'Brien (1969: 275). For Empedocles' language of limbs denoting the four elements of the cosmos in their different aspects as separate and joined-together, see Wersinger (2008: 63 n.1; cf. 66–7).
11 This physiological account complements the parallel imagery in the poem that evokes Empedocles' teachings as seeds to be pressed down under our "thinking organs," the *prapides* (B110 DK) or the *splancha* (B4 DK), and nurtured by the "assurances" of the senses (which bring in the elements that are aptly called "roots") at B4 DK, see Kingsley (2003: 554); Picot (2009: esp. 80).
12 For later classifications of speech as a sense in Philo of Alexandria (once in the context of an enumeration of seven senses), and several medieval writers, see Howes (2009: 3–6).
13 For the sense of the hot and the cold as an *aisthēsis*, see Pl. *Tht.* 156b. Cf. Presti (2007: 141); Jouanna (1999: 280).
14 For Hippocratic enumerations of the five senses (sight, hearing, smell, touch, taste) alongside *gnōmē* or *logismos*, as sources of knowledge for the physician, see Jouanna (2003: 17–18, 20); Presti (2007); Lee (2005: 229–47) discusses Democr. B11 DK.
15 Lee (2005: 156–7), and esp. 157 on 186b11–c5, d2–5 for the passivity of sense perception and the activity of thinking.
16 Cf. *Symp.* 210a4–12a7, esp. 212a4–5 (physical beauty as an *eidōlon*, "image" or "phantom," of the Beautiful itself); *Rep.* 598b with Paton (1922: 85) for sensible appearances as *phantasmata* and *eidōla*; and see also Nightingale (2004: 164–6) on *Phdr.* 250a–e for the philosophic soul's instant recollection of the Form of Beauty upon the visual perception of beauty; *Rep.* 509d–511e, 533a–34d for the soul's use of perceptible things as "images" or "likenesses" (*eikones*) in order to progress toward intelligibles; wider role of "likenesses" (*eikones*) in stimulating dialectical reflection, see Smith (1985).

17 I reverse the order of Aristotle's discussion; this question, explored in the first part of *DA* III.2, precedes the issue of complex perception.
18 I omit Augustine of Hippo (*c*. 354–430 CE), whose eclectic theory of perception, well known to medieval Latin authors, incorporates Aristotelian, Neoplatonic, Stoic, and ancient medical ideas.
19 Sharples and van der Eijk (2008: 9–10), with 25, 121–2 n.607 for Nemesius' likely debts to Posidonius of Byzantium; van der Eijk (2008); cf. Green (2003: 137–41). Nemesius does not use the term "inner senses", see Wolfson (1935: 72, esp. n.18); (cf. Fletcher and 1993: 562).
20 Wolfson (1935: 71–6) hypothesizes a Galenic source for the classifications of these Arab and Hebrew thinkers; for the transmission to the East of Galen's and Aristotle's ideas *via* the translation of Nemesius' treatise into Arabic in the ninth century CE, see Kahana-Smilansky (2011: 232); his influence on Avicenna, van der Eijk (2008); a different view, Heller-Roazen (2007: 145–6, and 321–2, n.10).

Chapter Seven

1 Translations from Greek and Latin are sometimes my own, sometimes borrowed from the Loeb editions of classical texts (unless otherwise indicated).
2 The first etymology is recorded by the lexicographer Hesychius (736.2) while the second appears in Plato *Cratylus* 420a–b.
3 The twelfth-century Byzantine commentator of Homer Eustathius argues that Nausicaa's compliments to Odysseus before and after he bathes ("you do not seem a bad man," 6.187; "Oh, if he wished to stay here! He looks like the gods!", 6.245 ff.) betray similar feelings, but that in the first instance she is understated because she is talking to him directly, whereas in his absence she finds the courage to praise him more exuberantly (*Commentary on the Odyssey* 1.251.40–3).
4 *Aeneid* 4.83: *illum absens absentem auditque videtque*. Thanks to Jim McKeown for the translation of this untranslatable line.
5 See, respectively, Athenaeus *Wise Men at Dinner* 13.564e; *Palatine Anthology* 5.141; 5.121; 5.69. Of a prized courtesan we read a similar compliment: "with voice and conversation she was well supplied" (Athenaeus 13.578c). *Peithô* and "sweetness of speech" appear also at *Palatine Anthology* 5.137. See also, in the same collection, 5.140; 5.148; 5.155; 5.158; 5.195; 5.241.
6 Aristaenetus 1.12.20. More sources (especially Roman) on the ancient erotics of smell are in Classen (1994: 27–30).
7 Lucian *Affairs of the Heart* 53. See also Achilles Tatius *Leucippe and Clitophon* 4.7.8: "I want to hear her voice, hold her hand, touch her body."
8 The novels are conveniently assembled in Reardon (1989), from where I borrow the translations with a few exceptions.
9 Daphnis and Chloe are the exception, and perhaps also the heroine of Achilles Tatius' novel; see below.
10 See *War and Peace*, Book 2, Part 3, Chapters 2 and 19; *L'enfant maudit*, pp. 194–5 (in the edition by François Germain, Paris, Les Belles Lettres, 1965). Dolar (1996a: 134) refers to these episodes as examples of "love at first hearing."

11 Scenes of first encounter can be accompanied by verbal exchanges: see the examples and the discussion in Rousset (1989).
12 In Achilles Tatius the hero's father and the heroine's mother are present at their children's first encounter.
13 In his recent *The Great Gatsby*, Luhrmann has filmed the encounter of Gatsby and Daisy in about this way.
14 See especially Morgan (1996: 188). The exception is *Daphnis and Chloe*, which tells the story of two children discovering love and its needs.
15 The bibliography on Greek and Roman conceptions of selfhood is vast. Concerning the novel see, most recently, the lucid treatment in Whitmarsh (2011: 41). Fundamental works on the topic of character are Pelling (1990) and Gill (2006).
16 In *An Ephesian Story*, two more stories of perfectly mutual love, parallel to the protagonists', also begin as love at first sight (3.2; 5.1).
17 The episodes are countless. On Callirhoe's epiphanies see Hägg (2004) and Zeitlin (2003).
18 This topic would require a much more in-depth treatment than can be afforded here. See the incisive reflections, in a Lacanian perspective, of Dolar (1996b: 16–24).
19 Helen has verbal and vocal talents: she can imitate the voices of other women, as she recounts in *Odyssey* 4; in the same book she pours a drug to enhance the pleasure of telling and hearing stories; and in *Iliad* 3 she describes the Greek heroes one by one to Priam (as well as to the poem's audience).
20 The famous episode in Herodotus in which Candaules praises his wife's beauty to Gyges, then coerces him to watch her as she undresses to go to bed, also plays up the stronger erotic power of sight.
21 See respectively, *Leucippe and Clitophon* 2.13; 6.3.5; 6.4.4. For the last passage I borrow Whitmarsh's translation (Whitmarsh and Morales 2001), which renders *physei* by "natural," pointing up the effectiveness of artifice in creating an illusion of reality. When Thersander finally sees Leucippe, he is struck by lightning (6.6.3). But he was planning to go to her already as a lover. The servant has a point when he tells Leucippe that Thersander's love for her is his doing (6.11.4).

Chapter Eight

1 Further on this approach, see Butler and Purves (2013), the first of a series of volumes to be published by Acumen examining each of the ancient senses in turn.
2 Discussion and references: Panzanelli *et al.* (2008) on ancient, medieval, and modern sculptural polychromy; Brinkmann (2003) on archaic and early classical polychromy; Brinkmann and Wünsche (2007: 150–67) on the "Alexander Mosaic."
3 I have discussed this literary tradition at some length in Bradley (2009a: Chapter 6, esp. p. 161 with references; in general on ancient cosmetics, see Carannante and D'Acunto 2012; Stewart 2007).
4 See Ovid, *Ars Amatoria* 3.159–68, discussed in Bradley (2009a: 176–8). Cf. Propertius 2.18.23–30; Martial 3.43 on a man dyeing his grey hair. See also the Introduction to this volume.

5 See Pliny *Natural History* 13.18 on *regalium*, a perfume traditionally believed to have been used by the kings of Parthia, which consisted of twenty-five different ingredients.
6 See Csapo and Slater (1995: esp. 331–48); Plato *Republic* 398d–9d on the relationship between music and words. Cf. Pollux, *Onomasticon* 99–112 on different types of singing and dancing associated with the chorus.
7 Aristotle *Rhetoric* 1403b26–33; Vitruvius 5.4–5 on setting up inverted bronze urns in Greek theaters to improve resonance. See Wiles (1991: Chapter 8) on language and voice; Csapo and Slater (1995: 265–8) on voice; cf. McCart (2007: 249–50) on Pythagoean/Platonic dimensions and symmetry at Epidauros to achieve acoustic perfection.
8 See Csapo and Slater (1995: 301–6, 118ff.) on organized support and chanting. See Pollux 121–32 on spectators clucking, hissing, and banging their heels, and on the production of thunder effects, with McDonald and Walton (2007: 5).
9 See Aristotle *Poetics* 1455, 1462a and Aulus Gellius 1.5 on elaborate gestures associated with actors. See Plato *Laws* 814d–16e on different types of dance and their associations; in general, Zarifi (2007). In general on theater and visual art, see Green (2007: 163–83).
10 Csapo and Slater (1995: 256ff.). On stage machinery, see Aristophanes *Peace* 173–6; Plato *Cratylus* 425d; Aristotle *Poetics* 1454a36–65. Pollux 121–32 also gives a detailed description of typical props, machinery, trapdoors, etc.
11 Horace *Epistles* 6.28; cf. 14.1–5 on visual effects creating only "sensation" (*to teratōdes*), observing that performances of the Oedipus story should avoid showing violence on stage. On Aristotle's *Poetics* and dramatic theory, see Wiles (2007).
12 Vitruvius 7 pref. 11; cf. 5.6.8–9 on stage scenery in the planning of theaters. See Pliny, *Natural History* 35.23 on the first multi-colored *scaena* in Rome in the early first century BCE, employing illusionistic techniques of *skēnographia*, which deceived the eyes of spectators and suicidal birds alike.
13 See Wiles (1999) and Beacham (2007) for a summary of developments and analysis of the evidence. Awnings: described in graphic detail in Lucretius *On the Nature of Things* 4.75–83, discussed in Bradley (2009a: 83–5) and Beacham (2007: 217). See Pliny *Natural History* 36.114–15, deriding Scaurus' richly decorated temporary theatre in 58 BCE, discussed by Beacham (2007: 217–18).
14 On this vase, see Taplin and Wyles (2010); Csapo and Slater (1995: 69–70 and plate 8). See also Ley (2007: 279) on the characteristic importance of visual and auditory props in satyr plays, as well as food and drink. In general on interpreting drama in vase painting, see Green (2007).
15 Demosthenes *Against Meidias* 51–4. In general, see Graf (2007: esp. 60–4), who discusses the importance of libations, sacrifice, and incense in dramatic performances. On the senses in religion, see Ashbrook Harvey, this volume.
16 See Csapo and Slater (1995: 106). See Plutarch *On the love of wealth* 527d on wine and figs; Pollux 6.75 and Athenaeus 3.111b on bread; Suda, s.v. "askophorein" on wineskins; cf. Scholion to Aristophanes *Acharnians* 241, discussing the "first fruits." On drama and festivals in general, see Rehm (2007).

17 See Beacham (2007: 202–4 and 218–23) for further details; cf. Csapo and Slater (1995: 49–50). See Gleason (1994) on the gardens. See Propertius 2.32.30 for a description of the portico, with its shady columns, plane trees and elaborate water features. Cf. Beacham (2007: 217) on stages decorated with silver, gold, and ivory. On the gardens, see Totelin (2012: esp. 134–5).

Chapter Nine

1 I am grateful to Jerry Toner for the invitation to write and for comments on drafts. Much of the writing was done in the congenial sensory settings of Taste Budd's Café in Red Hook, NY and Otherlands Café in Memphis, TN. The approach may also be called "sensorial anthropology." (See Carterette and Friedman 1978; Classen 1993: 1–14, 79–105, 121–38; Classen *et al.* 1994: 1–10; Howes 2003, 2005; Smith 2008; Stoller 1989; Synnott 1991. For "the five senses" see Serres 2009 and Vinge 1975.)
2 For "defamiliarization" see Shklovskij (1998).
3 Translations are Robert Fagles' (2006). On the first books of the *Odyssey* consult Heubeck *et al.* (1990). For discussions of Homer I am grateful to the students in my fall 2011 literature seminar in the Bard Prison Initiative.
4 Telemachus' question preoccupies the first four books. More generally the question of recognition centers around Odysseus: see above all Eurycleia's recognition of his scar (19.438–575, with Auerbach's essay, 2003).
5 Symbolically the wool links Helen to Penelope, whose weaving is both deception (of the suitors) and sign of fidelity (to Odysseus). But Helen is not pictured using the wool (*contra* Heubeck *et al.* 1990 *ad* 201, comparing *Il.* 3.125ff.). Likewise her emergence is different from Penelope's first appearance (1.380f.; cf. 21.390f.), where Penelope is "radiant" but veiled and dissolves into tears.
6 Helen's appearance to Telemachus must therefore be "striking" indeed, and her recognition of his paternity the more so.
7 See Heubeck *et al.* (1990) *ad loc.* 206–7. Unmixed wine in antiquity may have been sweet and thick. The connection between memory and sense-perception is pervasive in the epic; cf., e.g., the Lotus-eaters (9.95), and the dead drinking blood in order to speak (11.165).
8 On the difficulty of describing smells see Stevens (2008: 168), with sources in n. 17.
9 This affords poetry a suggestive power that is incompletely matched in visual arts (see e.g. Turner 2004 on problems casting an actress to play Helen).
10 Translations are Robin Waterfield's (2002). On the *Phaedrus*, see Ferrari (1987) and Rossetti (1992). For conversations about Plato I am grateful to Prof. Thomas Bartscherer of Bard College.
11 The *locus classicus* is of course the *Republic*. A "counter-argument" is offered in the *Symposium* by "Diotima": physical beauty may conduce to appreciation of beauty as such.

12 Cf. Homer *Il.* 6.169, where "baleful signs," the only writing in Homeric epic, are set to cause Bellerophon's death, but only via contiguity with his person (6.169). On the *Phaedrus'* sexual suggestiveness see Partridge (1999); cf. *Charmides* and *Symposium* 177d, 198d.
13 Cf. Homer *Il.* 3.150–2, where the Trojan old men, watching the war from a tower, are compared to cicadas in a tree; see Stanford (1969).
14 Socrates actually lived outside the walls (Osborne 1999 n. 9 observes that Socrates may have passed this "secluded spot" daily); cf. 229bc.
15 Translations from Horace are my own. On the *Odes* consult Commager (1995) and Nisbet and Hubbard (1989). For first and lasting lessons on *Ode* 1.9 I am grateful to Prof. Richard Tron of Reed College.
16 For wine cf., e.g., *Ode* 1.37.1: "now we must drink"; and the phrase *carpe diem*, meaning to "pluck each day" like a grape from the bunch; see Davis (2007).
17 Translations from Catullus are my own. A standard commentary is Thomson (2003). For discussions of Catullus I am grateful to students in various classes at Bard College, to Prof. David Wray of the University of Chicago, and to Prof. Ernst Fredricksmeyer of the University of Colorado, Boulder.
18 This literary practice (cf., e.g., Ovid *Amores* 1.1) is matched by a social practice of "circulating" a person with a letter of introduction. Books and persons could thus be figured as "guests" (e.g., Cicero *Off.* 3.121) and as "blemished" skins (with Fredrick 1997; cf. MacKendrick 2004).
19 Cf. modern debate about "purity" in the arts, e.g., Greenberg (1940) (after Lessing [1776] 1984) and Mitchell (1989).
20 On shadows in art see Stevens (2010: 3), with sources there.
21 Translations are Robert Fagles' (in *The Oresteia* [1984]). For conversations on *Agamemnon* I am grateful to the students in my fall 2011 literature seminar in the Bard Prison Initiative and to Lucy Schmid, Bard College 2012, whose honors thesis treated the play.
22 These terms are from information theory; see Hayles (1999). For "signals" in ancient intelligence activities see Sheldon (2007: 199–249).
23 Loss of "conversation" was central to exile: cf. Cicero *Att.* 3.12.3 (with Beard 2003: 133); and Ovid *Tr.* 1.3.69 and 5.7.61 (with Stevens 2009).
24 This is true even if, as seems possible, the sun crested the theater's horizon in time with the watchman's apostrophe to "fire of the night, that brings my spirit day."

BIBLIOGRAPHY

Adam, J-P., 1994, *Roman Building: materials and techniques*, Bloomington, IN: Indiana University Press.
Adams, J. N., 1995, *Pelagonius and Latin Veterinary Terminology in the Roman Empire*, Leiden: E. J. Brill.
Aldrete, G. S., 1999, *Gestures and Acclamations in Ancient Rome*, Baltimore, MD: Johns Hopkins University Press.
Aldrete, G. S., 2007, *Floods of the Tiber in Ancient Rome*, Baltimore, MD: Johns Hopkins University Press.
Aldrete, G. S., 2008, *Daily Life in the Roman City: Rome, Pompeii, and Ostia*, Norman, OK: University of Oklahoma Press.
Arbesmann, R., Joseph Daly, E., and Quain, E., 1959, *Tertullian: Disciplinary, Moral and Ascetical Works*, FC 40, New York: Fathers of the Church, Inc.
Atkins, M. and Osborne, R. (eds), 2006, *Poverty in the Roman World*, New York: Cambridge University Press.
Auerbach, E., 2003. *Mimesis: the representation of reality in western literature*, Princton, NJ: Princeton University Press.
Babbit, F. C. (ed. and trans.), 1972, Plutarch, *Moralia: table-talk*, LCL, 16 vols, Cambridge, MA: Harvard University Press.
Baldovin, J., 1987, *The Urban Character of Christian Worship: the origins, development, and meaning of stational liturgy*, OCA 228, Rome: Pontificum Institutum Studiorum.
Barbet, A., Fuchs, M., and Tuffreau-Libre, M., 1997, "Les divers utilisations des pigments et leurs contenants," in H. Béarat *et al.* (eds), *Roman Wall Painting: materials, techniques, analysis and conservation*, Freiburg: Institute of Mineralogy and Petrography.
Bardill, J., 2012, *Constantine, Divine Emperor of the Christian Golden Age*, Cambridge: Cambridge University Press.

Barker, A., 2000, "Timaeus on music and the liver," in M. R. Wright (ed.), *Reason and Necessity: essays on Plato's Timaeus*, London: Duckworth.

Barnard, L. W. (trans.), 1997, *Justin Martyr, The First and Second Apologies*, New York: Paulist Press.

Baynes, N. H. and Dawes, E., 1948, *Three Byzantine Saints: contemporary biographies*, Oxford: Blackwell.

Beacham, R., 1999, *Spectacle Entertainments of Early Imperial Rome*, New Haven, CT: Yale University Press.

Beacham, R., 2007, "Playing places: the temporary and the permanent," in M. McDonald and J. M. Walton (eds), 2007, *The Cambridge Companion to Greek and Roman Theatre*, Cambridge: Cambridge University Press.

Béarat, H., 1997, "Quelle est la gamme exacte des pigments romains? Confrontation des résultats d'analyse avec les textes de Vitruve et Pline," in H. Béarat *et al.* (eds), *Roman Wall Painting: materials, techniques, analysis and conservation*, Freiburg: Institute of Mineralogy and Petrography.

Beard, M., 2003, "Ciceronian correspondences: making a book out of letters," in T. P. Wiseman (ed.), *Classics in Progress*, Oxford: Oxford University Press.

Beard, M., North, J., and Price, P. (eds), 1998, *Religions of Rome*, 2 vols, Cambridge: Cambridge University Press.

Beare, J. I., 1906, *Greek Theories of Elementary Cognition From Alcmaeon to Aristotle*, Oxford: Clarendon Press.

BeDuhn, J. D., 2000, *The Manichean Body: in discipline and ritual*, Baltimore, MD: Johns Hopkins University Press.

Beer, M., 2010, *Taste or Taboo: dietary choices in antiquity*, Devon: Prospect Books.

Bell, A., 2004, *Spectacular Power in the Greek and Roman City*, New York: Oxford University Press.

Betts, E., 2011, "Towards a multisensory experience of movement in the City of Rome," in R. Laurence and D. J. Newsome (eds), *Rome, Ostia and Pompeii: movement and space*, Oxford: Oxford University Press.

Betz, H. D. (ed.), 1992, *The Greek Magical Papyri in Translation, including the Demotic spells*, Chicago: University of Chicago Press.

Bodel, J., 1986, "Graveyards and groves," *American Journal of Ancient History*, 11, 1–133.

Bodel, J., 2000, "Dealing with the dead: undertakers, executioners and potter's fields in ancient Rome," in V. Hope and E. Marshall (eds), *Death and Disease in the Ancient City*, pp. 128–51, New York: Routledge.

Bowie, E., and Elsner, J. (eds), 2009, *Philostratus*, Cambridge: Cambridge University Press.

Bradbury, S., 2004, *Selected Letters of Libanius from the Age of Constantius and Julian*, TTH 41, Liverpool: Liverpool University Press.

Bradley, K., 1994, *Slavery and Society at Rome*, New York: Cambridge University Press.

Bradley, M., 2004, "The colour blush in ancient Rome," in L. Cleland and K. Stears (eds), *Colour in the Ancient Mediterranean World*, Oxford: BAR.

Bradley, M., 2006, "Colour and marble in early Imperial Rome," *Proceedings of the Cambridge Philological Society*, 52, 1–22.

Bradley, M., 2009a, *Colour and Meaning in Ancient Rome*, Cambridge: Cambridge University Press.

Bradley, M., 2009b, "The importance of colour on ancient marble sculpture," *Art History*, 32, 427–57.

Bradley, M. (ed.), 2012a, *Rome, Pollution and Propriety: dirt, disease, and hygiene in the Eternal City from antiquity to modernity*, Cambridge: Cambridge University Press.

Bradley, M., 2012b, "Approaches to pollution and propriety," in M. Bradley, (ed.), *Rome, Pollution and Propriety: dirt, disease, and hygiene in the Eternal City from antiquity to modernity*, Cambridge: Cambridge University Press.

Bradley, M., 2013, "Colour as synaesthetic experience in antiquity," in S. Butler and A. Purves (eds), *Synaesthesia and the Ancient Senses*, Durham: Acumen.

Bremmer, J. N., 1994, *Greek Religion*, New York: Oxford University Press.

Brinkmann, V., 2003, *Die Polychromie der archaischen und frühklassischen Skulpturen*, Munich: Biering & Brinkmann.

Brinkmann, V. and Wünsche, R. (eds), 2007, *Gods in Color: painted sculpture of classical antiquity*, Munich: Stiftung Archäologie Glyptothek.

Brothwell, D. and Brothwell, P., 1998, *Food in Antiquity*, Baltimore, MD: Johns Hopkins University Press.

Brown, P., [1988] 2008, *The Body and Society: men, women, and sexual renunciation in early Christianity*, New York: Columbia University Press.

Bryan, J., 2012, *Likeness and Likelihood in the Presocratics and Plato*, Cambridge: Cambridge University Press.

Burkert, W., 1985, *Greek Religion*, trans. J. Raffan, Cambridge, MA: Harvard University Press.

Burnyeat, M. F., 1976, "Plato on the grammar of perceiving," *Classical Quarterly*, 26, 29–51.

Butler, S. and Purves, A. (eds), 2013, *Synaesthesia and the Ancient Senses*, Durham: Acumen.

Cameron, A. and Hall, S. G. (ed. and trans.), 1999, Eusebius, *Life of Constantine*, Oxford: Clarendon Press.

Carannante, A. and D'Acunto, M. (eds), 2012, *I profumi nelle societá antiche: produzione, commercio, usi, valori simbolici*, Paestum: Pandemos.

Carroll, M., 2006, *Spirits of the Dead: Roman funerary commemoration in Western Europe*, Oxford: Oxford University Press.

Carterette, E. C. and Friedman, M. P. (eds), 1978, *Tasting and Smelling*, New York: Academic Press Inc.

Cartledge, P., 1997, *Democritus*, London: Phoenix.

Caseau, B., 2001, "Les usages médicaux de l'encens et des parfums: un aspect de la medicine populaire antique et de sa christianisation," in S. Bazin-Tacchella, D. Quéruel, and É. Samama (eds), *Air, Miames, et Contagion: Les épidémies dans l'Antiquité au Moyen Age*, Langres: Dominique Guéniot.

Casson, L., 1989, *The Periplus Maris Erythraei: text with introduction, translation, and commentary*, Princeton: Princeton University Press.

Chadwick, H., 1991, *Saint Augustine, Confessions*, Oxford: Oxford University Press.
Cima, M. and La Rocca, E. (eds), 1998, *Horti Romani*, Rome: L'Erma di Bretschneider.
Clarke, E. C., Dillon, J. M., and Hershbell, J. P. (trans.), 2004, Iamblichus, *De mysteriis*, Leiden: Brill.
Classen, C., 1993, *Worlds of Sense: exploring the senses in history and across cultures*. London: Routledge.
Classen, C., 1994, "The aromas of antiquity," in C. Classen, D. Howes, and A. Synott (eds), *Aroma: the cultural history of smell*, London: Routledge.
Classen, C., Howes D., and Synnott, A. (eds), 1994, *Aroma: the cultural history of smell*, London: Routledge.
Coldstream, J. N., 2003, *Geometric Greece: 900–700 BC*, London: Routledge.
Colson, F. H. (ed. and trans.), 1984, Philo, *Works*, 9 vols, LCL, Cambridge, MA: Harvard University Press.
Commager, S., 1995, *The Odes of Horace: A Critical Study*, Norman, OK: University of Oklahoma Press.
Corbeill, A., 2004, *Nature Embodied: gesture in ancient Rome*, Princeton, NJ: Princeton University Press.
Costantini, M., Graziani, F., and Rolet, S., 2006, *Le défi de l'art: Philostrate, Callistrate et l'image sophistique*, Rennes: Presses Universitaires de Rennes.
Crow, J., 2008, *The Water Supply of Byzantine Constantinople*, JRS Monograph 11, London: Society for the Promotion of Roman Studies.
Csapo, E. and Slater, W., 1995, *The Context of Ancient Drama*, Ann Arbor, MI: University of Michigan Press.
Cunningham, A., 2002, "The pen and the sword: recovering the disciplinary identity of physiology and anatomy before 1800—I: old physiology—the pen," *Studies in History and Philosophy of Science*, 33, 631–5.
Curd, P., [1998] 2004, *The Legacy of Parmenides. Eleatic monism and later presocratic thought*, Las Vegas: Parmenides Publishing.
Curd, P., 2011, "Thought and body in Parmenides," in N-L. Cordero (ed.), *Parmenides: vulnerable and awesome*, Las Vegas: Parmenides Publishing.
D'Ambra, E., 2006, *Roman Women*, New York: Cambridge University Press.
D'Arms, J. H., 1998, "Between public and private: the *Epulum Publicum* and Caesar's *Horti trans Tiberim*," in M. Cima and E. La Rocca (eds), *Horti Romani*, Rome: "L'Erma" di Bretschneider.
D'Arms, J. H., 2000, "P. Lucilius Gamala's feasts for the Ostians and their Roman models," *JRA*, 13, 192–200.
Dalby, A., 2000, *Dangerous Tastes: spices in world history*, London: British Museum Press.
Dalby, A., 2002, *Empire of Pleasure*, New York: Routledge.
Davis, G., 2007, "Wine and the symposium," in S. Harrison (ed.), *The Cambridge Companion to Horace*, Cambridge: Cambridge University Press.
Denard, H., 2007, "Lost theatre and performance traditions in Greece and Italy," in M. McDonald and J. M. Walton (eds), *The Cambridge Companion to Greek and Roman Theatre*, Cambridge: Cambridge University Press.

Dillon, S., 2006, "Women on the columns of Trajan and Marcus Aurelius and the visual language of Roman victory," in S. Dillon and K. E. Welch (eds), *Representations of War in Ancient Rome*, Cambridge: Cambridge University Press.
Dodge, H. and Ward-Perkins, J. B. (eds), 1992, *Marble in Antiquity: collected papers of J.B. Ward-Perkins*, London: British School at Rome.
Dolar, M., 1996a, "At first sight," in R. Salecl and S. Zizek (eds), *Gaze and Voice as Love Objects*, Durham, NC: Duke University Press.
Dolar, M., 1996b, "The object voice," in R. Salecl and S. Zizek (eds), *Gaze and Voice as Love Objects*, Durham, NC: Duke University Press.
Donahue, J. F., 2004, *The Roman Community at Table During the Principate*, Ann Arbor, MI: University of Michigan Press.
Donato, G. and Seefried, M., 1989, *The Fragrant Past: perfumes of Cleopatra and Julius Caesar*, Rome: Istituto Poligrafico e Zecca dello Stato.
Douglas, M., 1996, *Purity and Danger: an analysis of concepts of pollution and taboo*, London: Routledge & Kegan Paul.
Dunbabin, K., 2004, *The Roman Banquet: images of conviviality*, Cambridge: Cambridge University Press.
Durand, J. L., 1989, "Greek animals: toward a topology of edible bodies," in M. Detienne and J-P. Vernant (eds) *The Cuisine of Sacrifice Among the Greeks* (trans. P. Wissing), Chicago: University of Chicago Press.
Dyck, A., 2004, *A Commentary on Cicero, De Legibus*, Ann Arbor, MI: University of Michigan Press.
Edmondson, J., 1996, "Dynamic arenas: gladiatorial presentations in the city of Rome and the construction of Roman society during the early empire," in W. J. Slater (ed.), *Roman Theater and Society*, Ann Arbor, MI: University of Michigan Press.
Edmondson, J. and Keith, A. (eds), 2008, *Roman Dress and the Fabrics of Roman Culture*, Toronto: University of Toronto Press.
Elliott, J. K., 1993, *The Apocryphal New Testament*, New York: Oxford University Press.
Elsner, J., 2003, "Archaeologies and agendas: reflections on late antique Jewish art and early Christian Art," *Journal of Roman Studies*, 93, 114–28.
Elsner, J., 2007, *Roman Eyes: visuality and subjectivity in art and text*, Princeton, NJ: Princeton University Press.
Elsner, J. and Rutherford, I. (eds), 2005, *Pilgrimage in Graeco-Roman and Early Christian Antiquity: seeing the gods*, Oxford: Oxford University Press.
Fagan, G., 1999, *Bathing in Public in the Roman World*, Ann Arbor, MI: University of Michigan Press.
Fagles, R. (trans.), 1984, Euripides, *The Oresteia*, London: Penguin.
Fagles, R. (trans.), 2006, Homer, *The Odyssey*, New York: Penguin.
Fantham, E., 2012, "Purification in ancient Rome," in M. Bradley (ed.), *Rome, Pollution and Propriety: dirt, disease, and hygiene in the Eternal City from antiquity to modernity*, Oxford: Clarendon Press.
Fantham, E., Peet Foley, H., Boymel Kampen, N., Pomeroy, S., and Shapiro, H. A., 1994, *Women in the Classical World*, New York: Oxford University Press.

Farrar, L., 1998, *Ancient Roman Gardens*, Stroud: Sutton Publishing Ltd.

Favro, D., 1996, *The Urban Image of Augustan Rome*, Cambridge: Cambridge University Press.

Ferguson Smith, M. (trans.), 2001, Lucretius, *On the Nature of Things*, Indianapolis, IN: Hackett Publishing Co.

Ferrari, G. R. F., 1987, *Listening to the Cicadas: a study of Plato's Phaedrus*, Cambridge: Cambridge University Press.

Flower, H., 1996, *Ancestor Masks and Aristocratic Power in Roman Culture*, Oxford: Clarendon Press.

Foster, B. O. et al. (ed. and trans.), 1961–84, Livy, *History of Rome*, 14 vols, LCL, Cambridge, MA: Harvard University Press.

Fredrick, D., 1997, "Reading broken skin: violence in Roman elegy," in J. Hallett and M. Skinner (eds), *Roman Sexualities*, Princeton, NJ: Princeton University Press.

Fremantle, W. H., Lewis, G., and Martley, W. G. (trans.), 1989, Jerome, *Letters and Select Works*, NPNF[2] 6, Grand Rapids, MI: Wm. Eerdmans.

Garnsey, P., 1999, *Food and Society in Classical Antiquity*, New York: Cambridge University Press.

Gill, C., 2006, *The Structured Self in Hellenistic and Roman Thought*, Oxford: Oxford University Press.

Gleason, K. L., 1994, "Porticus Pompeiana: a new perspective on the first public park of ancient Rome," *Journal of Garden History*, 14, 13–27.

Gold, B. and Donahue, J. (eds), 2005, *Roman Dining: a special issue of the American Journal of Philology*, Baltimore, MD: Johns Hopkins University Press.

Goody, J., 1982, *Cooking, Cuisine and Class: a study in comparative sociology*, Cambridge: Cambridge University Press.

Gordon, R., 1992, "The healing event in Graeco-Roman folk-medicine," in Ph. J. van der Eijk, H. F. J. Horstmanshoff, and P. H. Schrijvers (eds), *Ancient Medicine in its Socio-cultural Context*, 2 vols, Amsterdam: Rodopi.

Gowers, E., 1993, *The Loaded Table: representations of food in Roman literature*, Oxford: Clarendon Press.

Graf, F., 2007, "Religion and drama," in M. McDonald and J. M. Walton (eds), *The Cambridge Companion to Greek and Roman Theatre*, Cambridge: Cambridge University Press.

Green, C., 2003, "Where did the ventricular localization of mental faculties come from?" *Journal of History of the Behavioral Sciences*, 39, 131–42.

Green, D., 1997, "To '... Send up, like the smoke of incense, the works of the law' – the similarity of views on an alternative to temple sacrifice by three Jewish sectarian movements of the late Second Temple period," in M. Dillon (ed.), *Religion in the Ancient World: new themes and approaches*, Amsterdam: A. M. Hakkert.

Green, D. A., 2011, *The Aroma of Righteousness: scent and seduction in rabbinic life and literature*, Philadelphia, PA: University of Pennsylvania Press.

Green, R., 2007, "Art and theatre in the ancient world," in M. McDonald and J. M. Walton (eds), *The Cambridge Companion to Greek and Roman Theatre*, Cambridge: Cambridge University Press.

Greenberg, C., 1940, "Towards a newer *Laocoon*," *Partisan Review*, 7(4), 296–310.
Greer, R., 1979, *Origen: an exhortation to martyrdom, prayer, and selected works*, New York: Paulist Press.
Gregoric, P., 2006, *Aristotle on the Common Sense*, Oxford: Oxford University Press.
Grierson, P., Mango, C., and Ševenko, I., 1962, "The tombs and obits of the Byzantine emperors (337–1042); with an additional note," *Dumbarton Oaks Papers*, 16, 4–5, 20, 39–40.
Griffith, M., 2007, "'Telling the tale': a performing tradition from Homer to Pantomime," in M. McDonald and J. M. Walton (eds), *The Cambridge Companion to Greek and Roman Theatre*, Cambridge: Cambridge University Press.
Grmek, M. D., 1989, *Diseases in the Ancient Greek World*, trans. M. Muellner and L. Muellner, Baltimore, MD: Johns Hopkins University Press.
Grocock, C. and Grainger, S., 2006, *Apiciu: a critical edition with an introduction and an English translation of the Latin recipe text*, Totnes: Prospect.
Gross, N. P., 1979, "Rhetorical wit and amatory persuasion in Ovid," *Classical Journal* 74.4, 305–18.
Habinek, T. and Schiesaro, A., 1998, *The Roman Cultural Revolution*, Cambridge: Cambridge University Press.
Hadot, R., 1982, "Décret de Kymèen l'honneur de Prytane Kléanax," *The J. Paul Getty Museum Journal*, 10, 165–80.
Hägg, T., 2004, "Epiphany in the Greek novels: the emplotment of a metaphor," in L. B. Mortensen and T. Eide (eds), *Parthenope: studies in ancient Greek fiction (1969–2004)*, Copenhagen: Museum Tusculanum Press.
Harmon, A. M. (ed. and trans.), 1968, Lucian, *Works*, 8 vols, LCL, Cambridge, MA: Harvard University Press.
Harrak, A., 2009, *Jacob of Sarug's Homily the Partaking of the Holy Mysteries*, Piscataway, NJ: Gorgias Press.
Harris-McCoy, D. E., 2012, *Artemidorus' Oneirocritica: text, translation and commentary*, Oxford: Oxford University Press.
Hartranft, C. D. (trans.), 1989, Sozomen, *Ecclesiastical History*, NPNF[2] 2, Grand Rapids, MI: Wm. Eerdmans.
Harvey, S. A., 1998, "The Stylite's liturgy: ritual and religious identity in late antiquity," *Journal of Early Christian Studies*, 6, 523–39.
Harvey, S. A., 2006, *Scenting Salvation: ancient Christianity and the olfactory imagination*, Berkeley, CA: University of California Press.
Hayles, N. K., 1999, *How We Became Posthuman*, Chicago: University of Chicago Press.
Heller-Roazen, D., 2007, *The Inner Touch: archaeology of a sensation*, New York: Zone Books.
Heubeck, A., West, S., and Hainsworth, J. B. (eds.), 1990, *A Commentary on Homer's Odyssey, Vol. 1: Introduction and Books I–VIII*, Oxford: Oxford University Press.
Hill, J. E., 2009, *Through the Jade Gate to Rome: A study of the Silk Road during the later Han Dynasty 1st to 2nd centuries CE. An annotated translation of the Chronicle of the "Western Regions" from the Hou Hanshu*, Charleston, VA: BookSurge Publishing.

Hobson, B., 2009, *Latrinae et Foricae: toilets in the Roman world*, London: Duckworth.
Hodge, A. T., 2002, *Roman Aqueducts and Water Supply*, 2nd edn, London: Duckworth.
Hope, V., 2000, "Contempt and respect: the treatment of the corpse in ancient Rome," in V. Hope and E. Marshall (eds), *Death and Disease in the Ancient City*, New York: Routledge.
Hopkins, K., 1978, *Conquerors and Slaves*, Sociological Studies in Roman History, Vol. 1, New York: Cambridge University Press.
Hopkins, K., 1983, *Death and Renewal*, Sociological Studies in Roman History, Vol. 2, Cambridge: Cambridge University Press.
Horden, P. (ed.), 2000, *Music as Medicine: the history of music therapy since antiquity*, Aldershot: Ashgate.
Horstmanshoff, M., King, H., and Zittel, C. (eds), 2012, *Blood, Sweat, and Tears: the changing concepts of physiology from antiquity into early modern Europe*, Leiden: Brill.
Howes, D., 2003, *Sensual Relations: engaging the senses in culture and social theory*, Ann Arbor, MI: University of Michican Press.
Howes, D. (ed.), 2005, *Empire of the Senses: the sensual culture reader*, Oxford: Berg.
Howes, D. (ed.), 2009, *The Sixth Sense Reader*, Oxford: Berg.
Huby, P. and Steele, C. (trans.), 1997, *Priscian on Theophrastus' On Sense Perception, Simplicius on Aristotle's On the Soul 2.5–12*, London: Duckworth.
Hussey, E., 1990, "The beginnings of epistemology: from Homer to Philolaus," in S. Everson (ed.), *Companions to Ancient Thought, I. Epistemology*, Cambridge: Cambridge University Press.
Ierodiakonou, K., 2005, "Empedocles on colour and colour vision," *Oxford Studies in Ancient Philosophy*, 29, 1–37.
Iskandar, A. Z., 1988, *On Examinations by which the Best Physicians are Recognized*, CMG Suppl. Or. IV, Berlin: Akademie-Verlag.
Jones, C., 1996, "Plague and its metaphors in early modern France," *Representations*, 53, 97–127.
Jones, C. P., 1987, "Stigma: tatooing and branding in Graeco-Roman antiquity," *Journal of Roman Studies*, 77, 139–55.
Jones, C. P. (ed. and trans.), 2006, *Philostratus, The Life of Apollonius of Tyana*, LCL, Cambridge, MA: Harvard University Press.
Joshel, S., 2010, *Slavery in the Roman World*, New York: Cambridge University Press.
Jouanna, J., 1999, *Hippocrates*, Baltimore, MD: Johns Hopkins University Press.
Jouanna, J., 2003, "Sur la dénomination et le nombre des sens d'Hippocrate à la médecine impériale: réflexions à partir de l'énumération des sens dans le traité Hippocratique du *Régime*, c. 23," in I. Boehm and P. Luccioni (eds), *Les cinq sens dans la médecine de l'époque impériale: sources et développements*, Lyon: Université Jean Moulin.
Kahana-Smilansky, H., 2011, "The mental faculties and the psychology of sleep and dreams," in G. Freudenthal (ed.), *Science in Medieval Jewish Cultures*, Cambridge: Cambridge University Press.
Kahn, C. H., 1979, *The Art and Thought of Heraclitus: an edition of the fragments with translation and commentary*, Cambridge: Cambridge University Press.

Kemp, S. and Fletcher, G. J. O., 1993, "The medieval theory of the inner senses," *The American Journal of Psychology*, 106, 559–76.

King, H., 1998, *Hippocrates' Woman: reading the female body in ancient Greece*, London: Routledge.

King, H., 2004, *The Disease of Virgins: green sickness, chlorosis and the problems of puberty*, London: Routledge.

King, H. (ed.), 2005, *Health in Antiquity*, London: Routledge.

King, H., 2013, "Female fluids in the Hippocratic corpus: how solid was the humoral body?" in P. Horden and E. Hsu (eds), *The Body in Balance: humoral medicines in practice*, Oxford and New York: Berghahn.

Kingsley, P., 1999, *In the Dark Places of Wisdom*, Inverness, CA: The Golden Sufi Center Publishing.

Kingsley, P., 2002, "Empedocles for the new millennium," *Ancient Philosophy*, 22, 333–413.

Kingsley, P., 2003, *Reality*, Inverness, CA: The Golden Sufi Center Publishing.

Kirsopp Lake, H. J. et al. (eds and trans.), 1980, Eusebius, *Ecclesiastical History*, 2 vols, Cambridge, MA: Harvard University Press.

Knust, J. and Várhelyi, Z. (eds), 2011, *Ancient Mediterranean Sacrifice*, New York: Oxford University Press.

Kyle, D., 1998, *Spectacles of Death in Ancient Rome*, New York: Routledge.

Kyle, D., 2007, *Sport and Spectacle in the Ancient World*, Malden, MA: Blackwell Publishing.

Laks, A., 1990. "'The more' and 'the full': on the reconstruction of Parmenides' theory of sensation in Theophrastus, *De sensibus*, 3–4," *Oxford Studies in Ancient Philosophy*, 8: 1–18.

Laks, A., 1999, "Soul, sensation, and thought," in A. A. Long (ed.), *The Cambridge Companion to Early Greek Philosophy*, Cambridge: Cambridge University Press.

Lambert, S.D., 1993, *The Phratries of Attica*, Ann Arbor, MI: University of Michigan Press.

Lanciani, R., 1888, *Ancient Rome in the Light of Recent Discoveries*, New York: Houghton, Mifflin & Company.

Laurence, R., 2010, *Roman Passions: a history of pleasure in imperial Rome*, New York: Continuum.

Le Saint, W., 1951, *Tertullian: treatises on marriage and remarriage*, ACW 13, Westminster, MD: Newman Press.

Lee, M., 2005, *Epistemology after Protagoras: responses to relativism in Plato, Aristotle, and Democritus*, Oxford: Oxford University Press.

Lehoux, D., 2012, *What did the Romans Know? An inquiry into science and worldmaking*, Chicago: University of Chicago Press.

Lennon, J. J., 2014, *Pollution and Religion in Ancient Rome*, Cambridge: Cambridge University Press.

Lesher, J. H., 1999, "Early interest in knowledge," in A. A. Long (ed.), *The Cambridge Companion to Early Greek Philosophy*, Cambridge: Cambridge University Press.

Lessing, G. E., [1776] 1984, *Laocoon: an essay on the limits of painting and poetry*, trans. E. A. McCormick, Baltimore, MD: Johns Hopkins University Press.

Levine, L., 2005, *The Ancient Synagogue: the first thousand years*, 2nd edn, New Haven, CT: Yale University Press.
Levine, L. and Weiss, Z. (eds), 2000, *From Dura to Sepphoris: studies in Jewish Art and society in late antiquity, Journal of Roman Archaeology*, Supplementary Series 40, Portsmouth, RI: Journal of Roman Archaeology.
Ley, G., 2007, "A material world: costumes, properties and scenic effects," in M. McDonald and J. M. Walton (eds), *The Cambridge Companion to Greek and Roman Theatre*, Cambridge: Cambridge University Press.
Leyerle, B., 2001, *Theatrical Shows and Ascetic Lives: John Chrysostom's attack on spiritual marriage*, Berkeley, CA: University of California Press.
Liebeschuetz, J. H. W. G., 2005, *Ambrose of Milan: political letters and speeches*, TTH 43, Liverpool: Liverpool University Press.
Lilja, S., 1972, *The Treatment of Odours in the Poetry of Antiquity*, Helsinki: Societas Scientiarum Fennica.
Lindsay, H., 2000, "Death, pollution and funerals in the city of Rome," in V. Hope and E. Marshall (eds), *Death and Disease in the Ancient City*, New York: Routledge.
Lloyd, G. E. R., 1979, *Magic, Reason and Experience: studies in the origin and development of Greek science*, Cambridge: Cambridge University Press.
Long, A. A., 1966, "Thinking and sense-perception in Empedocles: mysticism or materialism?" *Classical Quarterly*, 16, 256–76.
MacCormack, S. G., 1981, *Art and Ceremony in Late Antiquity*, Berkeley, CA: University of California Press.
MacKendrick, K., 2004, *Word Made Skin: figuring language at the surface of flesh*, New York: State University of New York Press.
Magness, J., 2011, *Stones and Dung, Oil and Spit: Jewish daily life in the time of Jesus*, Grand Rapids, MI: William Eerdmans.
Mathews, T. F., 1999, *The Clash of the Gods: a reinterpretation of early Christian art*, rev. edn, Princeton, NJ: Princeton University Press.
Mattern, S. P., 2008a, "Galen's ideal patient," in L. Cilliers (ed.), *Asklepios: studies on ancient medicine*, Bloemfontein: Classical Association of South Africa.
Mattern, S. P., 2008b, *Galen and the Rhetoric of Healing*, Baltimore, MD: Johns Hopkins University Press.
Mattingly, D., 1990, "Paintings, presses, and perfume production at Pompeii," *Oxford Journal of Archaeology*, 9, 71–90.
Maxfield, V. and Peacock, D., [2001] 2007, *Roman Imperial Quarries: survey and excavation at Mons Porphyrites, 1994–1998*, 2 vols, London: Egypt Exploration Society.
Maxwell, J. L., 2006, *Christianization and Communication in Late Antiquity: John Chrysostom and his congregation in Antioch*, Cambridge: Cambridge University Press.
Mayer, W. and Allen, P., 2000, *John Chrysostom*, New York: Routledge.
McCart, G., 2007, "Masks in Greek and Roman theatre," in M. McDonald and J. M. Walton (eds.), *The Cambridge Companion to Greek and Roman Theatre*, Cambridge: Cambridge University Press.

McCauley, L. P. and Stephenson, A. (trans.), 1969–70, *The Works of Saint Cyril of Jerusalem*, Vol. 1, FC 61, Vol. 2, FC 64, Washington, DC: Catholic University of America Press.

McDonald, M. and Walton, J. M. (eds), 2007, *The Cambridge Companion to Greek and Roman Theatre*, Cambridge: Cambridge University Press.

McGovern, P., 2003, *Ancient Wine*, Princeton, NJ: Princeton University Press.

McKinnon, J., 1987, *Music in Early Christian Literature*, Cambridge: Cambridge University Press.

McLaughlin, R., 2010, *Rome and the Distant East: trade routes to the ancient lands of Arabia, India and China*, London: Continuum.

McVey, K., 1989, *Ephrem the Syrian: hymns*, Mahwah, NJ: Paulist Press.

Meijer, P. A., 1997, *Parmenides Beyond the Gates: the divine revelation on being, thinking, and the doxa*, Gieben: Amsterdam.

Miller, J. I., 1969, *The Spice Trade of the Roman Empire 29 B.C. to A.D. 641*, Oxford: Clarendon.

Miller, P. C., 2009, *The Corporeal Imagination: signifying the holy in late ancient Christianity*, Philadelphia, PA: University of Pennsylvania Press.

Minon, S., 2007, *Les inscriptions éléennes dialectales (vie-viie siècle avant J.-C.)*, Geneva: Droz.

Miola, R. S., 2000, *Shakespeare's Reading*, Oxford: Oxford University Press.

Mitchell, W. J. T., 1989, "Ut pictura theoria: abstract painting and the repression of language," *Critical Inquiry*, 15(2), 348–71.

Mols, S. and Moormann, E., 2008, *La villa della Farnesina: le pitture*, Milan: Electa.

Montiglio, S., 2000, *Silence in the Land of Logos*, Princeton, NJ: Princeton University Press.

Montiglio, S., 2013, *Love and Providence: recognition in the ancient novel*, New York: Oxford University Press.

Morales, H., 2004, *Vision and Narrative in Achilles Tatius' Leucippe and Clitophon*, Cambridge: Cambridge University Press

Morgan, J. R., 1996, "*Erotika mathemata*: Greek romance as sentimental education," in A. H. Sommerstein and C. Atherton (eds), *Education in Greek fiction*, Bari: Levante.

Morley, N., 1996, *Metropolis and Hinterland: the city of Rome and the Italian economy*, New York: Cambridge University Press.

Mourelatos, A. P. D., [1970] 2008, *The Route of Parmenides*, Las Vegas: Parmenides Publishing.

Munson, R. V., 2004, *Black Doves Speak: Herodotus and the languages of barbarians*, Cambridge: Cambridge University Press.

Musurillo, H., 1972, *The Acts of the Christian Martyrs*, Oxford: Clarendon Press.

Nagle, B. R., 1995, *Ovid's Fasti: Roman holidays*, Bloomington, IN: Indiana University Press.

Nightingale, A. W., 2004, *Spectacles of Truth in Classical Greek Philosophy: Theoria in its cultural context*, Cambridge: Cambridge University Press.

Nisbet, R.G.M. and Hubbard, M., 1989, *A Commentary on Horace: Odes, Book I*, Oxford: Oxford University Press.

Norman, A. F. (ed. and trans.), 1992, Libanius, *Autobiography and Selected Letters*, LCL, 3 vols, Cambridge, MA: Harvard University Press.
Norman, A. F., 2000, *Antioch as a Centre of Hellenic Culture as Observed by Libanius*, TTH 34, Liverpool: Liverpool University Press.
Nussbaum, M. C., 1972, "ΨYXH in Heraclitus, I," *Phronesis*, 17, 1–16.
Nutton, V., 1992, "Healers in the medical market place: towards a social history of Graeco-Roman medicine," in A. Wear (ed.), *Medicine in Society*, Cambridge: Cambridge University Press.
Nutton, V., 1993, "Galen at the bedside: the methods of a medical detective," in W. Bynum and R. Porter (eds), *Medicine and the Five Senses*, Cambridge: Cambridge University Press.
Nutton, V., 2004, *Ancient Medicine*, London: Routledge.
O'Brien, D., 1969, *Empedocles' Cosmic Cycle*, Cambridge: Cambridge University Press.
O'Brien, D., 1984, *Theories of Weight in the Ancient World. Four essays on Democritus, Plato and Aristotle. A study in the development of ideas, Vol. 2: Plato, weight and sensation. The two theories of the Timaeus*, Paris: Les Belles Lettres/Leiden: Brill.
Oakley, S. P., 2000, *A Commentary on Livy Books VI–X*, vol. 3, Oxford: Clarendon Press.
Oldfather, A. (trans.), 1925, *Epictetus, The Discourses as Reported by Arrion, The Manual, and the Fragments*, 2 vols, Cambridge, MA: Harvard University Press.
Oliver, J. H., 1971, "Epaminondas of Acraephia," *GRBS*, 12, 221–37.
Olson, K., 2008, *Dress and the Roman Woman: self-presentation and society*, London: Routledge.
Olson, S. D., 1998, *Aristophanes' Peace: edited with an introduction*. Oxford: Clarendon Press.
Olson, S. D. and Sens, A., 2000, *Archestratus of Gela: Greek culture and cuisine in the fourth century BCE*, Oxford: Oxford University Press.
Olyan, S. M., 2008, "Mary Douglas' holiness/wholeness Paradigm: its potential for insight and its limitations," *The Journal of Hebrew Scriptures*, 8, http://www.jhsonline.org/cocoon/JHS/a087.html.
Osborne, C., 1999, "The seduction of the world in Plato's *Phaedrus*," *Proceedings of the Boston Area Colloquium in Ancient Philosophy*, 15, 263–81.
Owens, E. J., 1991, *The City in the Greek and Roman World*, New York: Routledge.
Packer, J., 1971, *The Insulae of Imperial Ostia*, Rome: American Academy in Rome.
Palmer, J., 2009, *Parmenides and Presocratic Philosophy*, Cambridge: Cambridge University Press.
Panzanelli, R., Schmidt, E. D., and Lapatin, K. (eds), 2008, *The Color of Life: polychromy in sculpture from antiquity to the present*, Los Angeles: J. Paul Getty Museum/The Getty Research Institute.
Parker, R., 1983, *Miasma: pollution and purification in early Greek religion*, Oxford: Clarendon Press.
Parker, R., 2005, *Polytheism and Society at Athens*, Oxford: Oxford University Press.

Partridge, J., 1999, "Socratic dialectic and the art of love: *Phaedrus* 276e–277a," *Ancient Philosophy*, 19, 121–32.
Paton, H. J., 1922, "Plato's Theory of εικασια," *Proceedings of the Aristotelian Society*, 22, 69–104.
Patterson, J. R., 2000, "On the margins of the city of Rome," in V. Hope and E. Marshall (eds), *Death and Disease in the Ancient City*, New York: Routledge.
Peignard-Giros, A., 2000, "Habitudes alimentaires grecques et romaines à Délos à l'époque hellénistique: la témoignage de la céramique," *Pallas*, 52, 209–20.
Peirce, C. S., 1991, *Peirce on Signs: writings on semiotic*, ed. J. Hoopes, Chapel Hill, NC: University of North Carolina Press.
Pelling, C. (ed.), 1990, *Characterization and Individuality in Greek Literature*, Oxford: Oxford University Press.
Phillips, E. D., 1973, *Greek Medicine*, London: Thames & Hudson.
Picot, J-C., 2009, "Water and bronze in the hands of Empedocles' muse," *Organon*, 41, 5–84.
Pighi, J. P., 1965, *De ludis saecularibus populi Romani Quiritum*, Amsterdam: P. Schippers.
Pinault, J. R., 1992, *Hippocratic Lives and Legends*, Leiden: Brill.
Popham, M. R., Calligas, P. G., and Sackett, L.H., 1993, *Lefkandi II: The Protogeometric Building at Toumba pt 2: the excavation, architecture and finds*, Athens: British School of Archaeology at Athens.
Popper, K. R., 1963. *Conjectures and Refutations: the growth of scientific knowledge*, London: Routledge & Kegan Paul.
Potter, D. S., 1999, "Odor and power in the Roman empire," in J. I. Porter (ed.), *Constructions of the Classical Body*, Ann Arbor, MI: University of Michigan Press.
Potter, D. S., 2003, "Hellenistic religion," in A. Erskine (ed.), *A Companion to the Hellenistic World*, Oxford: Blackwell.
Potter, D. S., 2011, *The Victor's Crown: a history of ancient sport from Homer to Byzantium*, London: Quercus.
Potter, D. S., 2012, *Constantine the Emperor*, Oxford: Oxford University Press.
Presti, R., 2007, "The ambiguous role of perception: empiricist views and biological perspectives on sense perception among the Hippocratics," *Acta Classica*, 50, 129–46.
Price, R. M. (trans.), 1985, Theodoret of Cyrrhus, *History of the Monks of Syria*, Kalamazoo, MI: Cistercian Publications.
Price, S. R. F., 1993, "From noble funerals to divine cult: the consecration of Roman emperors," in D. Cannadine and S. R. F. Price (eds), *Rituals of Royalty: power and ceremonial in traditional societies*, Cambridge: Cambridge University Press.
Pritzl, K., 1985, "On the way to wisdom in Heraclitus," *Phoenix*, 39, 303–16.
Purcell, N., 1999, "The populace of Rome in late antiquity," *Journal of Roman Archaeology*, Supplementary Series no. 33, 135–62.

Quasten, J., 1983, *Music and Worship in Pagan and Christian Antiquity*, trans. B. Ramsey, Washington, DC: National Association of Pastoral Musicians.

Rashed, M., 2007, "The structure of the eye and its cosmological function in Empedocles: reconstruction of fragment 84 D.-K," in K. Corrigan and S. Stern-Gillet (eds), *Reading Ancient Texts: presocratics and Plato, vol. I: essays in honor of Dennis O'Brien*, Leiden: Brill.

Ratcliffe, M., 2008, *Feelings of Being: phenomenology, psychiatry, and the sense of reality*, Oxford: Oxford University Press.

Rathbone, D., 2000, "The Muziris papyrus," *BSAA*, 46, 39–50.

Raventós, X. D. and Remolà, J-A. (eds), 2000, *Sordes Urbis: La Eliminación de Residuos en la Ciudad Romana*, Rome: L'Erma di Bretschneider.

Reardon, B. (ed.), 1989, *Collected Greek Novels*, Berkeley, CA: University of California Press.

Rehm, R., 2007, "Festivals and audiences in Athens and Rome," in M. McDonald and J. M. Walton (eds), *The Cambridge Companion to Greek and Roman Theatre*, Cambridge: Cambridge University Press.

Reinhold, M., 1970, "History of purple as a status symbol in antiquity," *Collection Latomus*, 116, 48–73.

Rhees, R., 2004, *In Dialogue with the Greeks, vol I: The Presocratics and Reality*. Aldershot: Ashgate.

Rhodes, P. J. and Osborne, R., 2003. *Greek Historical Inscriptions 404–323 BC*, Oxford: Oxford University Press.

Rice, E. E., 1983, *The Grand Procession of Ptolemy Philadelphus*, Oxford: Oxford University Press.

Ridley, R. T. (trans.), 1982, Zosimas, *A New History*, Canberra: Australian Association for Byzantine Studies.

Rives, J., 2007, *Religion in the Roman Empire*, Malden, MA: Blackwell.

Robb, K., 1991, "The witness in Heraclitus," *The Monist*, 74, 638–76.

Rosivach, V. J., 2006, "The *Lex Fannia Sumptuaria* of 161 BC," *CJ*, 102, 1–15.

Rossetti, L. (ed.), 1992, *Understanding the Phaedrus*, St. Augustin: Academia Verlag.

Rousset, J., 1989, *Leurs yeux se rencontrèrent. La scène de première vue dans le roman*, Paris: José Corti.

Rowe, G. D., 2002, *Princes and Political Culture: the new Tiberian senatorial decrees*, Ann Arbor, MI: University of Michigan Press.

Ruden, S. (trans.), 2011, Apuleius, *The Golden Ass (Metamorphoses)*, New Haven, CT: Yale University Press.

Satlow, M., 2005, "Giving for return: Jewish offerings in late antiquity," in D. Brakke, M. Satlow, and S. Weitzman (eds), *Religion and the Self in Antiquity*, Bloomington, IN: Indiana University Press.

Scheid, J., 1990, *Romulus et ses frères: le college des frères aravles, modèle du culte public dans la Rome des empereurs*, Rome: École française de Rome.

Schied, J., 1998, "Commentarii Fratrum Arvalium Qui Supersunt: Les copies épigraphiques des protocols annuels de la confrérie Arvale (21 av.–304 ap. J.-C.)," *Recherches archéologiques á la Magliana Roman Antica*, 4.

Scheidel, W., 2003, "Germs for Rome," in C. Edwards and G. Woolf (eds), *Rome the Cosmopolis*, New York: Cambridge University Press.
Schiefsky, M. J. (ed.), 2005, *Hippocrates' On Ancient Medicine*, Leiden: Brill.
Schmitt Pantel, P., 1997, *La cité au banquet. Histoire des repas publics dans les cités grecques*, 2nd edn, Paris: École française de Rome.
Scobie, A., 1986, "Slums, sanitation, and mortality in the Roman world," *Klio*, 68, 399–433.
Sebeok, T., 1994, *Signs: an introduction to semiotics*, Toronto: University of Toronto Press.
Sebesta, J. L. and Bonfante, L. (eds), 2001, *The World of Roman Costume*, Madison, WI: University of Wisconsin Press.
Sedley, D., 2007, *Creationism and its Critics in Antiquity*, Berkeley, CA: University of California Press.
Segal, C., 1977, "Synaesthesia in Sophocles," *Illinois Classical Studies*, 2, 88–96.
Serres, M., 2009, *Five Senses: a philosophy of mingled bodies*, London: Continuum.
Sève, M., 1979, "Un décret de consolation à Cyzique," *BCH*, 103, 327–59.
Sharples, R. W. and van der Eijk, P. J. (eds.), 2008, *Nemesius On the Nature of Man: translated with an introduction and notes*, Liverpool: Liverpool University Press.
Shaw, G., 1995, *Theurgy and the Soul: the neoplatonism of Iamblichus*, University Park, PA: Penn State University Press.
Shaw, T. M., 1998, *The Burden of the Flesh: fasting and sexuality in early Christianity*, Minneapolis, MN: Fortress Press.
Sheldon, R. M., 2007, *Intelligence Activities in Ancient Rome: trust in the gods but verify*, London: Routledge.
Shklovskij, V., 1998, "Art as technique," in J. Rivkin and M. Ryan (eds), *Literary Theory: an anthology*, Oxford: Blackwell.
Sidebotham, S., 2011, *Berenike and the Ancient Mediterranean Spice Route*, Berkeley, CA: University of California Press.
Siegel, R. E., 1973, *Galen on Psychology, Psychopathology, and Function and Diseases of the Nervous System: an analysis of his doctrines, observations and experiments*, New York: Karger.
Skinner, M., 2003, *Catullus in Verona: A reading of the Elegiac Libellus, poems 65–116*, Columbus, OH: Ohio State University Press.
Smith, A. M., 1996, "Ptolemy's theory of visual perception: an English translation of the Optics with introduction and commentary," *Transactions of the American Philosophical Society*, 86(2).
Smith, J. E., 1985, "Plato's myths as 'likely accounts', worthy of belief," *Apeiron*, 19, 24–42.
Smith, M. J., 2008, *Sensing the Past: seeing, hearing, smelling, tasting, and touching in history*, Berkeley, CA: University of California Press.
Smith, M. M., 2007, *Sensing the Past: seeing, hearing, smelling, tasting and touching in history*, Berkeley, CA: University of California Press.
Spawforth, A., 2011, *Greece and the Augustan Cultural Revolution*, Cambridge: Cambridge University Press.

Squire, M., 2009, *Image and Text in Graeco-Roman Antiquity*, Cambridge: Cambridge University Press.
Squire, M., 2013, "Embodied ambiguities on the Prima Porta Augustus," *Art History*, 36, 243–79.
Stanford, W. B., 1967, *The Sound of Greek: studies in the Greek theory and practice of euphony*, Berkeley, CA: University of California Press.
Stanford, W. B., 1969, "The lily voice of the cicadas," *Phoenix*, 23(1), 3–8.
Stevens, B., 2008, "The scent of language and social synaesthesia at Rome," *Classical World*, 101(2), 159–71.
Stevens, B., 2009, "*Per gestum res est significanda mihi*: Ovid and language in exile," *Classical Philology*, 104(2), 162–83.
Stevens, B., 2010, "The beautiful ambiguity of *Blankets*: comic representation and religious art," *imageText*, 5(1).
Stevens, B., 2013, *Silence in Catullus*, Madison, WI: University of Wisconsin Press.
Stewart, S., 2007, *Cosmetics and Perfumes in the Roman World*, Stroud: Tempus.
Stoller, P., 1989, *The Taste of Ethnographic Things: the senses in anthropology*, Philadelphia, PA: University of Pennsylvania Press.
Sumi, G., 2006, *Ceremony and Power: performing politics in Rome between republic and empire*, Ann Arbor, MI: University of Michigan Press.
Swan, P. M., 2004, *The Augustan Succession: an historical commentary on Cassius Dio's Roman history books 55–56 (9 BC–AD 14)*, Oxford: Oxford University Press.
Syme, R., 1968, *Ammianus and the Historia Augusta*, Oxford: Clarendon Press.
Synnott, A., 1991, "Puzzling over the senses: from Plato to Marx," in D. Howes (ed.), *The Varieties of Sensory Experience*, Toronto: University of Toronto Press.
Taplin, O. and Wyles, R. (eds), 2010, *The Pronomos Vase and its Context*, Oxford: Oxford University Press.
Tchernia, A., 1986, *Le vin de l'Italie romaine: essai d'histoire économique d'après les amphores*, Rome: Ecole française de Rome.
Thomson, D. F. S., 2003, *Catullus*, Toronto: University of Toronto Press.
Tomber, R., 2008, *Indo-Roman Trade: from pots to pepper*, London: Duckworth.
Toner, J., 1995, *Leisure and Ancient Rome*, Cambridge: Polity Press.
Toner, J., 2009, *Popular Culture in Ancient Rome*, Cambridge: Polity Press.
Toner, J., 2013, *Roman Disasters*, Cambridge: Polity Press.
Toner, J., forthcoming, "The smell of Christianity," in M. Bradley (ed.), *Smell and the Ancient Senses*, Durham: Acumen Publishing.
Totelin, L., 2012, "Botanizing rulers and their herbal subjects: plants and political power in Greek and Roman literature," *Phoenix*, 66, 122–44.
Trombley, F. and Watt, J. W., 2000, *The Chronicle of Pseudo-Joshua the Stylite*, TTH 32, Liverpool: Liverpool University Press.
Tsouna, V., 1998, *The Epistemology of the Cyrenaic School*, Cambridge: Cambridge University Press.
Turner, J., 2004, "The many faces of Helen," *Slate*, May 13.
Ullucci, D., 2012, *The Christian Rejection of Animal Sacrifice*, New York: Oxford University Press.

van der Eijk, P. J., 2008, "The art of medicine: Nemesius of Emesa and early brain-mapping," *The Lancet*, 372, 440–1.
van Nijf, O. M., 1997, *The Civic World of Professional Associations in the Roman East*, Amsterdam: J. C. Gieben.
Varone, A., 1997, "Pittori romani al lavoro," in H. Béarat *et al.* (eds), *Roman Wall Painting: materials, techniques, analysis and conservation*, Freiburg: Institute of Mineralogy and Petrography.
Verhoogt, A., 2005, *Regaling Officials in Ptolemaic Egypt*, Leiden: Brill.
Vermes, G., 1997, *The Complete Dead Sea Scrolls in English*, London: Penguin Books.
Vernant, J. P., 1991, *Mortals and Immortals: selected essays*, Princeton, NJ: Princeton University Press.
Vinge, L., 1975, *The Five Senses: studies in a literary tradition*, Lund: LiberLäromedel.
Vivanto, B., 2008, *Daughters of Gaia: women in the ancient Mediterranean world*, Norman, OK: University of Oklahoma Press.
Vlastos, G., 1946, "Parmenides' theory of knowledge," *Transactions of the American Philological Association*, 77, 66–77.
Von Staden, H., 1989, *Herophilus: the art of medicine in early Alexandria*, Cambridge: Cambridge University Press.
Von Staden, H., 1992, "Women and dirt," *Helios*, 19, 7–30.
Walford, E. (trans.), 1855, Philostorgius, *Ecclesiastical History*, London: Henry G. Bohn.
Wallace-Hadrill, A., 1994, *Houses and Society in Pompeii and Herculaneum*, Princeton, NJ: Princeton University Press.
Wallace-Hadrill, A., 2008, *Rome's Cultural Revolution*, Cambridge: Cambridge University Press.
Walsh, P. G. (trans.), 1975, Paulinus of Nola, *Poems*, ACW 40, New York: Newman Press.
Ward-Perkins, J. B., 1974, *Cities of Ancient Greece and Italy: planning in classical antiquity*, New York: George Braziller.
Waterfield, R. (trans.), 2002, Plato, *Phaedrus*, Oxford: Oxford University Press.
Way, A. C. (trans.), 1963, *Basil of Caesarea, Homilies on the Hexaemeron: Saint Basil, Exegetical Homilies*, FC 46, Washington, DC: Catholic University of America Press.
Webb, R., 2008, *Demons and Dancers: performance in late antiquity*, Cambridge, MA: Harvard University Press.
Webb, R., 2009, *Ekphrasis: imagination and performance in rhetorical theory and practice*, Farnham: Ashgate.
Wersinger, A. G., 2008, *La sphère et l'intervalle: le schème de l'harmonie dans la pensée des Anciens Grecs d'Homère à Platon*, Grenoble: Editions Jérôme Millon.
West, M. L., 1971, "The cosmology of 'Hippocrates', De Hebdomadibus," *Classical Quarterly*, 21, 365–88.
Whitmarsh, T., 2011, *Narrative and Identity in the Ancient Greek Novel: returning romance*, Cambridge: Cambridge University Press
Whitmarsh, T. and Morales, H. (eds), 2001, *Achilles Tatius, Leucippe and Clitophon*, Translated with Notes by T. Whitmarsh, Introduction by H. Morales, Oxford: Oxford University Press.

Wild, J. P. and Wild, F., 2005, "Rome and India: early Indian cotton textiles from Berenike, Red Sea coast of Egypt," in R. Barnes (ed.), *Textiles in Indian Ocean Societies*, London: RoutledgeCurzon.

Wild, J. P. and Wild, F., 2008, "Early Indian textiles from Berenike," in E. M. Raven (ed.), *South Asian Archaeology 1999*, Groningen: Egbert Forsten.

Wild, J. P., Wild, F., and Clapham, A. J., 2008, "Roman cotton revisited," in C. Alfaro Giner and L. Karali (eds), *Purpureae Vestes II: Vestidos, Textiles y Tintes: Estudios sobre la Producción de Bienes de Consumo en la Antigüedad*, Valencia: University of Valencia.

Wiles, D., 1991, *Masks of Menander: sign and meaning in Greek and Roman performance*, Cambridge: Cambridge University Press.

Wiles, D., 1999, *Tragedy in Athens: performance space and theatrical meaning*, Cambridge: Cambridge University Press.

Wiles, D., 2007, *Mask and Performance in Greek Tragedy: from ancient festival to modern experimentation*, Cambridge: Cambridge University Press.

Wilkins, J., 2000, *The Boastful Chef: the discourse of food in ancient Greek comedy*, Oxford: Oxford University Press.

Wiseman, T. P., 1985, *Catullus and His World: a reappraisal*, Cambridge: Cambridge University Press.

Wolfson, H. A., 1935, "The internal senses in Latin, Arabic, and Hebrew philosophic texts," *Harvard Theological Review*, 28, 69–133.

Worman, N., 2002, *The Cast of Character: style in Greek literature*, Austin, TX: University of Texas Press.

Wright, R., 1981, *Empedocles: the extant fragments*, New Haven, CT: Yale University Press.

Wright, W. C. (ed. and trans.), 1959, Julian (emperor), *Works*, 3 vols, Cambridge, MA: Harvard University Press.

Wright, W. C. (ed. and trans.), 1968, Eunapius, *Lives of the Sophists*, Cambridge, MA: Harvard University Press.

Wycherley, R. E., 1963, "The scene of Plato's *Phaidros*," *Phoenix*, 17, 88–98.

Wynne-Tyson. E. and Taylor, T. (ed. and trans.), 1965, Porphyry, *On Abstinence from Animal Food*, New York: Barnes & Noble.

Yegül, F., 1992, *Baths and Bathing in Classical Antiquity*, New York and Cambridge, MA: The Architectural History Foundation and the MIT Press.

Zanker, P., 1988, *The Power of Images in the Age of Augustus*, Ann Arbor, MI: University of Michigan Press.

Zarifi, Y., 2007, "Chorus and dance in the ancient world," in M. McDonald and J. M. Walton (eds), *The Cambridge Companion to Greek and Roman Theatre*, Cambridge: Cambridge University Press.

Zeitlin, F. I., 2003, "Living portraits and sculpted bodies in Chariton's theater of romance," in S. Panayotakis, M. Zimmerman, and W. Keulen (eds.), *The Ancient Novel and Beyond*, Leiden: Brill.

Zenos, A. C. (trans.), 1989, Socrates Scholasticus, *Ecclesiastical History*, NPNF[2] 2, Grand Rapids, MI: Wm. Eerdmans.

NOTES ON CONTRIBUTORS

Gregory S. Aldrete is the Frankenthal Professor of History and Humanistic Studies at the University of Wisconsin—Green Bay. His particular areas of research interest are the social and economic history of the Roman Empire, rhetoric and oratory, military history, and urban problems in the ancient world. His publications include *Floods of the Tiber in Ancient Rome* (2007), *Gestures and Acclamations in Ancient Rome* (1999), and *Daily Life in the Roman City: Rome, Pompeii and Ostia* (2009).

Mark Bradley is Associate Professor of Ancient History at the University of Nottingham. He is author of *Colour and Meaning in Ancient Rome* (2009) and Editor of *Papers of the British School at Rome*. Together with Shane Butler (Bristol), he is co-editor of a series of volumes on "The Senses in Antiquity", for which he is contributing a volume on *Smell and the Ancient Senses* (2014), and he is currently writing a monograph on *Foul Bodies in Ancient Rome*.

Ashley Clements is Lecturer in Greek Literature and Philosophy at Trinity College, Dublin. He is author of *Aristophanes' Thesmophoriazusae: Philosophizing Theatre and the Politics of Perception in Late Fifth-Century Athens* (2014) and articles on the senses and perception in Greek literature. His research interests include the intersection of philosophy, literature and politics in the fifth and fourth centuries BCE, Greek wisdom literature, Platonic dialogue, and the anthropology of the Greeks.

Susan Ashbrook Harvey is the Willard Prescott and Annie McClelland Smith Professor of Religious Studies at Brown University. She specializes in late antique and Byzantine Christianity, with Syriac studies as her particular focus. She is the author of *Scenting Salvation: ancient Christianity and the olfactory imagination* (2006) and *Asceticism and Society in Crisis: John of Ephesus and the lives of the Eastern saints* (1990). She has published widely on topics relating to asceticism, hagiography, women and gender, hymnography, homiletics, and piety in late antique Christianity.

Helen King is Professor of Classical Studies at The Open University. She has published widely on ancient medicine, especially gynaecology, and its reception in Western Europe. Her books include *The One-Sex Body on Trial: the classical and early modern evidence* (2013); *Blood, Sweat and Tears: the changing concepts of physiology from antiquity into early modern Europe* (with Manfred Horstmanshoff and Claus Zittel, 2012); *Midwifery, Obstetrics and the Rise of Gynaecology* (2007); and *The Disease of Virgins: green sickness, chlorosis and the problems of puberty* (2004), as well as a short introductory book, *Greek and Roman Medicine* (Bloomsbury 2001).

Silvia Montiglio is Basil L. Gildersleeve Professor of Classics at Johns Hopkins University. Her publications include *Silence in the Land of Logos* (2000) which explores the meanings of silence in a variety of areas of the archaic and classical Greek world and *From Villain to Hero: Odysseus in ancient thought* (2011) which investigates the exploitation of Odysseus by Greek and Roman philosophers. Her book *Wandering in Ancient Greek Culture* (2005) studies the associations attached to wandering in Greek sources. Her latest book, *Love and Providence: recognition in the ancient novel* (2013) deals with the uses and meanings of recognition in the Greek and Roman novels in the context of their literary tradition.

David Potter is Francis W. Kelsey Collegiate Professor of Greek and Roman History and Arthur F. Thurnau Professor of Greek and Latin, at the University of Michigan. His research interests include Greek and Roman Asia Minor, Greek and Latin historiography and epigraphy, Roman public entertainment, and warfare.

Benjamin Eldon Stevens, Visiting Assistant Professor of Classics at Bryn Mawr College, has taught at Hollins University, the University of Colorado at Boulder, and Bard College. His research focuses on Latin poetry in connection with modern discourses including linguistics; and classical traditions in European epic, English poetry, and modern science fiction and fantasy. He is the author of *Silence in Catullus* (2013) and co-editor, with Brett M. Rogers, of *Classical Traditions in Science Fiction* (2014).

Jerry Toner is Fellow and Director of Studies in Classics at Churchill College, Universty of Cambridge. His book *Popular Culture in Ancient Rome* (2009) looked in part at the different sensory world the non-elite inhabited. His other books include *Roman Disasters* (2013), *Homer's Turk: how classics shaped ideas of the East* (2013), and *Leisure and Ancient Rome* (1995).

Andrew Wallace-Hadrill is Director of Research and Honorary Professor of Roman Studies at the University of Cambridge. He directs the Herculaneum Conservation Project, and his current research interests include Herculaneum, Pompeii, Roman urbanism, public and private space, and Roman cultural identity. His main publications include *Rome's Cultural Revolution* (2008), *Houses and Society in Pompeii and Herculaneum* (1994), *Augustan Rome* (1993), and *Herculaneum: Past and Future* (2011).

INDEX

Abraham 110
acclamation 14, 17, 42, 64–5
Achilles 174
acting 202–3
adornment 194–7
Aelius Aristides 152–4
Aelius Gallus 71
Aeneas 165
Aeschylus 199, 210, 222–4
Africa 72, 76, 82
Agrippa 50, 57
Alaric 74
Alcibiades 174
Alexander of Tralles 141
Alexander the Great 31, 32, 76
Alexandria 38, 65–6, 70–1, 79, 85, 89
amber 80–1, 82
amphitheaters 16–17, 28, 55
Anaxagoras 116
animals 12, 13, 14–15, 66–7, 159
Antioch 17, 38, 41, 96, 103, 108, 109, 112–13
Antiochus IV 34
Aphrodisias 17
Apicius 75–8, 88
apocalypse, 107
Appian Way 38, 45

applause *see* acclamation
Apuleius 96, 104, 204
aqueducts 50
Arabia 70–1, 77, 78, 88–9
architecture 185, 205–7
Aretaeus 141
Ariadne 166
Aristides Quintilianus 26–7
Aristippus 135
Aristophanes 30
Aristotle 25, 63, 122, 135–7, 144, 198, 199
Arius 10, 109, 111
art 183–208
  and distance 184–5
  and vision 185
Artaxerxes 173–4
Artemis 103
artwork 11, 12, 26, 27, 28, 51, 70, 86–7, 94
Arval Brethren 33
asceticism 99–100, 111
Asclepius 96, 152–4
astrology 159
astronomy 134
Athens 29, 31–2, 37, 62, 86, 139, 205, 206

augury 96
Augustine 25, 55, 108, 109
Augustus 12–13, 27, 34–5, 40, 50, 57, 70–1, 75, 81–2, 85, 104–5, 187, 189, 207, 217, 219
Averroës 136
Avicenna 137
awnings 14, 199, 207

Bacchanalia 103–4
bakers 53
Baltic trade 79–81
Balzac 168
baptism 97
barbarian 117–19
barley 59
Basil of Caesarea 98
bathing 11, 12, 20, 50, 54, 56, 88
beauty 27, 103, 108
belching 5
Berenike 71, 74, 75, 85
Bethlehem 97
Bible 101
body, the 3–4, 5, 6, 10, 19, 26, 39–40, 56, 98–9, 113, 140, 143, 145, 160–1, 185, 194–7
  and asceticism 100
  body parts 38
  female 108
  and Manichaeism 100
  and mental disorders 150
  and philosophy 117, 118, 120–4, 124–9, 129–31, 136
  and religion 91–100
boiling 32
branding 6
bread 40, 53, 97
breath 88, 100, 130–1, 156
butchers 6

cabbage 154
Caelius Aurelianus 141
Caligula (Gaius) 76, 79, 189
Calliope 166
Callistratus 186–7, 191

Campus Martius 12, 41, 207
candles 111
Carthage 38
catechumens 97
Cato the Elder 77, 154, 157
Catullus 210, 220–1, 222
Celsus 77, 141
Cerealia 34
ceremony 23–4, 28, 106
childbirth 108
children 27, 39
China 81–2
Christianity 2, 14, 18–21, 40, 97–100, 91–113, 160–1
  and accusations of cannibalism 104
  and accusations of child sacrifice 104
  pre-Constantinian 107
  and smell 109–10
Cicero 25, 27, 38, 64
circus 28, 36, 55, 64–5
citizenry 10
cleanliness 20, 25, 94
Clement of Alexandria 19
Cleopatra 29, 79
clothing 59, 63, 84–5, 89, 93–4, 185, 197
  and color 85, 87
cognition, and heat 129–31
coinage 74
color 4, 7, 10, 11, 15, 17, 26–7, 85–7, 89, 92, 94, 133, 135, 149, 155, 186–93
  and warmth 218
Colosseum, the 2, 35–6, 48, 65
comedy 100, 198
Commodus 76
comportment 5, 197
condiments 76
Constantine 19–20, 42–4, 48, 97, 104–5, 111
Constantinople 17
Constantius II 5, 24, 42–3
cookshops 88
corn dole 36
corpses 46–7

Cos, 83
cosmetics 87, 89, 185, 194–6
cosmology 116, 117–18, 121–2, 128, 130, 133, 135
costume 200–1
cotton 72, 84–5, 89
Crassus 34
cremation 37–8, 41–2, 46
crowds 13, 16, 17, 63–4
cultus 194–7
cushions 16
Cybele 104
Cyme 32
Cyril of Jerusalem 97
Cyrus 174

Daedalus 192
dance 8
death 36–44, 46
deception 117–19
decoration 4, 5, 26, 86–7, 89
defamiliarization 216–17, 226
Delos 29–30
Delphi 96
Democritus 131, 139, 115, 116
demons 10, 111, 159–61
Demosthenes 202
depilation 11
desire 27
Deuteronomy 26
diagnosis 143–5, 150
  and hearing 143, 144
  and sight 143, 144
  and speech 143, 144
  and taste 143, 144
  and touch 143, 144
diairesis 118, 119
dialectic 214
diamonds 78
Dido 165
Dio Chrysostom 7
Diocletian 23, 28, 43–4
  Price Edict 89
Dionysius of Halicarnassus 184
divination 142

doctors *see* physicians
Domitian 35, 74, 103
Donatists 109
dormice 76
drama 26, 63, 164, 185, 197–205, 223–4
  and audience 199
  and feasting 202–3
  festivals 202–3
  and hearing 198–9
  on pottery 201–2
  and smell 204–5
  and taste 202–3
  and the visual 199
dress *see* clothing
dyes 197

earrings 79, 84
education 3
Egypt 28–9, 70–1, 79, 85, 89, 214
ekphrasis 164, 166, 183–4, 185, 186, 191
elephants 12
elite, the 4, 6–7, 10, 12, 75
emotions 15, 26–7
  and age 27
  and gender 27
Empedocles 25, 116, 123, 124–9
  Love and Strife in 124–9
emperors 2, 11, 12–16, 17–18, 23–4
  and the poor 105
  and touch 24
empire 12, 17–18, 19–20
empiricism 117
empiricists 142
enargeia 164
Epictetus 102–3
Epicureanism 25, 27, 101, 135, 219
Epidauros 96, 152
epilepsy 147, 150
equestrians 42
Eros 165, 174
Ethiopia 84
Etruscans 31
Eucharist 40

euphony 163–4
Euripides 184, 191, 202
Eusebius 42–3, 105
excrement 47, 51
exorcism 160
eyebrows 87

fasting 95, 100
feasts 30–6, 88, 104
   and drama 202–3
   municipal 36
   and women 31–2, 35
festivals 93–4, 104, 105, 110–11, 112
fighting 6
fish 76
flamingos 76
flatulence 5
Fleshes 129–31
flowers 8, 12, 13–14, 78
food 24, 29–30, 31–2, 36, 59–61, 75–8
   mixing of 30
   and religion 93
   and status 36
forgery 7
Forma Urbis Romae 13
fowl 76
frankincense 72, 77, 78, 102, 107, 149
fullers 6, 53
funerals 36–44, 78
   in Homer 37
   and Rome 38–44
   and scents 78
   and status 38–44
   and touch 37

Galen 136, 141, 142, 144, 148, 150–2, 153, 155
   and pulse 144–5
   and touch 144–5
game 76
gameboards 17
games, the 2, 13–16, 34, 55, 64–5, 104
   and color 14–15
   and noise 14

garbage 46–7, 51
gardens 57–8
garlic 75, 77, 88
garum 59, 77, 88
gemstones 70, 78–9, 81, 89, 92
gender 4
   and emotions 27
Gérôme, Jean–Léon 192–3
gesture 63, 197
gladiators 13, 34, 107–8
God, nature of 102
gold 79
goose feathers, 81
graffiti 17–18
Greece 11
Gregory of Nyssa 98
grief 36

hagiography 111
hair dyes 87
hairstyles 17, 63, 196
halitosis 6, 7
hallucination 148
Han dynasty 82
handicrafts 185
healing events 159
health 140–2
hearing 26, 53–6, 110, 134, 166, 170–8, 213–14
   and the liver 134
heat 129–31
heaven 18, 97, 100, 107
Helen 172, 174, 210–13, 214, 216–17, 219, 225–6
hell 18, 107, 161
Heraclitus 116, 117–19, 124, 132
heralds 63
herbs 76–7, 87
Herculaneum 72–3, 79, 87
heresy 10, 111
Herodian 41
heterosexuality 170
Hippocrates, Hippocratic corpus 129–31, 139–40, 141–2, 143–4, 145, 151, 158

INDEX

Holy Land, the 97
holy men 10, 160
Homer 3, 31, 122, 163–4, 184, 210–13, 214, 217, 219, 221, 226
homilies 97, 111
homosexuality 170
Horace 199, 210, 217–20, 221, 222
horses 159
Hostius Quadra 27
housing 6, 61, 70
humor 154
humoral theory 3–4, 140–52, 153, 154
hygiene 88, 196
  dental 6
hymns 100, 102, 108–10, 111
hysteria 4, 150

Iamblichus 102
identity 17
illness 140–2, 154
impurity 25, 26, 37
incense 8, 13, 18–19, 20, 40, 66, 70, 72, 77, 78, 88, 92, 94, 97, 101, 106, 185, 202
India 70–1, 72, 74, 77, 78, 79, 82, 84, 88–9, 100
inhumation 38
insulae 48, 56
Intaglios 79
inversion 15
Isola Sacra 38
ivory 72

jade 82
jaundice 154–5
Jerome 111
Jesus 10, 97–8, 101, 160
John Chrysostom 97, 103, 109, 112–13, 196
Judaism 95, 99, 100–1, 102, 106, 110, 111, 112–13
Julian 96, 103, 104–5, 106, 109, 111
Julius Caesar 14, 34, 57, 64, 76
  funeral of 40–1

Justin Martyr 104, 105–6

kissing 166–7
knowledge 116, 131, 132
krasis 122–4, 129

landscape 217–18
language 118
law 30
  sumptuary 30, 34, 70, 88, 219
law courts 6
laxatives 150
leisure 12, 14
Leviticus 26
Libanius 96, 103
libitinarii 38
light 14, 18
literacy 3
literature 2, 3, 163–81, 210, 213, 217–20, 220, 226
  and hearing 213
  and translation 220–1
liturgy 97, 106, 108–10, 111
Livy 103–4
logos 119, 124, 134
love 163–81
  and hearing 170–81
  and rumor 174–9
  and sight 167–9, 172–3, 176, 181
  and smell 169–70, 181
  and touch 169–70, 181
Lucian 1–2, 184, 191
Lucretius 27, 101, 104
luxury 4, 10–12, 16, 19–20, 29, 34, 69–89, 100
  and medicine 87
  and the Orient 89
  and the senate 69–70
  and sight 78–88
  and social stratification 79
  and touch 78–88
luxury goods 69–89
  prices 69–70
  tax 74

madness 4
magic 7–8, 10, 155–9
   and sensory disorder 157–9
malingering 147
mania 5, 142
Manichaeism 98–9, 100
marble 11, 12–13, 45, 49–50, 51, 56,
     85–6, 89, 184–5, 187, 188, 189–91
Marcus Aurelius 82, 141
Mark Antony 29, 40
Marlowe, Christopher 210–11, 212, 213
marriage 95
Marseilles 87
martyrs 18, 100, 107–8, 113
masks 198, 199–200
mathematics 134
Maximian 23
meat 76
Medea, 165
media 209–26
medicine 3–4, 8, 77, 87, 116, 139–61
   and Christianity 159–61
   and demons 159–61
   folk 154–5
   humoral 140–52, 153, 154
   and luxury 87
   and magic 155–9
   and observation 139, 142
   and patients 147–8
   and philosophy 144
   and the physician 141–7
   "schools" of 141–3, 150
   and social status 151–2
   as technical skill 142
   use of herbs and spice in 77
   and women 145, 150–1
melancholia 5, 142
Melitians 109
memory 212, 215–16, 218–19, 222
mental disorders 148–51, 154, 159–60
   and body 150
   and women 150–1
metals 70, 82
meter 198
Methodists 142

middling sorts 75
millers 53
mime 28
mimesis 184
mind 116, 117, 120–4
Minucius Felix 104
Mithraism 106
morality 7, 10–12, 14, 18, 19, 103,
     106–7, 111, 219
mosaics 12, 56, 99
mourning 38
music 4, 8, 10, 11–12, 13, 14, 26–7, 33,
     92–3, 108–10, 134, 148, 170, 183,
     185, 198, 209
muslin 72
myrrh 77

nakedness 108
nature 86–7, 116
Nausicaa 165
Neo-Pythagoreanism 102
Neoplatonism 98, 101–2, 136
Nero 11, 14, 48, 52, 74, 78, 79
noise 14
novels 167–9
   protagonists in 179–80, 181

odor 5, 6, 95, 100, 169–70
   odor of sanctity 20, 100
   see also smell
Odysseus 163, 165, 171–2
oil 88, 97
oracles 96
oratory 197
   see also rhetoric
orgasm 27
Orient, the 11–12
   and luxury 89
   trade with 69–89
Origen 19, 98, 101
Ostia 36
Ovid 18, 78, 93–4, 95, 100, 195–7, 207

paganism 19, 20, 106, 110, 111
pain 147–8

INDEX

paint 86–7
paintings 183–4, 222
  on stage 199
Palmyra 81
Parmenides 116, 120–4, 126, 133
patients 147–8
  and social status 151–2
Paul of Aegina 141
pavements 12
pearls 72, 78, 79, 82
Pelagonius 159
Peloponnesian War 172
people, the 11–12
pepper 72–4, 76, 77, 78, 84, 88, 149
perception 24–8, 47–8, 116, 120–4, 128–9, 129–31, 132–5, 136–7, 209–10
performance *see* drama
perfume 4, 5, 11, 19, 59, 78, 92, 185, 196–7
  see also scent
perfumers 6
Pergamum 152
Periplus Maris Erythraei 71–2, 76
Perpetua 107
persecution 105
  see also martyrs
Persia 11, 23, 30, 31, 139, 179–80
Persian Gulf 84
persuasion 164, 166, 171–2, 180–1
Pertinax 41–2
Petra 81
Petronius 79
Philo 100–1
Philodemus 27
philosophy 115–37
Philostratus 102, 183–4, 186
phrenitis 4
physicians 141–7, 151, 154
  cost 151–2
placebo 153
plague 139, 160–1

Plato 25, 26, 27, 116, 117, 118, 132–5, 136, 210, 213–17
pleasure 26–7
Pliny the Elder 72, 74–5, 89, 139–40, 154–5, 191, 192
Plotinus 27
Plutarch 102, 103
poetry 3, 163–4, 165–6, 222
politics 16
pollution 6, 7, 38
Pollux 200, 204
Polycarp 40, 107
polychromy 185, 186–93
Pompeii 79, 86, 87
Pompey 34, 57
  Theater of 205–6
poor, the 38
popular culture 5–6, 7–8, 154
Porphyry 85
possession 160
Praxiteles 186
prayer 8, 92
priesthood 105
private life 30–44
processions 8, 13–14, 18, 28–9, 41–2, 66, 92, 111
proprioception 216, 218
prose 163–4
prostitution 7, 12
Protagoras 116
Ptolemy II 28–9, 66–7
public life 30–44
pulse 144–5, 150
punishment 2, 6, 15, 16, 62
purification 94–5
purple 17
Pygmalion 192
Pythagoras 102, 130

quarrying 85–6

Rationalists 142
reading 215–16
recipes 75–8
Red Sea ports 71

relics 111
religion 2, 8–10, 91–113
  and critique 100–5
  and daily life 95–6
  and food 93
  and "foreign" rites 104
  and philosophy 101
  and scents 94–5
  and sensory competition 105–13
  and social stratification 92
republic 12, 16, 70
resistance 16–18
revelry 183–4
rhetoric 11, 63, 103, 106–7, 111, 113
rhinoceros horn 72
riots 70
roasting 32
Romanization 17
Rome 6, 10, 11–12, 35–6, 45–67, 205–6, 219
  food supply 70
  gardens 57–8
  noise 53–6
  size 51
  smell 51–3
  social stratification 58–63
  street layout 64–5
rumor 174–9, 181

sacrifice 8, 13, 18–19, 26, 31, 33, 77, 88, 92, 101–2, 102–3, 111, 209
saints 111
sand 14, 16
Sappho 170–1, 220–1
Satan 107–8
satire 100
Saturnalia 35
sauces 76–7
scent 30, 31, 40, 52, 88, 93, 94, 196–7, 213
science 116, 142
sculpture 185, 186–93
Second Coming, the 18, 43, 107
seduction 165–6, 180

Segal, Eric 168
selfhood 168
senate, the 16, 42
  and luxury 69–70
Seneca 204
sense-perception, and truth 214
senses
  as cross-cultural 222–3, 224–6
  as deceptive 117–19, 145–7
  nature of 3, 19, 24, 115–37, 140, 142–3
  number of 3, 135–6, 142
  and order 11–12
  ranking of 24–5
  and truth 116
Septimius Severus 41–2
sex 7, 19, 26, 27, 167
  and impurity 26
shade 12, 14, 185
Shakespeare, William 137
sight 26, 27–8, 134, 143, 144, 145–6, 164–5, 167–9, 172–3, 176, 181
  and luxury 78–88
signal fires 209, 224–5, 226
silk 59, 69, 70, 72, 81–5, 89, 92
skin 6, 62, 78, 145, 170, 194–6
slaves 6, 11, 28, 38, 61–2, 70
smell 6, 7, 14, 19, 51–3, 75–8, 111, 140, 148, 150, 155, 166, 169–70, 181
  and Christianity 19–20
smoke 8, 13, 92
snorting 6–7
social stratification 2, 34–44, 48, 58–63, 75
  and luxury 79
  and religion 92
Socrates 132–5, 213–17
softness 10
Sophocles, 202
Soranus 141
soul 117–19, 132–5
sound 163–5
space, social 4
space travel 1–2

Sparta 31
speculum 146–7
speech 26, 27, 118, 130–2, 143, 144, 156, 214, 215–16
spice 11, 66, 70, 72, 76, 81, 88, 89
spinning 85
spitting 154, 155
statues 2, 8, 12, 13, 17, 48, 66, 92, 185, 186–93
  and color 186–93
  and touch 192–3
  see also sculpture
status 4–8, 48, 58–63
  and food 36
Stoicism 25, 102–3, 135
stone 12–13, 49–50, 51, 85–6
Strabo 75, 207
street layout 64–6
Sudan 71
Sulla 40
symmetry 27
synaesthesia 2–4, 164, 184, 211–14, 221–2, 225
synagogues 99, 112
Synesius of Cyrene 7
Syria 100
Syrian Goddess, the 8, 104

Tacitus 40, 50
tanners 6, 53
taste 4–5, 15, 75–8, 143, 144, 166
  popular 15
taverns 86, 88
Tertullian 19, 95, 104
textiles 72, 85, 100
theaters 28, 55, 109–10
  Theater of Pompey 205–6
Thecla 108
Theodoret of Cyrrhus 109
Theodosius I 17, 103, 104–5
Theophrastus 25
theurgy 98
Tiberius Sempronius Gracchus 34, 69–70, 74, 76, 89

togas 16, 58–9
toilet rituals 8
tombs 45–6
tortoiseshell 72
torture, 6, 62, 107
touch 6, 7, 16, 24–5, 144–5, 166, 170
  and emperors 24
  and healing 10, 160
  and luxury 78–88
trade 100
  with Baltics 79–81
  with the Orient 69–89
tragedy 199
Trajan 76
translation 220–1
Trier 85
Trimalchio 11
triumphs 28, 64
trompe l'oeil 191–2
Twelve Tables 40

underworld, the 120
urban life 11–12, 45–67, 75, 205–7

vegetables 76
Venus 165
Vespasian 75
Vestals 33, 95
Vesuvius 89
Vindolanda 72
Virgil 100, 184
vision *see* sight
Vitellius 76
Vitruvius 198
vividness 164
voice 165–6, 167–8, 170–4, 180–1, 197, 198–9
vomitives 150
votive offerings 99, 157
Vulcan 165

wall-painting 86–7, 89, 191–2
War and Peace 168
water 12, 50, 185, 216

wax images 41–2
wheat 59, 70
wigs 7, 87, 196
wind-charms 10
wine 8, 31, 60–1, 63, 66–7, 92, 97, 183, 212, 214, 217, 218–19
women 62–3, 145
  and mental disorders 150–1

work 7
worship 102–3
writing 130, 214–16

Xenophon 62

Zanzibar 72
Zosimas 105